1997
YEAR BOOK OF
SPORTS MEDICINE®

Statement of Purpose

The YEAR BOOK Service

The YEAR BOOK series was devised in 1901 by practicing health professionals who observed that the literature of medicine and related disciplines had become so voluminous that no one individual could read and place in perspective every potential advance in a major specialty. In the final decade of the 20th century, this recognition is more acutely true than it was in 1901.

More than merely a series of books, YEAR BOOK volumes are the tangible results of a unique service designed to accomplish the following:

- to *survey* a wide range of journals of proven value;
- to *select* from those journals papers representing significant advances and statements of important clinical principles;
- to provide *abstracts* of those articles that are readable, convenient summaries of their key points; and
- to provide *commentary* about those articles to place them in perspective.

These publications grow out of a unique process that calls on the talents of outstanding authorities in clinical and fundamental disciplines, trained literature specialists, and professional writers, all supported by the resources of Mosby, the world's preeminent publisher for the health professions.

The Literature Base

Mosby and its editors survey more than 1,000 journals published worldwide, covering the full range of the health professions. On an annual basis, the publisher examines usage patterns and polls its expert authorities to add new journals to the literature base and to delete journals that are no longer useful as potential YEAR BOOK sources.

The Literature Survey

The publisher's team of literature specialists, all of whom are trained and experienced health professionals, examines every original, peer-reviewed article in each journal issue. More than 250,000 articles per year are scanned systematically, including titles, text, illustrations, tables, and references. Each scan is compared, article by article, with the search strategies that the publisher has developed in consultation with the 270 outside experts who form the pool of YEAR BOOK editors. A given article may be reviewed by any number of editors, from one to a dozen or more, regardless of the discipline for which the paper was originally published. In turn, each editor who receives the article reviews it to determine whether or not the article should be included in the YEAR BOOK. This decision is based on the article's inherent quality, its probable usefulness to readers of that YEAR BOOK, and the editor's goal to represent a balanced picture of a given field in each volume of the YEAR BOOK. In addition, the editor indicates when to include figures and tables from the article to help the YEAR BOOK reader better understand the information.

Of the quarter million articles scanned each year, only 5% are selected for detailed analysis within the YEAR BOOK series, thereby assuring readers of the high value of every selection.

The Abstract

The publisher's abstracting staff is headed by a seasoned medical professional and includes individuals with training in the life sciences, medicine, and other areas, plus extensive experience in writing for the health professions and related industries. Each selected article is assigned to a specific writer on this abstracting staff. The abstracter, guided in many cases by notations supplied by the expert editor, writes a structured, condensed summary designed so that the reader can rapidly acquire the essential information contained in the article.

The Commentary

The YEAR BOOK editorial boards, sometimes assisted by guest commentators, write comments that place each article in perspective for the reader. This provides the reader with the equivalent of a personal consultation with a leading international authority—an opportunity to better understand the value of the article and to benefit from the authority's thought processes in assessing the article.

Additional Editorial Features

The editorial boards of each YEAR BOOK organize the abstracts and comments to provide a logical and satisfying sequence of information. To enhance the organization, editors also provide introductions to sections or individual chapters, comments linking a number of abstracts, citations to additional literature, and other features.

The published YEAR BOOK contains enhanced bibliographic citations for each selected article, including extended listings of multiple authors and identification of author affiliations. Each YEAR BOOK contains a Table of Contents specific to that year's volume. From year to year, the Table of Contents for a given YEAR BOOK will vary depending on developments within the field.

Every YEAR BOOK contains a list of the journals from which papers have been selected. This list represents a subset of the more than 1,000 journals surveyed by the publisher and occasionally reflects a particularly pertinent article from a journal that is not surveyed on a routine basis.

Finally, each volume contains a comprehensive subject index and an index to authors of each selected paper.

The 1997 Year Book Series

Year Book of Allergy, Asthma, and Clinical Immunology: Drs. Rosenwasser, Borish, Gelfand, Leung, Nelson, and Szefler

Year Book of Anesthesiology and Pain Management®: Drs. Tinker, Abram, Chestnut, Roizen, Rothenberg, and Wood

Year Book of Cardiology®: Drs. Schlant, Collins, Gersh, Kaplan, and Waldo

Year Book of Chiropractic®: Dr. Lawrence

Year Book of Critical Care Medicine®: Drs. Parrillo, Balk, Calvin, Franklin, and Shapiro

Year Book of Dentistry®: Drs. Meskin, Berry, Kennedy, Leinfelder, Roser, Summitt, and Zakariasen

Year Book of Dermatologic Surgery®: Drs. Greenway, Papadopoulos, and Whitaker

Year Book of Dermatology®: Drs. Sober and Fitzpatrick

Year Book of Diagnostic Radiology®: Drs. Federle, Gross, Dalinka, Maynard, Rebner, Smirniotopolous, and Young

Year Book of Digestive Diseases®: Drs. Greenberger and Moody

Year Book of Drug Therapy®: Drs. Lasagna and Weintraub

Year Book of Emergency Medicine®: Drs. Wagner, Dronen, Davidson, King, Niemann, and Roberts

Year Book of Endocrinology®: Drs. Bagdade, Braverman, Horton, Kannan, Landsberg, Molitch, Morley, Nathan, Odell, Poehlman, Rogol, and Ryan

Year Book of Family Practice®: Drs. Berg, Bowman, Davidson, Dexter, and Scherger

Year Book of Geriatrics and Gerontology®: Drs. Beck, Burton, Ostwald, Rabins, Reuben, Roth, Shapiro, and Whitehouse

Year Book of Hand Surgery®: Drs. Amadio and Hentz

Year Book of Hematology®: Drs. Spivak, Bell, Ness, Quesenberry, Wiernik, and Blume

Year Book of Infectious Diseases®: Drs. Keusch, Barza, Bennish, Poutsiaka, Skolnik, and Snydman

Year Book of Medicine®: Drs. Klahr, Cline, Petty, Frishman, Greenberger, Malawista, Mandell, and Utiger

Year Book of Neonatal and Perinatal Medicine®: Drs. Fanaroff, Maisels, and Stevenson

Year Book of Nephrology, Hypertension, and Mineral Metabolism: Drs. Schwab, Bennett, Emmett, Hostetter, Kumar, and Toto

Year Book of Neurology and Neurosurgery®: Drs. Bradley and Wilkins

Year Book of Nuclear Medicine®: Drs. Gottschalk, Blaufox, Neumann, Strauss, and Zubal

Year Book of Obstetrics, Gynecology, and Women's Health: Drs. Mishell, Herbst, and Kirschbaum

Year Book of Occupational and Environmental Medicine®: Drs. Emmett, Frank, Gochfeld, and Hessl

Year Book of Oncology®: Drs. Ozols, Cohen, Glatstein, Loehrer, Tallman, and Wiersma

Year Book of Ophthalmology®: Drs. Wilson, Augsburger, Cohen, Eagle, Flanagan, Grossman, Laibson, Maguire, Nelson, Penne, Rapuano, Sergott, Spaeth, Tipperman, Ms. Gosfield, and Ms. Salmon

Year Book of Orthopedics®: Drs. Sledge, Poss, Cofield, Dobyns, Griffin, Springfield, Swiontkowski, Wiesel, and Wilson

Year Book of Otolaryngology–Head and Neck Surgery®: Drs. Paparella and Holt

Year Book of Pathology and Laboratory Medicine: Drs. Mills, Bruns, Gaffey, and Stoler

Year Book of Pediatrics®: Dr. Stockman

Year Book of Plastic, Reconstructive, and Aesthetic Surgery®: Drs. Miller, Cohen, McKinney, Robson, Ruberg, Smith, and Whitaker

Year Book of Podiatric Medicine and Surgery®: Dr. Kominsky

Year Book of Psychiatry and Applied Mental Health®: Drs. Talbott, Ballenger, Breier, Frances, Meltzer, Schowalter, and Tasman

Year Book of Pulmonary Disease®: Dr. Petty

Year Book of Rheumatology®: Drs. Sergent, LeRoy, Meenan, Panush, and Reichlin

Year Book of Sports Medicine®: Drs. Shephard, Alexander, Drinkwater, Eichner, George, and Torg

Year Book of Surgery®: Drs. Copeland, Bland, Deitch, Eberlein, Howard, Luce, Seeger, Souba, and Sugarbaker

Year Book of Thoracic and Cardiovascular Surgery®: Drs. Ginsberg, Wechsler, and Williams

Year Book of Urology®: Drs. Andriole and Coplen

Year Book of Vascular Surgery®: Dr. Porter

1997

The Year Book of SPORTS MEDICINE®

Editor-in-Chief
Roy J. Shephard, M.D., Ph.D., D.P.E.
Professor Emeritus of Applied Physiology, Faculty of Physical Education and Health, and Department of Public Health Sciences, University of Toronto; and CTAL Resident Scholar in Health Studies, Brock University, St. Catharine's, Ontario

Editors
Marion J.L. Alexander, Ph.D.
Professor, Faculty of Physical Education and Recreation Studies; Research Associate, Health, Leisure and Human Performance Research Institute, University of Manitoba, Winnipeg

Barbara L. Drinkwater, Ph.D.
Research Physiologist, Department of Medicine, Pacific Medical Center, Seattle

Edward R. Eichner, M.D.
Professor of Medicine, University of Oklahoma Health Sciences Center, Oklahoma City

Francis J. George, A.T.C., P.T.
Head Athletic Trainer, Brown University, Providence

Joseph S. Torg, M.D.
Professor of Orthopedic Surgery, and Director, Sports Medicine Center, Allegheny University—Hahnemann, Philadelphia

American College of Sports Medicine Liaison Representative
Kent B. Pandolf, Ph.D.
Director, Environmental Physiology and Medicine Directorate, U.S. Army Research Institute of Environmental Medicine, Natick, Massachusetts

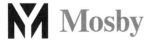

St. Louis Baltimore Boston Carlsbad Naples New York Philadelphia Portland London
Madrid Mexico City Singapore Sydney Tokyo Toronto Wiesbaden

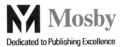

Mosby

Dedicated to Publishing Excellence

A Times Mirror Company

Publisher: Terry Van Schaik
Acquisitions Editor: Gina G. Byrd
Developmental Editor: Jaime Chatman
Manager, Periodicals Editing: Kirk Swearingen
Manuscript Editor: Amanda Maguire
Project Supervisor, Production: Joy Moore
Project Assistant, Production: Laura Bayless
Manager, Literature Services: Idelle Winer
Illustrations and Permissions Specialist: Steve Ramay

1997 EDITION
Copyright © January 1988 by Mosby–Year Book, Inc.

Printed in the United States of America
Composition by Reed Technology and Information Services, Inc.
Printing/binding by Maple-Vail

Mosby–Year Book, Inc.
11830 Westline Industrial Drive
St. Louis, MO 63146

International Standard Serial Number: 0162-0908
International Standard Book Number: 0-8151-9739-X

Table of Contents

Journals Represented

Mosby and its editors survey more than 1,000 journals for its abstract and commentary publications. From these journals, the editors select the articles to be abstracted. Journals represented in this YEAR BOOK are listed below.

Acta Paediatrica
American Heart Journal
American Journal of Cardiology
American Journal of Clinical Nutrition
American Journal of Emergency Medicine
American Journal of Epidemiology
American Journal of Hypertension
American Journal of Medicine
American Journal of Ophthalmology
American Journal of Orthopedics
American Journal of Otolaryngology
American Journal of Physical Medicine & Rehabilitation
American Journal of Physiology
American Journal of Public Health
American Journal of Respiratory and Critical Care Medicine
American Journal of Sports Medicine
Annals of Internal Medicine
Archives of Orthopaedic and Trauma Surgery
Archives of Pediatrics and Adolescent Medicine
Archives of Physical Medicine and Rehabilitation
Arthroscopy
Athletic Therapy Today
Australian Journal of Science and Medicine in Sport
British Journal of Sports Medicine
Canadian Family Physician
Chest
Circulation
Clinical Biomechanics
Clinical Orthopaedics and Related Research
Clinical Science
Diabetes Care
Diabetic Medicine
Ergonomics
European Heart Journal
European Journal of Nuclear Medicine
Foot & Ankle International
Hypertension
Injury
International Journal of Cancer
International Journal of Sports Medicine
Journal of Adolescent Health
Journal of Applied Physiology: Respiratory, Environmental, and Exercise
    Physiology
Journal of Athletic Training
Journal of Biomechanics
Journal of Bone and Joint Surgery (American Volume)
Journal of Bone and Joint Surgery (British Volume)

Journal of Bone and Mineral Research
Journal of Clinical Endocrinology and Metabolism
Journal of Computer Assisted Tomography
Journal of General Internal Medicine
Journal of Gerontology
Journal of Heart and Lung Transplantation
Journal of Hypertension
Journal of Internal Medicine
Journal of Orthopaedic Research
Journal of Orthopaedic and Sports Physical Therapy
Journal of Pediatrics
Journal of Rheumatology
Journal of Shoulder and Elbow Surgery
Journal of Spinal Disorders
Journal of Sports Medicine and Physical Fitness
Journal of Sports Sciences
Journal of Sports Traumatology and Related Research
Journal of Trauma: Injury, Infection, and Critical Care
Journal of the American Academy of Dermatology
Journal of the American Academy of Orthopaedic Surgeons
Journal of the American College of Cardiology
Journal of the American Geriatrics Society
Journal of the American Medical Association
Journal of the American Society of Nephrology
Journal of the Louisiana State Medical Society
Lancet
Medicine and Science in Sports and Exercise
Metabolism: Clinical and Experimental
Neurology
New England Journal of Medicine
New Zealand Medical Journal
Ophthalmology
Orthopedics
Pain
Pediatrics
Physical Therapy
Physician and Sports Medicine
Research Quarterly for Exercise and Sport
Spine
Sports Medicine
Thorax

STANDARD ABBREVIATIONS

The following terms are abbreviated in this edition: acquired immunodeficiency syndrome (AIDS), cardiopulmonary resuscitation (CPR), central nervous system (CNS), cerebrospinal fluid (CSF), computed tomography (CT), deoxyribonucleic acid (DNA), electrocardiography (ECG), health maintenance organization (HMO), human immunodeficiency virus (HIV), intensive care unit (ICU), intramuscular (IM), intravenous (IV), magnetic resonance (MR) imaging (MRI), and ribonucleic acid (RNA).

NOTE

The YEAR BOOK OF SPORTS MEDICINE is a literature survey service providing abstracts of articles published in the professional literature. Every effort is made to assure the accuracy of the information presented in these pages. Neither the editors nor the publisher of the YEAR BOOK OF SPORTS MEDICINE can be responsible for errors in the original materials. The editors' comments are their own opinions. Mention of specific products within this publication does not constitute endorsement.

To facilitate the use of the YEAR BOOK OF SPORTS MEDICINE as a reference tool, all illustrations and tables included in this publication are now identified as they appear in the original article. This change is meant to help the reader recognize that any illustration or table appearing in the YEAR BOOK OF SPORTS MEDICINE may be only one of many in the original article. For this reason, figure and table numbers will often appear to be out of sequence within the YEAR BOOK OF SPORTS MEDICINE.

Publisher's Preface

With the publication of the 1997 edition of the YEAR BOOK OF SPORTS MEDICINE, the publisher is pleased to welcome Marion J.L. Alexander, Ph.D, Professor, Faculty of Physical Education, of the University of Manitoba, Winnipeg, Canada. Dr. Alexander has contributed insightful selections and commentary to this edition, primarily in the area of biomechanics.

We welcome Dr. Alexander to our distinguished editorial board and look forward to her future contributions.

Introduction

Once again, the new edition of the YEAR BOOK OF SPORTS MEDICINE offers its readers an outstanding overview of major research in the many subdisciplines of sports medicine. The articles presented here range in their focus from the epidemiology, prevention and treatment of injuries and subsequent rehabilitation, through the monitoring of the athlete's environment, to an understanding of the body's physiological and biomechanical responses to physical activity in both health and disease. The development of structured abstracts now allows the reader to gain quick assess to key points that she or he may wish to verify in all of the papers which have been selected.

This year, we are pleased to welcome a second female to our editorial panel, Dr. Marion Alexander, of the University of Manitoba in Winnipeg. Despite the disastrous floods that coursed through the Red River Valley this spring, she has found time to bring us an outstanding collection of papers in her assigned area of biomechanics. This year's edition also marks the move of the Year Book's home base from Chicago to St. Louis as the consolidation of Mosby–Year Book operations progresses. I much appreciate the dedication of our technical editors, who have maintained a timely production schedule despite the inevitable problems associated with this relocation of offices and equipment.

In terms of exciting new developments in sports medicine, I am always most conscious of the ever-growing understanding of the inter-relationships between physical activity and the prevention and treatment of chronic disease. The question of just how much activity we should encourage sedentary patients to take continues to attract vigorous debate; Blair and his associates have argued recently that several major epidemiological studies point to the health benefits of quite low levels of physical activity, exercise prescriptions that would be insufficient to increase traditional markers of fitness such as maximal oxygen intake. But is participation in high-level competition disadvantageous to long-term health? A new Finnish study shows that long-term hospital usage is actually less in former national athletes than in the general population. Another supposed bogeyman of intense competition is an increase in free radical levels. However, a study completed on participants in the Hawaian Ironman Triathlon demonstrates that this event induced substantial reductions in lipid peroxidation. Regular vigorous exercise has a tendency to become addictive, and the health problems associated with exercise deprivation are the subject of a well-documented review.

Exercise causes a release of many chemicals that in theory might be expected to increase the risk of abnormal heart rhythms, but disaster is avoided because these substances interfere with one another. A study of this mutual antagonism offers potential new insights into the mechanisms of cardiac arrest. Chronotropic incompetence is shown to be a useful independent predictor of all-cause mortality and future coronary events in a recent analysis of data from the Framingham study. Cooper Clinic data indicate that prognostic significance can also be attached to peak heart rate and the systolic blood pressure response to exercise, although another study shows that an excessive hypertensive response to exercise is not necessarily a harbinger of future hypertension in athletes. A low level of personal fitness is a strong marker of poor prognosis, and an important new paper shows a substantial differential of mortality with fitness, even in those who are smokers or who have a high cholesterol level. Myocardial ischemia is shown to cause a prolonged local stunning of the myocardium.

The NHANES studies asked only one very simple question about each of recreational and non-recreational activity, and it is thus intriguing that responses to these two items showed significant associations with the future risk of stroke. The value of exercise in the control of hypertension continues to be debated. Time series analysis suggests that exercise brings about a reduction in both resting and exercise pressures, with a synergistic effect between exercise and weight loss.

Endurance performance sometimes depends on peripheral factors rather than aerobic function. de Groote and associates suggest that peripheral influences can be examined in terms of the speed of repayment of the oxygen debt, and they illustrate the contribution of this factor to prognosis in dilated cardiomyopathy. Magnusson and associates show the value of local muscle training in enhancing performance in chronic heart failure. Debate continues as to whether peripheral factors are responsible for the large and early accumulation of lactate when patients with an orthotopic cardiac transplant commence a progressive exercise test. Weight training is shown to improve the walking endurance of the elderly, even if there is no increase of aerobic power. Again, the mechanism is likely an improvement of the peripheral circulation. A comparison of walking while carrying a 10–15 kg load with the moderately paced ascent of 3–4 flights of stairs suggests that the former imposes a less dangerous circulatory load on older adults.

New insights into a congenital predisposition to obesity are provided by a study of plasma leptin levels in relation to body fat in endurance athletes.

A study of intestinal water flux shows similar results whether the flux is estimated following oral ingestion or whether the more traditional method of duodenal infusion is adopted. Medium-chained triglycerides have proven superior to 10% glucose as a means of improving performance in sustained cycling trials. The gain in performance is a substantial 2.5%.

A decrease in the gastrointestinal barrier to bacteria is demonstrated following a combination of aspirin treatment and endurance exercise. The hypothesis that overtraining suppresses immune function by reducing plasma levels of glutamine has been challenged by a study of elite Australian swimmers.

The need of the asthmatic athlete for salbutamol is questioned by a study which shows that intensive effort itself produces almost as large a bronchodilation as salbutamol. Those who suffer from exercise-induced asthma may profit from a recent demonstration that inhaled heparin is more effective than cromolyn in reversing bronchospasm. Obstructive sleep apnea syndrome is shown to be linked to abnormalities in the circadian rhythm of tumor necrosis factor alpha, thus opening a potential door to normalization of both cytokines and sleep patterns by an exercise program.

A paper on chronic fatigue syndrome suggests that affected patients can undertake a maximal oxygen intake test without serious detriment to their clinical status. A case study of myopathy proposes treatment by a combination of progressive exercise and dichloracetate, the latter being used to boost the activity of pyruvate dehydrogenase.

Prolonged treatment of urinary infections with pivalic acid-conjugated antibiotics is shown to cause a loss of left ventricular mass and a substantial decrease in maximal oxygen intake. Hyperkalemia has been suggested as one possible danger of exercise in patients with end-stage renal disease, but a study by Clark and associates found that extra-renal methods of regulating body mineral levels were well-preserved in such individuals.

In the first few weeks after a sudden ascent to high altitude, body water content may be reduced, but with the more gradual climb of the typical Himalayan trekker, a normal body water is regained while the person remains at altitude. High altitudes are shown to cause problems in many of the simple chromogen tests used to regulate blood sugar in diabetes. A large proportion of those who are particularly vulnerable to heat illness can be identified from two simple pieces of information: the body mass index and the time taken to run a distance of 2.4 km (1.5 miles). The determination of those individuals who will succumb to neurological complications of decompression sickness is important to the after-care of divers; hematological changes, including an increase of hematocrit, may offer advanced warning of an adverse response.

These are but a few of the exciting papers you will find in this year's edition. I hope you will enjoy reading them as much as I have.

Roy J. Shephard, M.D., Ph.D., D.P.E.

Issues in the Testing and Training of Prepubescent Children

ROY J. SHEPHARD, M.D., PH.D., D.P.E.
School of Physical and Health Education, University of Toronto; Department of Preventive Medicine and Biostatistics, Faculty of Medicine, University of Toronto; Health Studies Programme, Brock University, St. Catharine's, Ontario

The testing of endurance fitness in the child follows essentially the same principles as testing of the adult, although it is more difficult to demonstrate an oxygen consumption plateau in a young child, and lactate levels are lower in submaximal effort. It was once suggested that endurance training had little influence on the aerobic fitness of a prepubescent child; this review stresses that the twin explanations of the supposed phenomenon (a high intrinsic level of physical activity and an immaturity of biochemical systems) have little foundation in fact. Critical examination of the original training experiments shows a number of problems in experimental design, often including an inadequate sample size, a lack of a control group, an inappropriate pattern of exercise relative to the initial fitness of the child, and too short a period of observation. Recent, well-designed studies all show a training response in prepubescent children. Comparison with adults is hampered by difficulties in matching training intensity, but there is no immediate evidence that the response is less than that found in an older person. The main basis for the increase of oxygen transport seems an increase of cardiac stroke volume. Plainly, the development of athletic performance and the attack on cardiac risk factors may begin before puberty, although for the average prepubescent it may be more important that school programs aim to develop positive, lifelong attitudes toward physical activity rather than to seek a maximizing of immediate aerobic function.

Introduction

This article looks briefly at some issues of endurance testing and training in young children. Methods of assessment and the training response of the prepubescent child have considerable practical importance, given that athletic training programs are being developed for ever younger children. For the average, supposedly "well" child, endurance training also may control cardiac risk factors, which are also being noted at an ever younger age. Finally, many children with chronic disease face unnecessary physical restrictions, irrespective of the possible therapeutic value of training in such conditions as asthma, obesity, myopathies, hypertension, cerebral palsy, cystic fibrosis, and diabetes mellitus.

Exercise Testing

Problems of Testing

Most exercise tests were originally developed for adults, and young children often lack either the attention span or the motivation to reach peak effort. A lessening of anxiety after training may allow a child to make a better effort at a second test. Moreover, greater contact with the investigators may improve scores more for experimental than for control subjects. However, the reduction of peak heart rates is similar in experimental and control subjects if each visit the test laboratory the same number of times. The problem of test anxiety is greatest in short-term experiments, and it decreases as subjects make repeated visits to the laboratory.

Difficulty also arises from intra-individual variability of test scores relative to the size of any training response. Direct measurements of maximal oxygen intake have a coefficient of variation of at least 5%, and the variation in submaximal predictions is 10% to 15%. Thus, unless a substantial sample of subjects is tested, a 10% to 15% increase of maximal oxygen intake could prove statistically insignificant. On the other hand, a 15% gain in maximal oxygen intake would have substantial implications for both athletic performance and health.

Field Testing

Much field testing is carried out in schools, using simple physical performance tests: sit-ups performed in 1 minute, the time to run 1 km. But such tests are heavily influenced by maturity, height, and body mass. Too often, such measurements become only a difficult way of determining a child's physical dimensions. The scores relative to population norms reflect performance rather than health and can have a negative effect on the exercise behavior of a child with a poor genetic endowment.

Performance tests work a little better if subjects are compared with themselves. Several authors have seen an improvement in running times over several months of training, even though not all were able to demonstrate an increase of maximal oxygen intake. In some cases, there was also a decrease of heart rate during submaximal exercise or an increase of the calculated PWC_{170} or both. Bar-Or[1] argued that an increase of speed without a significant change of maximal oxygen transport was caused by an increase in the efficiency of running. Efficiency certainly improves with

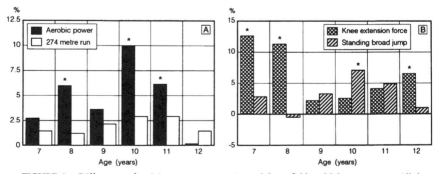

FIGURE 1.—Differences of training response as estimated from field and laboratory tests. All data expressed as percent differences between scores for experimental and control students over a 6-year program of enhanced physical education. (Courtesy of Shephard RJ and Lavallée H: Changes of physical performance as indicators of the response to enhanced physical education. *J Sports Med Phys Fitness* 34:323–335, 1994.)

deliberate track training, but such an effect is less likely with a general endurance training program for young children. Alternative explanations are that there was a functional gain specific to the speed of running or that training was more easily detected with a stopwatch because it is difficult to measure maximal oxygen intake in young children.

Another possible justification of field testing is to evaluate an entire program by using a large sample of students. Still, the correlation between laboratory and field test findings is quite weak. Fig 1 illustrates gains of maximal oxygen intake and muscle strength vs. gains in field test performance when primary school children participated in a 6-year program of enhanced physical education.

Laboratory Testing

Before a child reaches the age of 7 or 8 years, laboratory scores are reliable and valid only for measurements that require little cooperation from the subject: height, body mass, skinfold readings, and lean tissue mass. A young child might perform a simple step test if the observer climbs and descends the staircase with the child, or an ergometer can be attached to a pedal car. However, the resulting estimates of aerobic performance are crude. No commercial cycle ergometer has appropriate dimensions for very young children. Children of 5 or 6 years wearing a safety harness can run on a treadmill, but fear accelerates their heart rates and makes it difficult for us to decide when maximal effort has been reached. Likewise, it is difficult to persuade young children to make consistent maximal muscular efforts against any type of dynamometer.

An International Biological Programme working group looked at methods of evaluating the various components of physical working capacity in older primary school children. In general, their recommended methodology did not differ from that for adults. Maximal oxygen intake is best determined by means of uphill treadmill running, although because most children are accustomed to riding a bicycle, the discrepancy between cycle ergometer and treadmill maxima (around 7%) is less than in adults. Oxygen plateaus are not seen in about half of students, but some observers claim that the peak value is a stable measure of performance in a child and that average values are similar for children with and without a plateau. Early studies found maximal heart rates of around 195 beats/min, but more recently 200 beats/min has been accepted as a more accurate maximum value for maximum heart rate. Muscle and blood lactate concentrations equilibrate more rapidly than in adults, within 1–2 minutes, and the peak value is about 8 mmol/L rather than 10–11 mmol/L. This reflects a smaller muscle mass and immaturity of anaerobic mechanisms.

If there is recourse to submaximal testing, endurance fitness scores can be influenced by both test learning and habituation. Young children take a considerable time to learn the operation of exercise test equipment and to become at ease in the laboratory environment. Further problems can arise if the equipment is too large and heavy to be operated with the anticipated mechanical efficiency. The classical submaximal measurements have been the PWC_{170} test and the Åstrand nomogram prediction of maximal oxygen intake, both developed for adults rather than for children. In 10- to 12-year-old children, predictions show a rather unsatisfactory 15% coefficient of variation relative to direct maximal measurements, and predictions are even less reliable in younger individuals. There have been suggestions that fitness be compared in terms of the "anaerobic threshold," but blood sampling is traumatic for children, and ventilatory measurements are distorted as a result of anxiety. Probably because of changes in anxiety in their subjects, Rotstein et al.[2] found no change of "anaerobic threshold" after training, even when maximal oxygen intake had increased.

Exercise at any given submaximal intensity also elicits somewhat lower lactate values in children than in adults. Some authors have recommended adopting a lactate threshold as low as 2.5 rather than 4.0 mmol/L. Children are technically capable of performing a Wingate test of anaerobic capacity and power, although actual scores may be below potential because of problems in motivation and pacing. Muscle strength can be determined by means of cable tensiometers and dynamometers or with isokinetic devices. Skinfold determinations of body levels measure the same skinfolds as in adults, but conversion to body density and levels of body fat requires age-specific equations that allow for differences in the distribution of body fat and the density of the lean compartment. Underwater weighing is also possible, although there is often difficulty in having the child sit still on the weighing sling. If the lungs are disease free, residual volume can be predicted from vital capacity.

Training Response

Do children need endurance training, and can it be accomplished? Many authors have claimed that the prepubescent child does not respond to such programs.[3] If true, this certainly weakens the case for the special sports schools that many nations have developed for athletically gifted young students. Equally, it counters the call of many physical educators for a daily program of vigorous physical education at the primary school.

Bailey[4] drew attention to a progressive decline of aerobic fitness scores in Canadian schoolboys. He claimed that deterioration began when a child sat at a school desk, and he blamed the decrease in scores on an inadequate school physical education program. Many authors have noted such a trend in girls, but Bailey's data have less often been replicated in boys. Bailey's measure of aerobic fitness was the directly measured maximal oxygen intake, expressed in milliliters per kilogram·minute. In fact, his data do not show any substantial decline until around the age of 12 years. Moreover, the decline in score is shown by both active and inactive students. This is puzzling, and we may question Bailey's implicit assumption that peak oxygen transport per kilogram of body mass should remain constant throughout childhood. Fitness scores change in a different manner if oxygen consumption is scaled in relation to height or weight[2]. Nevertheless, the oxygen cost of many endurance tasks is approximately proportional to body mass, and the commonly adopted milliliters per kilogram·minute units thus offer a reasonable basis of data standardization. In such terms, the aerobic potential of the Canadian boy worsens on moving from childhood into adolescence.

Would this loss of aerobic function be checked if children devoted more time to physical education at school? In Canada, the curricular time allocated to physical education varies widely, depending on the interest and the enthusiasm of parents, local school boards, and school principals. Recommended minimums for elementary and junior high schools range from 150 min/week in Saskatchewan to only 30 min/week in Prince Edward Island. At primary schools, specialist physical education teachers are found in only two of ten Canadian Provinces. Usually, classes are taught by the homeroom teacher (who may have had a limited amount of training in physical education). Key issues are whether young children can respond to such training, and whether the teacher uses the allocated curricular time effectively. The long-term effect of required physical education programs is particularly controversial. While habit seems an important determinant of both the intention to exercise and its realization, school physical education programs too frequently engender negative attitudes, and physical activity quickly ceases when physical education is no longer a required subject.

Response of Young Children to Endurance Training

Early investigators claimed that young children did not respond to endurance training because of either a high inherent level of physical activity or some unexplained immaturity of biological response mechanisms.

Casual observation of play patterns suggested almost continual movement of the young child. Such impressions have not been supported by systematic measurement of daily physical activity patterns, use of Holter monitors or Sport testers, and other devices for monitoring heart rates and body motion. Young children may spend little time completely at rest, but physiologically significant intensities of activity occur only in quite short bursts. Further, the average child rarely reaches that combination of exercise intensity and duration when an aerobic training effect might be anticipated. Atomi et al.[5] found that 9- to 10-year-old boys spent only 18 minutes per day at the lactate threshold, and 34 minutes per day at the 60% of maximal oxygen intake. Armstrong et al.[6] measured heart rates of 12 8-year-old students over 12 waking hours; values above 159 beats/min were seen only 1.8% of the time in girls and 2.6% in boys; over 85% of girls and 70% of boys did not show a single 20-minute period of the day when they were exercising at more than 70% of maximal oxygen intake.

The immaturity hypothesis also lacks objective support. Zauner et al.[7] noted some metabolic differences in very young children but concluded that aerobic energy systems were well developed by 6 years of age.

Some early longitudinal studies of prepubescent children found no increase of aerobic power in response to deliberate increases of habitual activity. In contrast, a dozen or more cross-sectional comparisons show high values for aerobic power in youngsters selected and trained for endurance sports.[3] Is the advantage of the athletes a result of initial selection, or can it be attributed to prolonged aerobic training? The difference between untrained and trained children widens in older age groups, but it remains unclear whether this is caused by more intense selection or heavier training. Sunnegardh and Bratteby[8] noted a correlation of 0.41 between maximal oxygen intake and activity measurements in 8-year-olds—significant in boys but not in girls.

Flaws of Experimental Design

Given the conflict between cross-sectional observations on prepubescent children and some apparently negative longitudinal training studies, we should look at possible flaws in experimental design. These include a nonrandom allocation of subjects, inadequate sample size, heterogeneity of the students tested, an inadequate intensity, frequency or duration of exercise sessions, a high level of initial fitness in the experimental subjects, and an inadequate total volume of training. Each of these criticisms will be examined relative to the design of our study of primary school students, which did demonstrate a training response. Our main study was conducted in Trois Rivières.[9] It compared the responses of prepubescent children to either a standard program (a single 40-minute activity period per week) or an enhanced physical education program (five additional 1-hour classes per week, taught by a physical education specialist).

Subject Allocation

Few authors have used true experimental designs, and many studies have had no controls. Some authors compared the development of trained students with other samples of students who were presumed to be sedentary, or were following a standard physical education program.[3]

Three previous experimental studies had major problems. Ekblöm[10] noted that 3 of 13 subjects defected from their allocated regimen. Stewart and Gutin[11] admitted an 18% difference of body mass between their experimental and control students, and Gatch and Byrd[12] made no measurements of maximal oxygen intake.

The Trois Rivières study included an equal number of control students by allocating immediately preceding and succeeding school classes to the control regimen.[9] Subject allocation was thus determined simply by year of birth. All study participants were exposed to the same school, the same teachers, and the same community environment.

Sample Size

Many investigators have tested very small groups, heterogenous in age and unrepresentative of the base population. In 18 published studies, sample size ranged from 9 to 90 students, with an average of 34. Several of the larger studies were poorly controlled comparisons between students undergoing athletic training and their sedentary peers, and sometimes the apparent sample size was boosted by a preponderance of control subjects (in one example, 43 to 7 subjects).

The Trois Rivières study recruited a large, relatively homogenous and representative sample of 546 students, beginning at age 6 years. This allowed stratification of response by program (experimental or control), sex, and area of residence (urban vs. rural school).

Sample Heterogeneity

In some longitudinal studies (both negative and positive) the age spread of the participants was such that students were either very young or entered puberty before data collection was completed.

In the apparently negative study of Yoshida et al.,[13] students were only 5 years old. Their motor development required an exercise program focused on skill acquisition rather than on specific cardiorespiratory training. Our data support the view that it is difficult to train children so young they do not know how to exercise. We saw no substantial training response before 8 years of age, but we believe this reflects problems with the mechanics of exercising rather than an inherent lack of trainability.

The inclusion of older students potentially causes a problem from training-induced differences in the timing and magnitude of the pubertal growth spurt, with resulting differences of body size. Although physiologic data can be scaled relative to an exponent of standing height or body mass, there is still no consensus on an appropriate method of making such adjustments.

The Trois Rivières study followed students from the ages of 6–11 years, and with the exception of a few of the oldest girls there was no evidence that participants had begun their pubertal growth spurt.

Intensity

The threshold intensity needed to train a prepubsescent child is probably higher than in an adult, because the child has a higher peak heart rate. Massicotte and MacNab[14] suggested a threshold heart rate of 170–180 beats/min in 11- to 13-year-old students. Washington et al.[15] also noted that the heart rate at the anaerobic threshold was 167–169 beats/min, substantially higher than in adults. Kanaely and Boileau[16] likewise placed the anaerobic threshold at 68.6% of peak oxygen intake, compared with their value of 58.5% for adults; 68.6% would correspond to a heart rate of 150–160 beats/min.

We saw an aerobic training response with a physical education program that developed telemetrically recorded heart rates of 150–160 beats/min for 20–30 minutes per class. Only two other studies of the prepubescent child have reported the heart rates attained during training. Sometimes, the intensity of activity has seemed quite high, but several authors have relied on ice hockey games (not strictly an endurance sport) or normal school physical education as their source of aerobic conditioning. Goode et al.[17] demonstrated that unless programming maximized use of class time, physical education was unlikely to improve physical condition. Often, too large a fraction of class was devoted to changing, preparation, explanations of simple techniques, and administrative matters. In more deliberate longitudinal experiments, the activity has commonly been running, but in five studies where no training was seen, the students undertook brief bouts of interval work (runs of 145–800 m, 1- to 4-minute bursts of activity), rather than prolonged, moderate intensity endurance exercise.

Frequency

In several supposedly negative training studies, the frequency of exercise sessions was only once or twice per week—well below the usually accepted threshold frequency for adults. There is no reason to expect such activity would be effective in training a young child. In contrast, our Trois Rivières experiment used five 1-hour sessions of required physical education per week.

Duration

A substantial part of any activity program for young children is occupied with changing, waiting, and verbal instruction. Such time loss sometimes precludes a training effect. Other training studies have used running programs; here, the duration of activity is more certain, but with the distances chosen (commonly 750–800 m) the total time per session has been rather short for a training response to occur. The uncontrolled studies of Brown et al.[18] are an exception. They had 8- to 9-year-old girls run 6.4–11.2 km 4 to 5 times per week, and found gains in maximal oxygen intake of up to 33% in as little as 6 weeks.

The Trois Rivières experiment offerred a nominal hour of physical activity per class session, and telemetry showed that children spent at least 20–30 minutes of class time in the usually accepted heart rate training zone.

Initial Fitness

Initial fitness is one of the main determinants of training response. In some supposedly negative studies, subjects had too high an initial level of fitness; they had been selected for summer endurance training camps or belonged to track or swimming clubs. A substantial increase over baseline activity would be needed to train such persons. However, from the viewpoint of the family physician and the physical educator, the relevant issue is the response of the average sedentary school student rather than any additional gains that can be induced in children who are already highly athletic.

Training Volume

Most negative studies involved only limited volumes of training, measurements covering periods of 7–9 weeks. Such times are too brief to elicit a response from young children who must develop motor skills before serious training can begin. A short observation period causes complications from seasonal variations of aerobic power. Fitness peaks during the hockey season in some Canadian communities and then often deteriorates over the summer vacation. Such seasonal effects are a particular problem in uncontrolled studies.

Proving the Trainability of Prepubescent Children

General Considerations

There are many obstacles to proving the trainability of prepubescent children, including concerns about the safety of tests and training programs, concomitant effects of growth, issues of human experimentation with young children, test learning and habituation, sample attrition, poor program compliance, altered patterns of physical activity outside the experimental training program, contamination of control children by an interest in exercise, and secular changes in physical activity patterns.

Human Experimentation

Committees on human experimentation are increasingly reluctant to sanction any type of experiment involving prepubescent children, because of difficulties in ensuring that subjects understand the nature of the experiment and give their consent freely. One approach is to solicit the cooperation of entire school boards. By making physical activity a part of the normal academic day for certain school classes, the only part of the study requiring cooperation and formal consent becomes participation in annual clinical and physiologic evaluations.

Test and Program Safety

Test and program safety is of less concern in children than in an adult. On rare occasions, endurance training has induced a cardiac emergency or even death.[19] Potential causes include aortic stenosis, viral myocarditis, an anomalous origin of the coronary arteries, and a berry aneurysm of the circle of Willis. However, young children generally halt physical activity before they have induced a dangerous level of fatigue.

In a very young child, lack of coordination may increase the risk of injury from falling (for example, during a treadmill test). Moreover, because understanding of the nature of the experiment is limited, children may be more nervous than adults. Training-induced musculoskeletal injuries become increasingly prevalent in older children. Factors include excessive competition, undue pressure from coaches or parents, and a poor matching of opponents for size, skill, and maturity. Nevertheless, effective forms of aerobic conditioning such as progressive distance running have an extremely low risk of injury.

Allowance for Growth

If growth differs between experimental and control subjects, it becomes difficult to decide whether any training-associated gains of aerobic power are due to exercise per se or an acceleration of growth. However, acceleration of growth is not an inevitable consequence of endurance training. In the Trois Rivières sample, we saw 4 months' delay in maturation of the wrist bones among the exercised students, but training had no impact on height or other major body dimensions. In such circumstances, aerobic fitness scores can safely be compared in terms of maximal oxygen intake per kilogram of body mass, irrespective of theoretical arguments for alternative treatments of the data.

Sample Attrition

Attrition of the subject pool is a major problem in any long-term training experiment, in children as in adults. However, only three studies have commented on this issue.

If the exercise program is arranged in the child's leisure hours, there may be some exchange of students between control and experimental groups (as in Ekblöm's study[10]). Again, if the basis of treatment is the school class, subjects may be lost to investigation through their removal by the parents, by accelerated or retarded academic progress, and by voluntary withdrawal from the associated clinical and physiologic testing program. Given a stable community and good cooperation by the local school board, such losses can be held to 4% to 5% per annum, an acceptable limitation of longer-term investigations.

Compliance With Training Program

Program compliance is less of an issue in prepubescent children than in adults. Coaches usually insist that a child participate regularly in sport practices, and equally, the young child must attend required school physical-activity programs. However, there is some risk that sedentary students will defect from a strenuous training program and that active students will resent their allocation to a control group. This could increase scores in the experimental group and reduce scores in the control group. Laboratory stress testing is also popular with fit students, defections biasing data for both experimental and control groups in an upward direction.

The use of video cameras and pulse rate recordings by researchers has further emphasized that required attendance by no means guarantees effective participation in a physical activity program. An apparent lack of response to endurance training could reflect a dilution of data by children who attend exercise classes, but who do not participate effectively.

Contamination of Control Subjects

Where control students are drawn from the same school or the same families, there is a possibility of contamination by personal contact with the subjects who are undergoing training. We compared control children who had relatives participating as experimental subjects with those did not, and we found no evidence of contamination. However, it is difficult to rule out a more general contamination of the community by an increased interest in endurance training. Such an effect would reduce the apparent training response.

Compensating Changes of Behavior

If a child becomes tired as a result of participating in a vigorous training program, he or she may curtail voluntary leisure activity by a compensating amount. However, if the physical demands of the program exceed the likely volume of spontaneous activity, there is no possibility that the program effect could be entirely annulled. If the child has a positive attitude toward exercise, it is also likely that physical activity will be voluntarily increased rather than decreased on days when participation in the experimental program is not required.

Most investigators have not considered this issue. Detailed diary records for students at Trois Rivières support the hypotheses proposed above. The experimental students curtailed their leisure activity on school days, but not enough to negate the effect of the physical education program. Moreover, on weekend days, vigorous voluntary activity was more prevalent in the experimental subjects than in control subjects.

Secular Trends

Secular trends to an increase of body size distort both cross-sectional and longitudinal curves illustrating the growth of performance capability, limiting their generality. Secular changes in body size affect both maximal oxygen intake and the ability to perform aerobic tasks. There have also been secular changes in the activity patterns of many communities, leading to progressive changes in the baseline fitness of both experimental and control subjects. Until recently, the secular trend was for a progressive decrease in the habitual amount of physical activity. Television came to occupy 25–30 hrs/week that had previously been allocated to active pursuits. Lower baseline fitness level could be one reason why training responses have been demonstrated more readily in recent than in earlier studies. Now, there is a growing public awareness of fitness, and a secular tendency for control subjects to become more active, again complicating data interpretation.

In the Trois Rivières study, the initiation of our training experiment in a small village led to the development of new community exercise facilities that were inevitably available to both experimental *and* control students. Construction of a new auto-route also led to an inward migration of higher-income families who had a greater interest in health and fitness.

Magnitude of Prepubescent Response to Endurance Training

Theoretical Arguments

There are several theoretical arguments concerning why the training response might be reduced in a young child: a hypokinetic circulation, a limited secretion of male sex hormones, a low enzyme level, and a lack of physical skills.

Hypokinetic Circulation

In an adult, the increase of maximal oxygen intake with endurance training normally involves both a widening of the arteriovenous oxygen difference and an increase of stroke volume with a resultant augmentation of maximal cardiac output. However, the circulation of the prepubescent child is "hypokinetic," with a low cardiac output relative to oxygen transport in both submaximal and maximal exercise. The maximal arteriovenous oxygen difference is typically wider than in an adult; thus, there is little scope to broaden this by training. Further, it is unclear whether the myocardium can increase maximal stroke volume as in a highly trained adult.

Male Sex Hormones

Some authors have argued that secretion of the male sex hormones is important to the synthesis of muscular protein during training. However, training-related gains of muscle strength are as great in prepubescent boys as in adults, and such responses seem unrelated to blood levels of testosterone or dihydroepiandrosterone. Opinions are divided as to whether training-related increments of aerobic power are greatest when hormone levels are maximal, immediately following the peak pubertal growth spurt, or are relatively independent of peak height velocity.

Enzyme Activities

There have been suggestions that both the intramuscular stores of anaerobic substrates and the activity of anaerobic enzymes are lower in prepubescent than in pubertal children. However, anaerobic training can increase both the peak and the mean power output of prepubescent children as measured on such tests as the Margaria staircase sprint and the Wingate all-out cycle ergometer test. Further, aerobic function is centrally limited. Thus, an immaturity of muscle enzyme systems could limit function only through a weakening of myocardial performance.

Skill Levels

There is little information on the minimum level of skill that a child needs for endurance training to be effective. Plainly, it is not necessary to run efficiently to train—indeed, an inefficient subject will be stimulated more by a given pace of activity. On the other hand, data from the Trois Rivières study shows little training response before the age of 8 years. Possibly, the younger subjects lacked the physical and psychosocial skills needed to sustain vigorous physical activity.

Matching Training Stimuli

To compare training responses between young children and adolescents or adults, it is necessary to match training stimuli. This is difficult. If a child does not show a clear-cut oxygen consumption plateau, how can we express the intensity of training as a fraction of maximal oxygen intake? Likewise, heart rate does not provide a reliable guide to intensity because of high but variable heart-rate maxima (210–215 beats/min) and the effect of anxiety on heart rates.

Results of Training Experiments

Despite a substantial number of reviews suggesting that prepubescent children cannot be trained, the only *long-term* experiment that failed to elicit a training response in primary school children was that of Yoshida et al.[13] Possibly, their children, at age 5 years, were too young to run effectively. The pattern of exercise adopted, a single run of 750 or 1500 m, one or five times per week, was also not optimal from the viewpoint of endurance training. Positive responses have generally been associated with prolonged and intensive training, and with an optimal experimental design. One 12-week study and three other studies of 30-, 260-, and up to 300-weeks' duration, all with four to five vigorous training sessions per week, have shown substantial training responses relative to matched control students, the gain in the first experiment being seen despite a high initial level of fitness.

The magnitude of response averaged around a 15% gain in the three long-term studies. All had used relatively fit subjects (initial aerobic power in milliliters per kilogram·minute: 47.3 [M + F], 47.5 [M], 45.3 [M], and 43.3 [F]). Such gains are approximately what would be anticipated if adults who were initially of moderate fitness participated in an optimal training program, although the response may be a little less than would be seen in sedentary grown-ups.

Basis of Aerobic Training Response

An increase of maximal oxygen intake could theoretically arise from a greater peak effort, an increase of cardiac stroke volume, a more effective distribution of cardiac output, or a more efficient extraction of oxygen in the working muscles. Which explanation is relevant to the prepubescent child?

Intensity of Peak Effort

We found that the peak heart rate decreased by an average of 4 beats/min after training, with similar changes in experimental and control subjects. Thus, there is little evidence of a spurious training response caused by a greater effort in the second trial, although it remains just as conceivable that a lessening of anxiety at a second visit could have offset the tachycardia associated with a greater physical effort.

Cardiac Stroke Volume

Limited published information suggests that the cardiac stroke volume of the prepubescent child increases by an average of 6.2 mL (about 10%) over 8–12 weeks of training. The published data also show an increase of some 3.3 mL in control subjects, suggesting that a lessening of anxiety or a contamination of the controls may have contributed to these gains. In support of the contamination hypothesis, the control subjects also showed small gains of peak oxygen intake (1.2%, 1.5%, and 5.9%, respectively). The parallel between the increase of stroke volume and the increase of peak oxygen transport suggests that this is the main basis of the prepubescent training response.

Unfortunately, technical reasons led to the collection of data during submaximal exercise. From the viewpoint of peak oxygen transport, the key issue remains whether training allows a larger stroke volume to be developed during maximal effort. In the absence of good maximal data, no strong conclusions may be drawn.

Peripheral Oxygen Extraction

The data of Saltin (1973)[20] suggest that during vigorous exercise, oxygen extraction is fairly complete in normal working muscles. Thus, it is unlikely that training could induce any great gains in oxygen extraction through adaptations in either the enzyme systems or the capillary bed of the working muscles. There may be some redirection of blood flow from the skin and viscera to the active muscles with training, but the potential to increase the peak arteriovenous oxygen difference seems quite small in the young child.

By exclusion, an increase of maximal stroke volume is the most logical explanation of the training response that is seen in the prepubescent child.

Conclusions

Although many early reports suggested that prepubescent children did not respond to aerobic training, this hypothesis seems to have been based on poorly designed experiments with an inadequate training stimulus relative to the initial fitness of the subjects. If an adequate endurance program is continued for 12 weeks or more, the maximal oxygen intake of the prepubescent child is increased by about 15%, much as an older person. The main mechanism for this gain seems to be an increase of cardiac stroke volume. One issue that investigators have yet to resolve is whether early training increases the likelihood of lifelong activity patterns that will protect the individual against future cardiac disease. It may be much more important to have programs that engender positive attitudes than to seek an immediate maximization of aerobic power.

*References**

1. Bar-Or O: Trainability of the pre-pubescent child. *Physician and Sports Medicine* 17:64–82, 1989.
2. Rotstein A, Dotan R, Bar-Or O, et al: Effects of training on anaerobic threshold, maximal aerobic power and anaerobic performance of preadolescent boys. *Int J Sports Med* 7:281–286, 1986.
3. Shephard RJ: Effectiveness of training programmes for prepubescent children. *Sports Med* 13:194–213, 1992.
4. Bailey DA: Exercise, fitness and physical education for the growing child, in Orban WAR (ed): Presented at the National Conference on Fitness and Health. Ottawa, 1974, pp 13–22.
5. Atomi Y, Ohnishi H, Watanabe C, et al: Daily physical activity levels in preadolescent boys related to VO_2max and lactate threshold. *Eur J Appl Physiol* 55:156–161, 1986.
6. Armstrong N, Balding J, Gentle P, et al: Estimation of coronary risk factors in British schoolchildren: A preliminary report. *Br J Sports Med* 24:61–66, 1990.
7. Zauner CW, Maksud MG, Melichna J: Physiological considerations in training young athletes. *Sports Med* 8:15–31, 1989.
8. Sunnegardh J, Bratteby LE: Maximal oxygen uptake, anthropometry and physical activity in a randomly selected sample of 8- and 13-year-old children in Sweden. *Eur J Appl Physiol* 56:266–272, 1987.

*A more detailed list of references is given in Shephard.[3]

9. Jéquier J-C, LaBarre R, Shephard RJ, et al: Externe und interne Fehlerquellen einer Längsschnitt-untersuchungen, Bauss R, Roth K (eds): *Motorische Entwicklung, Probleme und Ergebnisse von Längschnittuntersuchungen.* Darmstadt, Institüt für Sportwissenschaft, 1977, pp 383–393.
10. Ekblöm B: Effect of physical training in adolescent boys. *J Appl Physiol* 27: 350–355, 1969.
11. Stewart KJ, Gutin B: Effects of physical training on cardiorespiratory fitness in children. *Res Q* 47:110–120, 1976.
12. Gatch W, Byrd R: Endurance training and cardiovascular function in 9- and 10-year-old boys. *Arch Phys Med Rehabil* 60:574–577, 1979.
13. Yoshida TI, Ishiko I, Muraoka I: Effect of endurance training on cardiorespiratory functions of 5-year-old children. *Int J Sports Med* 1:91–94, 1980.
14. Massicotte DR, MacNab RBJ: Cardiorespiratory adaptations to training at specified intensities in children. *Med Sci Sports* 6:242–246, 1974.
15. Washington RL, Van Gundy JC, Cohen C, et al: Normal aerobic and anaerobic exercise data for North American school-age children. *J Pediatr* 112:223–233, 1988.
16. Kanaely JA, Boileau RA: The onset of the anaerobic threshold at three stages of physical maturity. *J Sports Med* 28:367–374, 1988.
17. Goode RC, Virgin A, Romet T, et al: Effects of a short period of physical activity in adolescent boys and girls. *Can J Appl Sport Sci* 1:241–250, 1976.
18. Brown CH, Harrower JR, Deeter MF: The effects of cross-country running on preadolescent girls. *Med Sci Sports* 4:1–5, 1972.
19. Shephard RJ: Exercise and sudden death: An overview. *Sports Sci Reviews,* 1:1–13, 1995.
20. Saltin … . Vaccaro P, Mahon AD: Cardiorespiratory responses to endurance training in children. *Sports Med* 4:352–363, 1987.

1 Prevention, Prevalence, Treatment, Head Injuries

Is Prevention of Sports Injuries a Realistic Goal? A Four-Year Prospective Investigation of Sports Injuries Among Physical Education Students

Twellaar M, Verstappen FTJ, Huson A (Univ of Limburg, Maastricht, The Netherlands)

Am J Sports Med 24:528–534, 1996   1–1

Introduction.—The risk of getting injured is part of sports participation; however, little is known about the absolute and relative number of injuries of different sports. The reliability of prospective and retrospective sports injury registration in physical education students during their 4-year education was established. The injury incidence in intramural (program of the institution) and extramural (leisure time) sports activities was determined.

Methods.—A group of 136 physical education students participated in having information on their sports injuries prospectively recorded for 4 years. Every 3 weeks, registration forms were completed and medical consultations were recorded. To establish the reliability of retrospective injury registration, in the last year 50 students were asked to recall all injuries sustained.

Results.—There were 525 sports injuries recorded in the prospective study, with 58% reported in intramural activities and 42% in extramural activities. There were 183 injuries reported by women (3.3 per person); 342 injuries were reported by men (4.3 per person). There was a significantly lower incident rate per 1000 hours of intramural activities (1.26) when compared with the extramural activities (1.77). A decreasing compliance during the study period was noted by the gradual decline in response rate from 98.4% in the first year to 87.7% in the last year. The students did not report 18% of all injuries with recorded medical consultation. Up to 54% of the recorded injuries were forgotten by students at the retrospective injury registration in the last year of the study. The highest number of injuries were sustained in gymnastics (17%), soccer

(15%), and athletics (13%). The risk of injury in ball games and martial arts is lower than for extramural sports activities.

Conclusion.—Prospective injury registration is not complete, even in a well-supervised population, with the reliability of retrospective injury registration being even poorer. Preventive programs will probably not be successful in reducing the number of injuries sustained during physical education lessons.

▶ Clearly, the only conclusion that can be drawn from this study is that the authors are really not good clinical scientists. The basic principal in injury prevention is to first identify the problem, delineate the causative factor or factors, modify the causative variable or variables, and document the results. To conclude that sports injuries cannot be prevented because of inability to collect adequate data is not logical. That is, prevention does not depend on data collection. Also, the conclusion that "sports activities always will result in a certain number of injuries, and the only way to completely avoid the risk is to stop participating" is not only not supported by the data, but, in my view, is rather absurd.

J.S. Torg, M.D.

Football Cleat Design and Its Effect on Anterior Cruciate Ligament Injuries
Lambson RB, Barnhill BS, Higgins RW (West Texas A&M Univ, Canyon; Panhandle Sports Medicine Inst, Amarillo, Tex)
Am J Sports Med 24:155–159, 1996   1–2

Introduction.—Foot fixation is a common factor in anterior cruciate ligament (ACL) injuries and is a primary cause of ankle and knee injuries in sports. These injuries are often the result of torsional forces transmitted to the knee when a player makes a sudden directional change while decelerating. There have been numerous cleat designs over the years promoted as enhancing performance. Sometime "enhanced performance" has been accompanied by serious knee injuries. A 3-year prospective investigation was conducted to determine (1) the torsional resistance of modern football cleat designs and (2) the incidence of surgically documented ACL tears in high school football players wearing varying cleat types.

Methods.—Four cleat designs were compared: (1) edge, longer irregular cleats placed at the peripheral margin of the sole with a number of smaller pointed cleats positioned interiorly (2231 players); (2) flat, cleats on the forefoot the same height, shape, and diameter (832 players); (3) screw-in, 7 screw-in cleats of 0.5-inch height and 0.5-inch diameter (46 players); and (4) pivot disk, a 10-cm circular edge on the sole of the forefoot, with 1 0.5-inch cleat in the center (10 players) (Fig 2). Shoes were evaluated with an apparatus with a prosthetic foot mounted on a steel shaft and loaded with 45.5 kg (Fig 1).

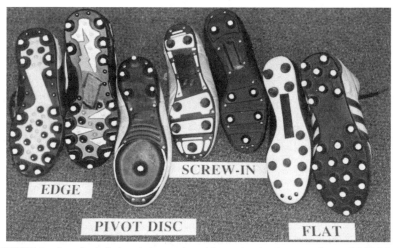

FIGURE 2.—Four football cleat designs evaluated for torsional resistance and rate of ACL injuries. (Courtesy of Lambson RB, Barnhill BS, Higgins RW: Football cleat design and its effect on anterior cruciate ligament injuries. *Am J Sports Med* 24:155–159, 1996.)

Results.—The edge design caused significantly higher torsional resistance than the other designs. The edge design was correlated with a significantly higher ACL injury rate compared with the other 3 designs combined.

Conclusion.—Findings suggest that cleat design has a significant influence on the risk of serious injuries. The edge design was significantly more

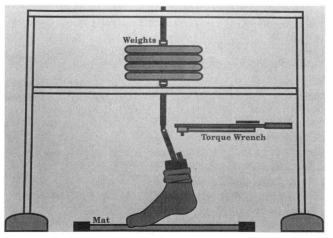

FIGURE 1.—The evaluating apparatus used with a 45.5 kg load to measure shoe-to-surface torsional resistance of different football cleat designs using a Vermont Release Calibrator torque wrench. (Courtesy of Lambson RB, Barnhill BS, Higgins RW: Football cleat design and its effect on anterior cruciate ligament injuries. *Am J Sports Med* 24:155–159, 1996.)

likely to contribute to serious knee injuries than the other designs combined.

▶ The conclusion that "this study suggests a cleat design for football shoes may have a significant influence on the risk of serious knee injury" is in keeping with our observations published 23 years ago.[1] Most unfortunate is the fact that during this intervening period there has been little, if any, interest on the part of responsible athletic administrators, equipment manufacturers, or the sports medicine "leadership" to effectively deal with the issue of the shoe-surface interface and serious knee injuries. Clearly, from a cost analysis standpoint, the interest of the latter group is best served in the treatment rather than prevention of ACL injuries.

J.S. Torg, M.D.

Reference

1. Torg JS, Quedenfeld TC, Landau BS: The shoe-surface interface and its relationship to football knee injuries. *J Sports Med* 2:261–269, 1974.

The Effect of Ambient Temperature on the Shoe-surface Interface Release Coefficient
Torg JS, Stilwell G, Rogers K (Univ of Pennsylvania, Philadelphia)
Am J Sports Med 24:79–82, 1996   1–3

Background.—Foot contact with the playing surface is known to be a possible element in the cause of sports-related knee injuries. Past researchers have studied the correlations between shoe-surface interface and cleat length, configuration, and material composition as well as turf type and surface conditions. The effect of temperature on the rotational torsion resistance of artificial turf football shoes was investigated.

Methods.—Five models of football shoe were investigated on dry artificial playing surface at 5 temperatures ranging from 52° F to 110° F. These included a flat-soled basketball-style turf shoe, a natural grass soccer-style shoe, and 3 multi-studded turf shoes. The force necessary to release a shoe from the turf surface was determined with an assay device—a prosthetic foot mounted on a loaded stainless steel shaft. A torque wrench was used to apply a rotational force to pivot each shoe counterclockwise through an arc of 60 degrees.

Findings.—Release coefficients differed within and among the shoe models at the different turf temperatures. An increase in turf temperature combined with cleat characteristics affected shoe-surface interface friction, which could put the athlete's knee and ankle at risk of injury.

Conclusions.—The flat-soled, basketball-style shoes are the only shoes that can be designated safe or probably safe at all 5 turf temperatures tested. Further research is needed to correlate shoe-surface interface data with the occurence of lower extremity injuries in certain playing conditions before shoe-sole parameters can be recommended definitively. The current data suggest that soft rubber sole shoes on a warm artificial playing surface may pose a risk.

▶ Of note is the conclusion of this paper, which states that to definitely recommend shoe-sole parameters, additional clinically supported research is necessary to correlate shoe-surface interface data with the occurrence of lower extremity injuries under playing conditions. Also of note is the observation that soft rubber-sole shoes worn on an artificial playing surface create a significant risk factor.

J.S. Torg, M.D.

Ultrasound Therapy in Musculoskeletal Disorders: A Meta-analysis
Gam AN, Johannsen F (Bispebjerg Hosp, Copenhagen)
Pain 63:85–91, 1995   1–4

Introduction.—Ultrasound therapy is used to relieve pain and joint immobility. A meta-analysis was performed to determine the effectiveness of therapeutic ultrasound in the treatment of pain in musculoskeletal disorders.

Methods.—The Index Medicus (1950–1966) and Medline (1966–1992) were used to locate papers on the therapeutic use of ultrasound. A total of 293 papers published since 1950 were reviewed to determine those that could be used in the meta-analysis.

Results.—Twenty-two of 293 papers met inclusion criteria. Many papers had to be excluded because of lack of appropriate data. Many variables have been used to assess the effectiveness of ultrasound, including pain, muscle strength, walking distance, and range of motion (ROM). Trials were placed in 1 of 2 categories: A) Trials included a sham-ultrasound-treated group; and B) Trials included only nonultrasound treatment or an untreated control group. Two standardized effect sizes ($d_{d/r}$ and $d_{d/s}$) were used to evaluate the effect of ultrasound treatment on pain. There were 16 category A trials and 6 category B trials. Thirteen of 16 trials in category A presented data in a way that made pooling possible using $d_{d/r}$. Nine of the 13 category A trials presented data in a way that made pooling possible using $d_{d/s}$. No reduction of pain was statistically evidenced in any of these trials. One trial reported a reduction in calcification in bursitis calcarea. There was no reason to analyze the remaining papers in category B because of the lack of evidence of therapeutic effect in category A patients. It was not possible to perform a dose-response analysis because of insufficient description of the methods used.

Conclusion.—Analysis of literature published since 1950 indicates that the use of ultrasound in the treatment of musculoskeletal disorders is based on empirical experience. Well-designed, controlled trials are lacking. Further investigation should evaluate the effect of ultrasound in conjunction with exercise therapy in the treatment of musculoskeletal disorders.

▶ The conclusion of this paper, that "... the use of ultrasound in treatment of musculoskeletal disorders is based on empirical experience, but lacks substantial support in controlled studies," is something that we have either known or suspected for a long time. However, it should be pointed out that there are fundamental problems with this study. Meta-analysis involves pooling of results involving both chronic and acute disorders, as well as results from the 2 modes of delivery, continuous and pulsed. Also to be answered is the question of whether there is any beneficial effect of ultra-sound when supplementing an exercise therapy program.

J.S. Torg, M.D.

Perioperative Compartment Syndrome: A Report of Four Cases
Seiler JG, Valadie AL III, Drvaric DM, et al (Emory Univ, Atlanta, Ga)
J Bone Joint Surg Am 78A:600–602, 1996   1–5

Introduction.—The use of pressurized devices to enhance fluid flow postoperatively is sometimes associated with acute compartment syndromes. The authors have encountered 4 patients in whom an acute compartment syndrome developed during surgery. An analysis of these 4 cases, including their functional outcomes, was reported.

Patients.—The patients were 3 men and 1 woman, 26 to 57 years of age. Intraoperative compartment syndrome developed in the forearm in 2 cases, the calf in 1, and the hand in 1. In each case, the affected extremity rapidly became swollen and tense. The compartment syndromes were linked to a pressurized pulsatile irrigation system in 2 patients, a fluid infusion pump during arthroscopy in 1, and a device for pressurized infusion of parenteral fluids in 1. Each patient was managed by appropriate fasciotomies, which revealed large amounts of extravasated fluid within the soft tissues. At follow-up, 3 of the patients had no neurologic abnormalities. One of the patients with forearm compartment syndrome had no recovery of ulnar nerve function, although median and radial nerve functions were intact.

Discussion.—Perioperative compartment syndromes can be related to the use of pressurized irrigation devices. These devices should be used with caution, and any extremity at risk of excessive fluid infiltration should be carefully examined during surgery. If perioperative compartment syndrome develops, immediate fasciotomy is warranted. Prompt recognition and treatment of this complication are essential.

▶ On the basis of my own experience with fluid extravasation into the thigh or calf during arthroscopic procedures as well as the several reports in the literature, I question the necessity of having performed fasciotomies. Simply put, with patience, and "tincture of time," these "perioperative compartment syndromes" would have resolved.

J.S. Torg, M.D.

Thromboembolic Complications in Arthroscopic Surgery: Experience of the Italian Arthroscopy Group and Review of the Literature
Adriani E, Conforti M (Ospedale S Pertini, Rome, Italy)
J Sports Traumatol Rel Res 18:159–172, 1996   1–6

Background.—Though arthroscopy appears to be a harmless procedure, the potentially fatal complications of pulmonary embolism and deep vein thrombosis (DVT) can occur. The incidence, risk factors, and prevention of thromboembolic complications in patients undergoing arthroscopic surgery were established by reviewing the literature.

Review.—Thromboembolic complications occur less often in arthroscopic than in open surgery. The incidence of DVT appears to be about 1%. However, most case series rely on clinical data. No prospective studies based on instrumental diagnosis and conducted with uniform groups of patients have been done to determine the risk factors of this complication. Authorities generally believe that patients at risk for thromboembolism should receive prophylaxis and that some risk factors should be decreased or eliminated. However, it is still not known which patients are at risk, which intraoperative parameters are most effective for decreasing the risk of DVT, and what type of prophylaxis is appropriate. It is also unclear whether the use of prophylaxis is more of a medicolegal necessity than a medical one.

Current Indications for Prophylaxis.—Currently it is believed that prophylaxis is indicated for patients with previous DVT episodes, patients older than 50 years, and patients with medical or surgical risk factors such as diabetes, hypertension, and vasculopathy. Prophylaxis is also deemed necessary for patients undergoing tibial plateau repairs; ligament surgery, especially acute and subacute cases; surgery with forseeably long operative and tourniquet times; and operations requiring slow rehabilitation. Treatment of infections also calls for prophylaxis.

▶ The authors present a comprehensive review of thromboembolic complications in arthroscopic surgery. Their conclusion that although deep vein thrombosis and thromboembolic phenomena occur less frequently in arthroscopic procedures than in open surgery, "they are nonetheless a real risk and must always be borne in mind by the surgeon." They fail to mention incomplete exsanguination of the involved extremity with tourniquet use as a contributing factor. Also deserving greater emphasis is the contributing role that oral contraceptives play in postoperative phlebitis.

J.S. Torg, M.D.

Roller-Blades: Should They Carry a Government Health Warning?
Spicer DDM, Mullins MM, Wexler DM (St Mary's Hosp, London)
Injury 27:401–403, 1996   1–7

Background.—Rollerblading is becoming increasingly popular in England. Injuries associated with rollerblading that were seen at St. Mary's Hospital in London during a 12 week-period are described.

Methods.—Between June 1 and August 31, 1995, all referrals from the emergency department to the orthopedics department related to roller-blading were recorded. Data were collected on age, sex, handedness, experience, protective equipment usage, injury, and treatment.

Findings.—During this study, 29 patients were treated for 30 injuries associated with rollerblading. Of these 29 patients, 9 required inpatient treatment and 10 required operative treatment. The patients ranged in age from 10–49 years. There were 13 injuries involving the dominant arm and 2 the nondominant arm. There were 23 fractures, 2 dislocations, and 5 soft tissue injuries. The most frequently injured bone was the radius. The majority of these patients were wearing protective gear while rollerblad-ing. The most serious injuries were sustained after striking an object at high speed.

Conclusions.—This study describes injuries associated with rollerblad-ing. Although there was a range of injuries, injuries to the radius were the most common. There was generally good compliance with current safety gear recommendations in the study group, but wrist guards appeared to be relatively ineffective against transmitted force injuries. Protective gear may be giving rollerbladers a false sense of security.

▶ Scheiber et al. have recently reported that 9.3 million individuals are estimated to have participated in inline skating in 1992, with 30,863 treated injuries documented by the National Electronic Injury Surveillance System.[1] Although it is difficult to translate available data in terms of injury rates, it appears that in-line skating is clearly an at-risk activity.

J.S. Torg, M.D.

Reference

1. Scheiber RA, Branche-Dorsey CM, Ryan GW: Comparison of in-line skating in-juries with roller-skating and skateboarding injuries. *JAMA* 271:1856–1858, 1994.

Risk Factors for Injuries From In-line Skating and the Effectiveness of Safety Gear

Scheiber RA, Branche-Dorsey CM, Ryan GW, et al (Centers for Disease Control and Prevention, Atlanta, Ga; Consumer Product Safety Commission, Washington, DC)
N Engl J Med 335:1630–1635, 1996   1–8

Background.—The popularity of in-line skating is growing fast in the United States, accompanied by an increase in the number of in-line skating injuries severe enough to necessitate care in the emergency department. The wrist is the most common site of injury among in-line skaters, ac-counting for 37% of all such injuries. The efficacy of currently available wrist guards, elbow pads, knee pads, and helmets in preventing skating injuries was investigated.

Methods.—Data from 91 emergency departments participating in the National Electronic Injury Surveillance System was analyzed. Persons seeking medical care for in-line skating injuries between December 1992 and July 1993 were identified and interviewed by telephone. Skaters who injured their wrists, elbows, knees, or heads were compared with skaters with injuries to other parts of their bodies in a case-control design.

Findings.—One hundred sixty-one of 206 eligible patients (78%) were interviewed; 32% of the injuries were to the wrist. Twenty-five percent of all injuries were wrist fractures. Seven percent of all patients wore all safety gear, and 46% wore none. Forty-five percent wore knee pads; 33%, wrist guards; 28%, elbow pads; and 20%, helmets. Patients not wearing wrist guards had a 10:4 odds ratio for wrist injury compared with patients who did wear wrist guards, after adjustment for age and sex. The odds ratio for elbow injury, after adjustment for number of lessons taken and whether the skaters trick-skated, was 9:5 for patients who did not wear elbow pads. The increase in risk of knee injury associated with nonuse of knee pads was nonsignificant. The efficacy of helmets cound not be determined, because too small a number of skaters sustained head injuries.

Conclusions.—In-line skaters should wear wrist guards, elbow pads, knee pads, and helmets. The current data clearly demonstrate the efficacy of wrist guards and elbow pads in preventing in-line skating injuries.

▶ The small number of skaters who sustained a head injury did not permit the authors to determine the degree of protection afforded by helmets. However, to this observer it appears that the recommendation for in-line skaters to wear the standard bicycle helmet is, so to speak, a no-brainer.

J.S. Torg, M.D.

Trauma Epidemiology in the Martial Arts: The Results of an Eighteen-year International Survey
Birrer RB (Catholic Med Ctr, Jamaica, NY)
Am J Sports Med 24:S72–S79, 1996   1–9

Background.—The martial arts have become extremely popular worldwide. The epidemiology of traumatic injury associated with the martial arts was determined using data from an 18-year international survey.

Trauma Epidemiology in the Martial Arts.—The risk of injury in the martial arts is significant. Most injuries are of mild to moderate severity and consist of contusions, sprains, strains, lacerations, and abrasions. The most common injury is contusion. Dislocations and fractures are least common. The lower extremity, especially the leg, is most often injured, and the neck is least at risk. Injuries to the arm and forearm are the mildest, whereas those to the face and head are most severe. Most injuries occur during fighting, particularly during noncompetitive training situations. The rate and severity of injury are significantly reduced by protective equipment. Most injuries go unreported. The rate and severity of injuries are significantly greater in men than women. Injury rate and severity are also greater among participants with less experience. The risk of a life-threatening injury is only 1 in 500 to 600 injuries. Increasing levels of contact during fighting are directly related to increasing rates and severity of injury. Also, the risk and severity of injury during competition are greater than during noncompetition. Several significant risk factors for injury in the martial arts have been identified, including failure to use protective equipment, lack of training experience, male sex, and competition.

Recommendations.—To reduce the number and severity of injuries in the martial arts, safety guidelines should be established to standardize and enforce rules across organizations and styles for all forms of competition, to mandate the use of protective equipment, to create and maintain safe environments for training and competition, to track injuries through a standardized registry, to develop a pre-bout clearance system for all fighters, to establish clinical protocols for return to play, and to create specific guidelines and plans for medical coverage at all competitive events. Certifiable medical standards should also be established for instructors, referees, and physicians. Finally, continued research is warranted.

▶ The author has produced an ambitious attempt to document martial arts injuries that occurred during an 18-year period. As may be expected, this study is beset with the problems incurred by the retrospective questionnaire method of data collection. However, their 41% response rate is certainly creditable. An interesting comparison can be made with data reported by the National Electronic Injury Surveillance System (NEISS) for the period 1979 through 1992, in which 5,617 cases were documented, having been seen in emergency facilities. Of these, 5% were considered to be severe injuries as compared to 1.7% in the Birrer study. With regard to anatomical location of the injuries, they were similar in both studies. It is interesting to note that the incidence and prevalence rates developed indicate that with regard to risk, martial arts compares favorably with other sports and recreational activities. Specifically, it is claimed that the injury rate for martial arts is one twentieth that of football, and the activity appears to be safer than golf and general exercise. Of course, the author's data do not support his contention and his reliance on data reported in the literature is to be questioned.

J.S. Torg, M.D.

Shoulder Injuries During Alpine Skiing

Kocher MS, Feagin JA Jr (Harvard Med School, Boston; Duke Univ, Durham, NC)
Am J Sports Med 24:665–669, 1996   1–10

Objective.—Possible reasons for the increase in upper extremity injuries among alpine skiers include changes in equipment, environment, and behavior. Although shoulder injuries account for 4.5% to 10% of all alpine skiing injuries, they have not been well studied. Results of an investigation to characterize the incidence and types of shoulder injuries during alpine skiing are presented.

Methods.—A retrospective review of records from 1990 to 1993 at the Jackson Hole Ski Resort ski clinic was conducted to determine the population at risk and the number of injuries per 1,000 skier-days.

Results.—There were 3,451 injuries in 3,247 patients for an incidence of 4.44 injuries per 1,000 skier-days. Upper extremity injuries represented 29.1% ($n = 1,004$) of all injuries with the most common injury being a sprained thumb. Shoulder injuries accounted for 11.4% of all injuries and 39.1% of upper extremity injuries for an incidence of 0.51 injuries per 1,000 skier-days. The most common shoulder injuries were rotator cuff strains (24.2%), anterior glenohumeral dislocations or subluxations (21.6%), acromioclavicular separations (19.6%), and clavicle fractures (10.9%), and most were due to falls (93.9%). The average age at injury was 35.4 years and the male-to-female ratio was 3:1. The incidence and total number of shoulder injuries is higher than in previous studies.

Conclusion.—Because the incidence and number of shoulder injuries appears to be increasing among alpine skiers, and because of the morbidity that can occur as a result of such injuries, additional studies should examine skiing surfaces, technique, education, exercise, and bracing.

▶ I certainly agree with the conclusion of the authors that "... the prevention of shoulder injuries during skiing through interventions in skiing surfaces, technique, education, exercise, and bracing is worthy of further consideration and study."

J.S. Torg, M.D.

Acute Injuries in Cross-country and Downhill Off-road Bicycle Racing
Kronisch RL, Pfeiffer RP, Chow TK (San Jose State Univ, Calif; Boise State Univ, Idaho; Loma Linda Univ, Calif)
Med Sci Sports Exerc 28:1351–1355, 1996   1–11

Introduction.—Acute injuries are common among participants in off-road (or mountain) bicycling, especially during the most popular forms of competition: cross-country (CC) and downhill (DH) races. One study found a greater than four-fold increased risk of injury in competitive versus noncompetitive riding situations. To further describe injury patterns in this rapidly growing sport, injured cyclists at 3 major off-road bicycle races were examined and interviewed.

Methods.—The study was conducted at 3 of 7 races in the 1995 national championship series of the National Off-road Bicycle Association (NORBA). Sites of these NORBA races were Mount Spokane, Wash., Vail, Colo., and Mammoth Mountain, Calif. Reportable injuries were those that occurred during competition and prevented the cyclist from completing the event. A standardized questionnaire was used to record demographic data and details of the injury.

Results.—The overall injury rates were 0.49% for CC races and 0.51% for DH events. For every hour of racing time there were 0.37 injured cyclists for CC versus 4.34 for DH—a significant difference. Women had a significantly higher injury rate (1.05%) than men (0.40%) in CC events. The most frequent types of injuries—abrasions, contusions, and lacerations—occurred in 95% of cyclists injured in CC and 73% of those injured in DH events. Musculoskeletal injuries, including sprains, strains, fractures, dislocations, and subluxations, occurred in 35% of injured CC cyclists and 55% of injured DH cyclists. Concussions occurred in 15% of injured CC cyclists and in 9% of injured DH cyclists. The need for emergency room treatment was significantly greater for those injured in DH versus CC events (8 of 11 versus 7 of 20 cyclists). Severity of injury was greater in injuries involving loss of control, mechanical failure, or collision with a stationary object than in injuries involving loss of traction or collision with another rider. Injuries were also more severe when cyclists fell forward over the handlebars than when they fell to the side in CC events.

Discussion.—Overall injury rates were similar for CC and DH events, but when rates were calculated for injuries per 100 hours the DH events had an increased risk of injury; and based on the need for emergency room treatment, DH-related injuries were more severe than CC-related injuries. Women, however, had a higher injury rate and more severe injuries in CC events.

Forearm and Wrist Fractures in Mountain Bike Riders
Rajapaske BN, Horne G, Devane P (Wellington School of Medicine, New Zealand)
N Z Med J 109:147–148, 1996   1–12

Introduction.—Mountain biking has been growing in popularity in New Zealand. An increase in the sale of mountain bikes and in the number of riders has been accompanied by a significant number of forearm fractures. In a review of forearm fractures treated at a single institution, researchers sought to identify the different types of fractures sustained by mountain bikers and to assess the physical and social consequences of these injuries.

Methods.—Between July 1992 and July 1994, 37 patients were treated at the Wellington (New Zealand) Hospital for forearm or wrist fractures sustained in mountain biking accidents. Twenty-five patients were located and agreed to participate in the study. Fractures were classified on the basis of radiographs. The patients completed questionnaires on the circumstances of the injury, time required off work, and functional outcome. Clinical examinations were designed to evaluate pain, dexterity, deformity, range of movement, and strength.

Results.—Patients were 21 men and 4 women with a mean age of 25.9 years at the time of the accident. One had a bilateral fracture, 4 had unilateral fractures in more than 1 location, and 20 had unilateral fractures at a single location. Seventeen fractures occurred in the distal third of the forearm and 10 at the radial head. In 16 cases the accident occurred while riding on the road. Eight patients had previous injuries to the affected arm and 11 had injuries in addition to the forearm fracture. Thirteen patients required time off work; the average time off was 28 days. Fifteen patients received an excellent rating on the functional assessment, 5 were graded as satisfactory, 4 as unsatisfactory, and 1 as poor. Twelve patients reported residual pain and stiffness from the injury.

Discussion.—The increase in fractures seen with mountain biking is similar to an increase reported in the mid-1980s when bicycles known as BMXs—also different from the conventional road bicycle—became quite popular. Mountain bike accidents can cause significant traumatic injury, usually in the distal third of the forearm, but most patients recover well.

▶ These two studies are in keeping with that of Chow,et al. (Abstracts 1–11 and 1–12).[1] This study of 268 members of California off-road bicycle associations found that extremity injuries such as abrasions, lacerations, and contusions occurred in 90% of the cyclists, and 12% sustained a fracture. Of note, Tucci and Barone[2] found radial head fractures to be the most common in cyclists, whereas Lofthouse[3] determined that most upper-extremity injuries involve carpal bones, with the scaphoid being most commonly fractured.

J.S. Torg, M.D.

References

1. Chow TK, Bracker MD, Patrick K: Acute injuries from mountain biking. *West J Med* 159:145–148, 1993.
2. Tucci JJ, Barone JE: Study of urban bicycling accidents. *A J SM* 16:181–184, 1988.
3. Lofthouse GA: Traumatic injuries to the extremities and thorax. *Clin Sports Med* 13:113–135, 1994.

Causes of Horse-related Injuries in a Rural Western Community
Thompson JM, von Hollen B (Univ of Calgary, Canada; Sundre Gen Hosp, Canada)
Can Fam Physician 42:1103–1109, 1996   1–13

Objective.—Horseback riding is common in rural Alberta, Canada, and so are related injuries. The role of horse behavior during injury incidents was examined to gain a better understanding of this problem.

Methods.—Physicians in the rural community of Sundre, population 5000, were asked to report horse-related injuries occurring between March 5, 1989, and July 30, 1991, on a special form. Retrospectively, the patients' age, sex, home town, management after diagnosis, transfer to a higher level of care, self-assessed riding experience, the horse's experience, and any contributing factors were determined. Primary causes of injuries were collected and classified.

Results.—During the study period 150 injuries were reported, and primary causes were ascertained in all but 5 cases. The horse was found to be at fault in 102 cases and not primarily at fault in 43 cases. One person was wearing a helmet. After treatment 127 patients were sent home, 11 were admitted to the local hospital, 11 transferred to an urban center, and 1 died. Most (103) were engaged in recreational activities, 107 were riding the horse, and 93 were intermediate or experienced at handling a horse. Most horses (70) were ridden daily or weekly. Sites of injuries included the head and neck in 18 patients, the trunk in 26, the upper extremities in 42, the lower extremities in 38, and multiple sites in 26. Injuries occurred much more frequently in the summer.

Conclusion.—Although the study was small and probably did not include all cases of injury, the reported horse-related injuries were found to be primarily the fault of the horse in 66% of cases. Only 1 patient wore a helmet, although head injuries were common.

▶ This comprehensive, interesting article is the first study to analyze the role of horse behavior in human injuries. Noteworthy is the fact that two thirds of the injuries were attributed to and caused by the horses. Although it was observed that head injuries were relatively common, certainly the horses cannot be blamed for the fact that helmets are rarely worn in the "western community."

J.S. Torg, M.D.

Major Injuries Occurring During Use of a Golf Cart
Kelly EG (South Hills Orthopaedic Surgery Associates, Pittsburgh, Pa)
Orthopedics 19:519–523, 1996   1–14

Objective.—Major injuries from golf cart use are largely unreported. A report of a poll of 280 orthopedic surgeons regarding their experience with major traumatic injuries occurring as a result of an accident while using a golf cart is presented.

Methods.—The surgeons were asked about the type of injury and treatment, age of the patients, adverse outcome, and number of years in practice. A total of 119 surgeons from 37 states responded and reported 111 injuries, including 11 to cart drivers younger than 16.

Results.—Patients sustained 49 fractured tibias, 10 fractured femurs, 2 dislocated knees, 6 fractured spines, 8 fractured pelvises, 8 fractured humeri, and 7 major ligamentous tears. Associated injuries included 1 lacerated liver, 2 lacerated spleens, 1 subdural hematoma, 3 spinal cord injuries, 2 full-thickness burns, and 2 patients with acute respiratory compromise. Adverse outcomes included 4 deaths, 2 patients with paraplegia, 5 with compartment syndrome, 7 with chronic osteomyelitis, 2 with ischemic contracture, 2 with pulmonary embolism, and 5 with reflex sympathetic dystrophy. Surgery was required in 81 patients; 10 needed more than 1 operation. Most injuries occurred when a foot or leg outside the cart was caught on an obstacle or the cleat of the shoe caught on the

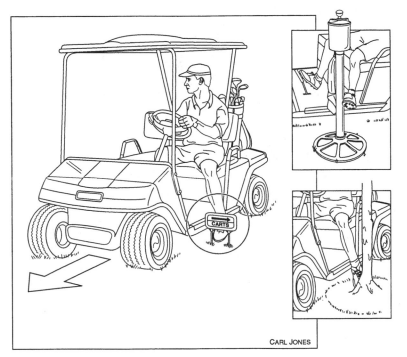

CARL JONES

FIGURE 2.—Leg catching on an obstacle. (Courtesy of Kelly EG: Major injuries occurring during the use of a golf cart. *Orthopedics* 19:519–523, 1996).

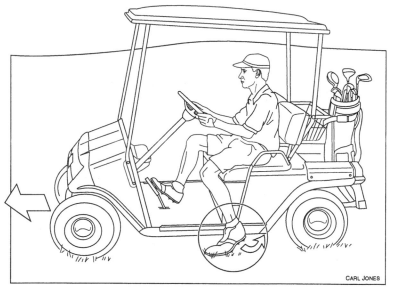

CARL JONES

FIGURE 3.—Cleat of shoe catching in turf. (Courtesy of Kelly EG: Major injuries occurring during the use of a golf cart. *Orthopedics* 19:519–523, 1996).

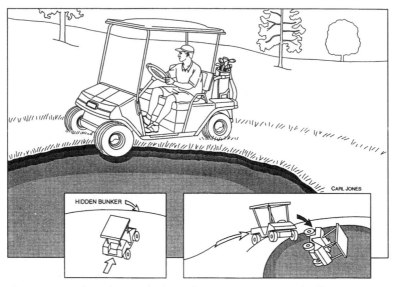

FIGURE 4.—Cart descending into bunker and overturning. (Courtesy of Kelly EG: Major injuries occurring during the use of a golf cart. *Orthopedics* 19:519–523, 1996.)

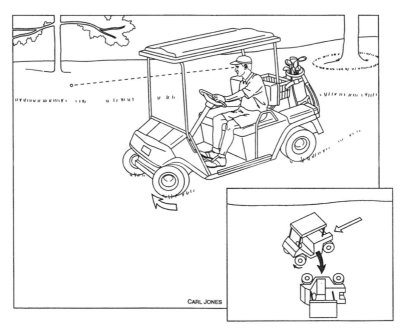

FIGURE 5.—Turning wheels of cart while descending a grade causing a cart to overturn. (Courtesy of Kelly EG: Major injuries occurring during the use of a golf cart. *Orthopedics* 19:519–523, 1996.)

turf (Fig 2 and Fig 3). All fatalities involved an overturned cart (Fig 4 and Fig 5).

Conclusion.—Golf cart injuries are serious and potentially fatal. They also can result in permanent disability. Preventive measures such as keeping feet inside the cart, being cautious on a slope particularly in wet conditions, strict enforcement of age requirements, and prohibition of alcohol would eliminate most of these accidents.

▶ Although the frequency of occurrence of these injuries is not given, the article clearly points out the potential for a significant trauma and morbidity during the operation of a golf cart. With regard to safety practices, feet should be kept in, caution should be observed on slopes during wet conditions, and alcohol consumption forbidden.

J.S. Torg, M.D.

The Effect of Nonablative Laser Energy on Joint Capsular Properties: An In Vitro Histologic and Biochemical Study Using a Rabbit Model
Hayashi K, Thabit G III, Vailas AC, et al (Univ of Wisconsin, Madison; Sports, Orthopedic and Rehabilitation Medicine Associates, Menlo Park, Calif)
Am J Sports Med 24:640–646, 1996   1–15

Introduction.—Collagen shrinks when heated in its hydrated state, with resultant significant changes in its chemical and physical properties. The nonablative application of laser energy from the holmium:yttrium-aluminum-garnet (Ho: YAG) laser to the joint capsule in patients with glenohumeral instability has been shown to shrink the joint capsule and stabilize the shoulder. The effect of laser energy at nonablative levels on the histologic and biochemical properties of joint capsular tissue was analyzed in an in vitro rabbit model.

Methods.—Twelve New Zealand White rabbits were killed and specimens were collected from the medial and lateral portion of the femoropatellar joint of each leg of each rabbit. The specimens were assigned to 5, 10, or 15 W treatment groups or a control group. The specimens were mounted in a custom-made jig and placed in a 37°C bath of lactated Ringer's solution. Laser energy was applied with a Ho:YAG laser at a velocity of 2 mm/sec. The handpiece was set 1.5 mm from the synovial surface, and 4 transverse passes were made across the tissue. Six specimens underwent histologic analysis and 6 underwent biochemical analysis.

Results.—Histologic evaluation showed thermal alteration of collagen at all laser energy densities; collagen was fused and there were pyknotic nuclear changes in fibroblasts. The higher laser energy was responsible for significantly greater morphologic changes over a significantly larger area. Biochemical analysis showed application of laser energy did not significantly alter type I collagen content or nonreducible crosslinks.

Conclusion.—The effect of nonablative laser energy on joint capsular tissue was primarily caused by thermal denaturation of collagen. The components of type I collagen and its nonreducible crosslinks were not changed. Fibroblasts demonstrated necrotic changes after application of laser energy. Findings should be interpreted with caution until in vivo investigations can evaluate the effect of tissue responses.

▶ The clinical relevance of this study relates to the current practice of using nonablative application of laser energy from the Holmium:YAG laser to shrink the glenohumeral joint capsule of patients with multidirectional or unidirectional instability. Of note, the authors caution that "the results of this study should be interpreted with caution until in vivo studies are performed to determine the effect of tissue response on these properties."

J.S. Torg, M.D.

Effect of Growth Factors on Matrix Synthesis by Ligament Fibroblasts
Marui T, Niyibizi C, Georgescu HI, et al (Univ of Pittsburgh, Pa)
J Orthop Res 15:18–23, 1997   1–16

Introduction.—The most common injuries found by orthopedists are ligamentous injuries of the knee joint, which cause significant joint instability and can lead to degenerative changes of the joint. Different growth factors can elicit different biologic responses during wound healing, such as cell proliferation, matrix synthesis, chemotaxis, and secretion of other growth factors. Wound healing has been shown to have been enhanced by transforming growth factor β1, epidermal growth factor, and fibroblast growth factor, which may also play a role in ligament healing. The effect of growth factors on ligament fibroblast was invesitgated to evaluate the potential to improve the healing processes of tissue.

Methods.—Using cultured fibroblasts from medial collateral ligament and anterior cruciate ligament in vitro, the effects of basic and acidic fibroblast growth factors, transforming growth factor β1, and epidermal growth factor on collagen and noncollagenous protein synthesis were examined. To measure synthesis of collagen and noncollagenous protein, uptake of tritiated proline was used. To analyze the type of collagens synthesized, sodium dodecyle sulfate-polyacrylamide gel electrophoresis was used.

Results.—On a dose-dependent basis, transforming growth factor β1 increased both collagen and noncollagenous protein synthesis by medial collateral and anterior cruciate ligament fibroblasts. Treatment with transforming growth factor β1 increased collagen synthesis by cultured fibroblasts from the medial collateral and anterior cruciate ligament by as much as 1.5 times when compared with controls that were untreated. The amounts of matrix proteins synthesized by anterior cruciate ligament fibroblasts were approximately half of that by medial collateral ligament fibroblasts, although the response to transforming growth factor β1 by anterior cruciate ligament fibroblasts was equal to that by medial collateral ligament fibroblasts. The increase was mostly seen in type I collagen.

Collagen synthesis was increased by about 25% with epidermal growth factor in the treatment of anterior cruciate ligament fibroblasts, but on the medial collateral ligament fibroblasts, there was little effect. Collagen or noncollagenous protein synthesis was not increased by basic or acidic fibroblast growth factor.

Conclusion.—The ligament may be potentially strengthened by topical application of transforming growth factor β1, alone or in combination with epidermal growth factor by increasing matrix synthesis during its remodeling and healing processes.

Systemically and Locally Administered Growth Hormone Stimulates Bone Healing in Combination With Osteopromotive Membranes: An Experimental Study in Rats

Hedner E, Linde A, Nilsson A (Göteborg Univ, Sweden)
J Bone Min Res 11:1952–1960, 1996   1–17

Background.—Transosseus "critical size" bone defects do not heal with bone, but fill with fibrous connective tissue. These defects will heal with bone if an artificial, biocompatible membrane covers the injury. Growth hormone (GH) stimulates postnatal longitudinal bone growth in a dose-dependent manner. Its effects on the healing of bone defects have not been as well investigated. It may be possible to combine the use of the artificial membrane and GH to improve bone regenration and healing. The effect of GH was investigated using transosseus defects in the mandibles of rats.

Methods.—Transosseus defects were created in the mandibles of 93 adult rats and covered with fitted e-PTFE (polytetrafluoroethylene) membranes. Rats were treated with either human GH at 0.2, 2, 20 and 200 μg/day, bovine GH at 200 μg/day, prolactin at 200 μg/day or saline, administered systemically or lcocally via subcutaneously implanted mini-osmotic pumps. Healing was determined after 2, 3, and 4 weeks.

Results.—Both human and bovine growth hormone stimulated local bone growth, as compared to prolactin and saline. Human GH significantly promoted bone growth after 3 weeks at concentration of at least 2 μg/day, whether administered locally or systemically. There were no detrimental or inflammatory reactions to the artificial membranes during the course of this study.

Conclusions.—The results of this study of a rat model of transosseus bone defects demonstrated that human growth hormone stimulates bone growth when administered either locally or systemically. Human GH can be used in conjunction with osteopromotive membranes, such as e-PTFE, to stimulate bone healing of transosseus defects. GH appears to exert specific, direct effects on bone tissue that are not mediated by the liver.

▶ These two articles (Abstracts 1–16 and 1–17) suggest that perhaps there will be a place in the future for gene therapy and molecular biology in the management of acute injuries to both ligaments and bone. Interesting!

J.S. Torg, M.D.

Techniques of Cartilage Growth Enhancement: A Review of the Literature

Wirth CJ, Rudert M (Med School of Hannover, Germany)

Arthroscopy 12:300–308, 1996   1–18

Background.—Joint cartilage is generally thought to have limited regenerative capacity. However, despite this belief, experience suggests that cartilage defects can heal with surgery, particularly arthroscopic surgery. Many questions remain about the potential for cartilage healing. The literature on techniques of cartilage growth enhancement is reviewed.

Cartilage Growth Enhancement.—The data suggest that cartilage cannot completely regenerate itself. Cartilage cells may increase production of cartilage matrix if stimulated to do so by injury. In superficial defects, this process leads to temporary repair of defects with fibrous cartilage. For deeper defects in the subchondral zone, only pluripotent progenitor cells can effect repair. These cells, taken from the bone marrow, perichondrium, or periosteum, are transplanted into the defect. The fibrous cartilage that fills the defect may subsequently be transformed into hyaline cartilage, depending on the functional conditions in the area. However, the collagen produced by these cells is not the same as the specific type II collagen found in cartilage. Primary healing is achieved with bone-cartilage autografts and allografts. However, these grafts are subsequently transformed into fibrous cartilage, thus losing their biomechanical properties over the long term. Laboratory studies have tried stimulating isolated chondrocytes in culture medium with growth hormones and vitamins. The result is increased production of extracellular matrix and increased cell growth. Because adult chondrocytes cannot multiply, this growth may take place through amitotic partition. Studies have shown that it is possible to preserve chondrocytes in a viable state for prolonged periods.

Summary.—Various reported techniques of cartilage growth enhancement are reviewed, including osteochondral autograft and allograft, perichondral and periosteal grafts, osteochondral progenitor cell transplantation, and chondrocyte transplantation. All of these techniques are designed to overcome the incomplete capacity of cartilage to repair itself. In the future, cartilage may be grown in the laboratory for subsequent transplantation into the same individual.

▶ This article is a concise review of current concepts regarding the known principles involved in articular cartilage cell transplantation. Actually, its main strength lies in an exhaustive bibliography that includes 96 citations. Although lacking in convincing clinical data, it is concluded that "chondrocyte viability can be preserved in the laboratory over extended periods. In the future, cartilage growth in the laboratory and replantation of explanted cartilage into cartilage defects of the same individual may make cartilage healing possible."

J.S. Torg, M.D.

Injection Techniques and Use in the Treatment of Sports Injuries
Scott WA (Kaiser Permanente Med Ctr, Santa Clara, Calif; Stanford Univ, Palo Alto, Calif)
Sports Med 22:406–416, 1996   1–19

Introduction.—This article describes therapeutic techniques for injectable medications commonly used to treat musculoskeletal problems. The data are derived from the author's experience and a review of the literature.

Overall Treatment Program.—The best results can be achieved only by a combined program. Before injection, the REST (*R*esume *E*xercise below *S*oreness *T*hreshold) concept should be applied to all activities. All injections should be both diagnostic and therapeutic. The characteristic injury pain should be provoked during physical examination and eliminated by the anesthetic portion of the injection. Needle penetration should not be very painful and must avoid neurovascular bundles. Medication should flow freely from the needle. Ten to 20 minutes afer injection, pain provocation procedures should be repeated, with approximately 90% pain relief if placement has been accurate. All injections are followed by a program of progressive stretching and strengthening.

Pain Reduction.—Many patients fear needles. The skin is heavily innervated and pain is proportional to the size of the needle and the tissue density injected. To partially anesthetize the skin, ice or a topical vapocoolant spray is applied or the injection site skin is firmly pinched for 3 to 4 seconds. After this temporary partial anesthesia, the needle should be inserted quickly and anesthesia applied into the lowest density tissue closest to the actual injury site. As the needle is withdrawn, a small amount of anesthesia is infiltrated into the skin. After 10 minutes, the corticosteroid/anesthetic mixture, diluted to pass through the needle, is injected. Complications of injection can include allergy, infection, and vasovagal syncope, but are rare.

Bone Tendon Injection Technique.—Either carefully penetrate the skin with a 25-gauge 1.5-inch needle and lightly deposit small amounts of steroid/anesthetic over the tender area or repeatedly pierce the periosteum. The second procedure is painful. Follow up all injections with ice and rest for several days. All bone-tendon injuries require counter-force compressive bracing, eccentric-type strengthening, and sports-specific functional progressive resistance programs. Recovery usually takes 3 to 6 months and can take 18 months.

Intraarticular Injections.—Intraarticular injections are easy to do and well tolerated. A 25-gauge 1.5-inch needle should be used to pierce the joint at its thinnest point, avoiding neurovascular bundles. The medicine should flow freely and there should be tolerable pain. As the joint fills, pressure will need to be increased on the syringe.

Joint Aspirations.—Aspirated joint fluid can be useful for diagnosis. Thick fluids may require an 18-gauge needle. Follow-up includes ice, gentle range-of-motion exercises, and supportive/protective bracing.

Bursae Sacs.—Acute olecrannon and prepatellar bursitis can result in a painful sac filled with blood. If the sac reaches 2 cm, draining is recommended. A 20-gauge 1.5-inch needle attached to a 20 ml syringe is used to penetrate nontraumatized skin. The sac is compressed to express the blood. After drainage, a pressure bandage is applied with ice. The bursa should be protected for 1 to 2 months. If the bursa becomes chronic, corticosteroid injection is an effective treatment.

Fan Blocks.—Fan blocks can be used to treat muscle spasms and painful knots. A 27-gauge 1.5-inch needle is used to inject each trigger site after inducing temporary skin anesthesia. For larger dorsal lumbar muscles, a 25-gauge 3.5-inch needle should be used after skin anesthesia to puncture at a low angle into the middle of the muscle. Slowly advance and withdraw the needle to fan out the medication. Significant temperature relief can occur within 20 minutes. Proprioceptic neuromuscular facilitation in a stretch-contract-stretch technique should be carefully performed after injection.

Perineural Injections.—Injection of a steroid-anesthetic mixture can be helpful or even curative in the case of nerve injuries. The goal is to bathe the soft tissues surrounding the nerve with the mixture. A 27- to 30-gauge 1.5-inch needle is used to search for the nerve. When the nerve is contacted, the patient will experience a heightened electrical transmission over the domain of the nerve. As soon as the nerve is located, the needle is removed 1 to 2 mm and left to mark the spot. A 25-gauge 1.5-inch needle is used to spread the steroid-anesthetic mixture along the pathway near the trigger point site. The anesthetic should temporarily eliminate the patient's pain. These injections may need to be repeated. Complete healing may take several months.

Sheath Technique.—A 25-gauge 1.5-inch needle is used to penetrate soft tissue to the middle of the tendon. Contact with the tendon may lead to a muscle reflex. If so, back off 1 mm and inject while palpating to feel the medicine fill the tendon sheath. Sheath injections are well tolerated and can be repeated.

Acromioclavicular Joint.—Multiple injections at 2- to 3-month intervals can halt joint degeneration. Each injection should produce a positive response of 1 to 3 months' duration.

Capsular Distention of the Shoulder.—Capsular distention with about 30 ml of anesthetic, corticosteroid, and saline can be used to break adhesions and mobilize the joint capsule. A 22-gauge 1.5-inch needle is positioned to scrape the humeral head and carefully worked into the joint. Ten milliliters of anesthetic is injected and then the syringe is removed, leaving the needle. Medication should drip if the needle is properly positioned. The needle is steadied and a 20 ml syringe filled with saline and corticosteroid is injected into the joint. The injection is followed by assisted-forceful range of motion to safely distend the joint and rupture the adhesions.

Ganglion Cysts.—The cyst is punctured multiple times with a 20-gauge 1.5-inch needle containing 2 to 3 ml anesthetic/corticosteroid mixture. Injection is followed by ice and protective splinting.

Plica Band.—The band is trapped between the fingers and 2 to 3 ml of anesthetic/corticosteroid is directly injected with a 25-gauge 1.5-inch needle. This procedure can be repeated several times at intervals of a few weeks.

Conclusions.—Corticosteroid injections are effective in the treatment of exercise-related musculoskeletal injuries that are resistant to conservative teatment. Pain provocation tests should always be performed before injection to localize the injury site and after injection to confirm injection accuracy. Injections should involve minimal pain and be well tolerated. Rehabilitation involves a combined approach of activity modification, protective bracing, progressive stretching and strengthening, and education.

▶ This is one of the few didactic articles dealing with soft tissue and joint injections for the treatment of sports injuries. Considering the effectiveness and widespread use of this treatment modality, this organized presentation of the subject matter is certainly appropriate. I certainly agree that all injections should serve the dual function of being both diagnostic and therapeutic. Also, the point that complications are rare and risk of infection virtually nonexistent is sound. Worth adding is the importance of diluting corticosteroid substances with 5 to 10 mL of 1% xylocaine to prevent residual deposits in soft tissue.

J.S. Torg, M.D.

Hyperbaric Oxygen Chambers and the Treatment of Sports Injuries
Staples J, Clement D (Allan McGavin Sports Med Centre, BC, Canada; Univ of British Columbia, Canada)
Sports Med 22:219–227, 1996   1–20

Introduction.—Hyperbaric oxygen therapy, or breathing 100% oxygen at elevated pressures, may potentiate healing of soft tissue injuries such as burns, crush injuries, compartment syndromes, and osteomyelitis.

Physiology of Hyperbaric Oxygen.—Hyperbaric oxygen therapy may confer benefits by increasing tissue oxygen tensions, such as enhancing oxygen dissolution in plasma and maintaining oxygen delivery. Oxygen at 3 atm can increase the risk of grand mal seizures and at 2 atm can result in pulmonary damage after prolonged exposure. At 2 to 2.4 atm, nausea, tooth and sinus pain, and blurred vision have been reported. Contraindications for hyperbaric oxygen therapy include pneumothorax and predisposition to tension pneumothorax.

Soft Tissue Injury Healing.—Hyperbaric oxygen potentiates wound healing by providing oxygen for collagen synthesis and hydroxylation of collagen for scar formation; promoting granulation tissue formation, revascularization, and epithelialization; and stimulating fibroblastic activity, fibroblast migration, and capillary budding. Hyperbaric oxygen appears to promote fracture healing by increasing the rate of bone mineralization and hematoma formation and to shorten healing times.

Hyperbaric Oxygen in Sports Medicine.—Although there are few studies in this area, an ankle inversion study found that patients treated with hyperbaric oxygen recovered 30% faster than the control group. Rat studies indicated that hyperbaric oxygen inhibited the inflammatory process in a running model and enhanced the recovery of human beings with exercise-induced muscle soreness. Both animal and human studies showed that ligamentous injuries healed faster with hyperbaric oxygen therapy. Hyperbaric oxygen appears to decrease the inflammatory response to injury and impair the adhesion of neutrophils and their subsequent release of free radicals that scavenge oxygen and promote destructive events after injury. Hyperbaric oxygen's vasoconstrictive properties, enhanced leukocyte killing, and hydroxyproline formation combine with these factors to promote healing.

Conclusion.—Prompt treatment of soft tissue injuries with hyperbaric oxygen promotes healing by reducing neutrophil adhesion, controlling edema and inflammation, enhancing collagen synthesis and scar formation, and mediating pain and soreness.

▶ As this review article points out, "persuasive anecdotal evidence exists which demonstrates the efficacy of hyperbaric healing." However, at this time, there are no credible data to support the use of hyperbaric oxygen chambers in the treatment of sports injuries other than in a controlled, experimental setting.

J.S. Torg, M.D.

Asphyxial Death of a Young Skier
Shephard RJ (Univ of Toronto; Brock Univ, St Catharines, Ont, Canada)
J Sports Med Phys Fitness 36:223–227, 1996   1–21

Purpose.—Downhill skiers sometimes die during their sport, most often because of blunt trauma. Death caused by immersion in powder snow has been reported in snowboarders. A downhill skier who died of asphyxiation in powdered snow is reported.

Case Report.—Boy, 11 years, an experienced skier, was skiing on his own on a day with 14 inches of fresh powdered snow. He was last seen headed off a groomed trail and down a steep slope. The boy was reported missing, and 4 hours after his last descent he was found immersed headfirst in 1 m of powdered snow. He had no vital signs when found; there was no evidence of an avalanche or a struggle. The boy did not respond to standard CPR, rewarming by bladder irrigation, and extracorporeal circulation. He had no ECG; rhythm radiographs showed pulmonary edema but no cervical fracture. Although his blood gases were normalized by emergency treatment, his heart did not start beating again. The official cause of death was congestive heart failure caused by hypothermia. However, the circumstances were more consistent with asphyxia in the snow after a mild concussion.

Discussion.—As previously reported in snowboarders, this young skier appears to have asphyxiated in powdered snow after having a concussion. Winter athletes need to be informed about the potential dangers of deep powdered snow. Preventive measures should include wearing helmets, not skiing alone on deep mountainsides, and wearing bright-colored clothing.

▶ The author describes a number of excellent measures that can be taken to prevent skiing and riding (snowboarding) accidents. Using helmets to prevent concussions, never skiing alone, wearing bright-colored equipment and clothes, closing lifts well before dark, and knowing the dangers of deep powder and off-trail skiing/riding all are important measures that can reduce the incidence of fatal injuries.

F.J. George, A.T.C., P.T.

Managing Successive Minor Head Injuries: Which Tests Guide Return to Play?
Putukian M, Echemendia RJ (Pennsylvania State Univ, University Park)
Physician Sportsmed 24:25–32,37–38, 1996   1–22

Background.—Close follow-up is crucial in the management of athletes who sustain a head injury. It is especially important in the return-to-play decision. One case of head injury in a female college basketball player was presented.

Case Report.—Woman, 21, was struck on the right side of her jaw during a game. She fell backward and struck the ground with the back of her head. The woman lost consciousness for 20 seconds. Examination on the court revealed mild anisocoria and an inability to move her left arm. She had had a grade 1 concussion 2 years previously. In the emergency department, her memory was fragmentary and her factual knowledge was impaired. In addition to loss of motion in the left arm, she had weakness with resisted left hip flexion and left knee extension. A CT scan of the head and cervical spine produced normal results. The next morning, the patient's left arm felt normal. She reported only general fatigue and a dull occipital headache. Findings of an electroencephalogram, MRI of the head and cervical spine, and a neurologic examination were normal. Results of MR angiogram of the circle of Willis was normal. About 2 1/2 weeks after the injury, (and 1 1/2 weeks of being asymptomatic) she was permitted to indulge in gentle cardiovascular activity. After 1 month, she was allowed to participate in full competitive play. However, on her second day back, the woman sustained another mild head injury. This resulted in persistent headache, cognitive difficulties, and a hand dominance reversal. She was kept from play for the rest of the season and eventually recovered completely.

Conclusion.—This report illustrates return-to-play issues for athletes with head injury, especially the risk of recurrent injury. The risk of recurrent head injury and second impact syndrome—in which fatal brain swelling can occur—needs to be discussed with head-injured athletes and their coaches and parents.

▶ This report covers the difficult clinical decisions physicians face in trying to decide when athletes with head injury can return to play. In this case the initial injury was diagnosed as a grade 3 concussion (despite a transient hemiparesis), but the many neurologic tests done all produced normal findings (including CT, electroencephalography, MRI, and angiogram), so she returned to full play in 1 month. The second head injury was milder, but the athlete's persistent subtle symptoms (and possibly the results of neuropsychological testing) may have been shaped by her anxiety about the risks of successive injuries. The authors discuss differences among various guidelines for handling concussions and the problems of telling postconcussive headache from trauma-induced migraine[1] and of picking the ideal medication for an athlete with headaches.

The controversy—and the fears of litigation—in this field are discussed in another article that compares the 2 concussion-management guidelines best known to sports medicine physicians: the Cantu and the Colorado.[2] More team physicians use the Cantu guidelines; the newer Colorado guidelines are more conservative but more restrictive and are called impractical by some team physicians. A lack of scientific evidence, i.e., of objective ways to grade concussion and recovery, is the chief reason for the differences in guidelines. Regardless of which guidelines they follow, all physicians agree that an athlete who still has symptoms or signs of a concussion should not return to play—and that the most dreaded risk is the second impact syndrome.[3]

E.R. Eichner, M.D.

References

1. Diamond S: Managing migraines in active people. *Physician Sportsmed* 24:41–53, 1996.
2. Roos R: Guidelines for managing concussion in sports: A persistent headache. *Physician Sportsmed* 24:67–74, 1996.
3. Cantu RC, Voy R: Second impact syndrome: A risk in any contact sport. *Physician Sportsmed* 23:27–34, 1995.

Migraine Precipitated by Head Trauma in Athletes

Plager DA, Purvin V (Indiana Univ, Indianapolis)
Am J Ophthalmol 122:277–278, 1996   1–23

Objective.—This report presents a case of migraine precipitated by trauma to the top of the head while participating in football.

> *Case Report.*—A college football player aged 21 years complained of incomplete binocular loss of vision after direct helmet-to-helmet contact with another player. Decreased vision persisted for 3 to 4 hours and was followed by severe headache. Both headache and decreased vision were eliminated after a night's sleep. The patient reported several similar episodes over several years. Each was precipitated by direct head-to-head trauma while playing football. There was no family history of migraine. Results of neurologic examination, magnetic resonance imaging, and ophthalmologic examination were unremarkable. The diagnosis was trauma-induced migraine.

Conclusions.—The onset of sensory or motor loss with severe headache after head trauma during athletic competition can be very alarming. In the setting of these characteristic symptoms after head trauma, coupled with normal examination findings, the diagnosis of trauma-induced migraine should be considered. Familiarity with migraine precipitated by head trauma will permit patients with these symptoms to avoid expensive examination.

▶ "Migraine" precipitated by head trauma in athletes had been reported by Matthews[1] in soccer players, Bennett et al.[2] in football, and by Ashworth[3] in rugby players. An unusual entity, a high index of suspicion appears necessary to ensure its recognition. However, I am not sure that I agree with the authors that "familiarity with this entity can obviate an expensive examination for patients with these classic symptoms."

J.S. Torg, M.D.

References

1. Matthews WB: Footballer's migraine. *BMJ* 2:326–7, 1972.
2. Bennett DR, Fuenning SI, Sullivan G, Weber J: Migraine precipitated by head trauma in athletes. *Am J Sports Med* 8:202–205, 1980.
3. Ashworth B: Migraine, head trauma and sport. *Scott Med J* 30:40–42, 1985.

Retinal Detachments by Squash Ball Accidents

Knorr HLJ, Jonas JB (Univ Erlangen Nürnberg, Germany)
Am J Ophthalmol 122:260–261, 1996   1–24

Objective.—The characteristics and anatomic and functional outcomes of retinal detachments as a complication of squash ball accidents are discussed.

Methods.—Twenty-six patients (9 women) had retinal detachments after being hit by a squash ball.

Results.—Retinal tears occurred parallel to the corneoscleral limbus and close to the ora serrata with a width of < 30 degrees in 10 eyes, 30 to 60 degrees in 7 eyes, and 60 degrees in 9 eyes. The retinal detachment was in the temporal superior fundus quadrant in 14 eyes, the temporal inferior quadrant in 7, the nasal superior quadrant in 3, and the nasal inferior quadrant in 2. Half the patients had an avulsion of the vitreous. After surgery, 22 (85%) eyes had complete retinal attachment and a visual outcome of 20/40 or better. This group had lower visual acuity than a comparable group of patients with retinal attachments after ordinary rhegmatogenous detachments.

Conclusion.—Squash players should wear protective eyewear to avoid retinal damage.

▶ This article clearly underlines both the value and necessity of protective eyewear when playing squash.

J.S. Torg, M.D.

Acute and Chronic Brain Injury in United States National Team Soccer Players

Jordan SE, Green GA, Galanty HL, et al (Univ of California, Los Angeles; Univ of Pittsburgh, Pa)
Am J Sports Med 24:205–210, 1996   1–25

Introduction.—The growing popularity of soccer in the United States has led to an increased awareness of potential injuries associated with the sport. Although considered relatively safe, soccer can lead to acute or chronic head injuries. Some studies suggest that repetitive heading of the ball might cause a chronic brain syndrome of the type seen in professional boxing. To determine the effects of repetitive heading of a soccer ball, elite soccer players and track athletes were studied with MRI scans of the brain.

Methods.—The soccer players were 20 members of the U.S. Men's National Soccer Team training camp. Their average age was 24.9 years, and the average duration of their soccer participation was 17.7 years. None of the 20 age-matched male track athletes—sprinters, middle- and long-distance runners—had played soccer. All participants completed a questionnaire on head injury symptoms and underwent MRI of the brain. Questions on current and past alcohol use also were included because of the effects of alcohol on MRI findings. An exposure index to headers was developed to assess the dose-response effect of chronic heading.

Results.—Compared with track athletes, soccer players had started their sport at an earlier age. Seven soccer players reported having head injuries during soccer play, and 5 experienced a complete loss of consciousness. Eight runners had received head injuries, 5 during sports other than track, and 3 during non–sports-related activities. Four of the runners had complete loss of consciousness. The mean total symptoms scores were similar for soccer (24.4) and track (25.3) groups. No correlations were found among the head injury symptoms or between symptoms and reported alcohol use. Positive MRI findings were present in 9 soccer and 6 track athletes, but overall differences between the 2 groups were not significant. Although symptoms and MRI findings in soccer players did not correlate with age, years of play, exposure index results, or number of headers, there was a correlation between reported head injury symptoms and history of acute head injury.

Conclusion.—This study of elite soccer players showed no evidence of a relationship between extensive heading and chronic encephalopathies. It is possible, however, that repetitive heading may exacerbate the effects of an acute head injury.

▶ The stated purpose of this study was to "compare 20 national team soccer players with 20 elite track athletes to determine whether repetitive heading of a soccer ball causes either symptoms of brain injury or changes on magnetic resonance imaging (MRI) scans of the brain." Unfortunately, this study did not show that cumulative brain injury was related to repetitive contact with a soccer ball.

Although their view is not supported by the data, the authors believe it appears that soccer does expose the player to substantial risk of acute head injury, which raises the possibility that repetitive heading may exacerbate the effects of an acute head injury. Compared with the mostly linear acceleration encountered when heading a soccer ball, it is the rotational acceleration in boxing that presumably is responsible for the chronic encephalopathies that occur in that activity.

J.S. Torg, M.D.

The Influence of Baseball Modulus and Mass on Head and Chest Impacts: A Theoretical Study
Crisco JJ, Hendee SP, Greenwald RM (Brown Univ, Providence, RI; Orthopaedic Biomechanics Inst, Salt Lake City, Utah)
Med Sci Sports Exerc 29:26–36, 1997   1–26

Introduction.—Injuries that result in death occur in amateur baseball, and those deaths caused directly by impact of the ball are almost entirely in the youth group (aged 5 through 14 years). Of 88 deaths reported in youth baseball from 1973 to 1995, 77% were attributed to being struck by the ball. The chest was hit in 38 cases and the head or neck in 30. Softer baseballs, now commercially available, are promoted as safer. A theoretical model was used to study the effect of lowering ball modulus and mass on the likelihood of reducing impact injury.

Methods.—Separate theoretical models were used to study the responses of the head and the chest to ball impacts. The model used to calculate the impact response of the head used the assumption of ideal elastic behavior. An existing viscoelastic lumped-element model of the chest was used to study the impact response of the ball and the chest. Ball models assumed a high modulus with a high or low mass and a low modulus with a high or low mass.

Results.—Varying the ball modulus and ball mass had considerable effect on impact. Head impacts with the high-modulus, high-mass ball resulted in the greatest peak impact forces at all velocities. Lowering the ball mass decreased peak impact forces by approximately 41% at each of the tested impact velocities, which ranged from 11.2 mph to 89.5 mph. Lowering the ball modulus had an even greater effect, decreasing the impact force by 66%. Reduction of both modulus and mass decreased the impact force of the high-modulus, high-mass ball by 80%. The contact time of the ball with the head also was affected by ball model. Studies of the impact response of the chest showed ball mass to have an even greater effect than ball modulus. Lowering modulus, for example, decreased peak sternal velocity but did not affect peak sternal displacement. The greatest peak velocity occurred with the high-modulus, high-mass ball; this was reduced by 71% by lowering both mass and modulus.

Discussion.—The impact response depends on baseball mass and modulus, the physical properties of the target, and the specific impact variable studied. A softer and lighter ball reduced all impact response variables and would thus be likely to minimize impact injuries.

▶ This is an excellent theoretical and laboratory study with potentially profound clinical implications. However, as the authors state, "the results suggest that 'softer than traditional' baseballs may be safer. How much safer is not known." They also suggest that the term *safer* is too ambiguous because the decrease in the impact response varied with both the specific impact variable and the specific target. However, this study does suggest that baseballs with a lower modulus and lower mass would most likely reduce all injuries caused by the impact of baseballs.

J.S. Torg, M.D.

Concussion Among Swedish Elite Ice Hockey Players
Tegner Y, Lorentzon R (Ermeline Clinic, Luleå, Sweden; Univ Hosp, Umeå, Sweden)
Br J Sports Med 30:251–255, 1996   1–27

Background.—Since 1963, when wearing a helmet became compulsory in Swedish ice hockey, no deaths have occurred from head injury among the players. However, concussions constitute 2% to 14% of all ice hockey injuries. Concussions are potentially dangerous and are associated with widespread microscopic changes in the brain. Lesions have been detected on MR images of the brain in individuals with concussion. The frequency of concussion among Swedish ice hockey players was determined.

Methods and Findings.—Two hundred twenty-seven Swedish Elite League players responded to a questionnaire (response rate, 86%). These players are semiprofessional and play 40–55 league games a year. Fifty-one players (22%) reported sustaining a total of 87 concussions during their entire career. Thirty-eight had 1 concussion, 11 had 2–5, and 2 had more than 5. The annual risk for sustaining concussion was about 5%. The most common cause of concussions was body contact. Injured players missed a mean of 6 days of full training and play.

Conclusion.—Concussion is a potentially dangerous injury that must be treated seriously. Athletes sustaining repeated concussions in the same season need to be kept from play for a longer period than is currently practiced. Those sustaining several concussions over the years should undergo a thorough medical examination, including an electroencephalogram, CT, MRI, and neuropsychological testing. If any abnormalities are found on these tests, the patient should be advised to quit playing ice hockey.

▶ Helmets have reduced fatal head injuries in hockey, but concussions still occur and represent 2% to 14% of all ice hockey injuries. Concussions are often regarded as minor injuries, but they can cause microscopic and MRI brain lesions, have a cumulative effect on cognitive function, and predispose to the second impact syndrome.[1] This study suggests that the risk of concussion in Swedish elite hockey may be about five 5% per year and 20% in a career, mainly from body contact, checking, or boarding. Nearly 6% of respondents to the survey had had 2 or more concussions.

A practical problem is that, after concussion, the player wants to come back too soon and the coach agrees, so the mean time out of play in this study was only 6 days, whereas the Swedish Medical Association recommends 1–3 weeks. These authors recommend that the player who has had several concussions undergo a thorough examination including electroencephalography, CT, MRI, and neuropsychological testing; if anything is abnormal, the player should be advised to quit the game. See also the next 2 abstracts.

E.R. Eichner, M.D.

Reference

1. Cantu RC, Voy R: Second impact syndrome. A risk in any contact sport. *Physician Sportsmed* 23:27–34, 1995.

Sparring and Cognitive Function in Professional Boxers

Jordan BD, Matser EJT, Zimmerman RD, et al (Hosp for Special Surgery, New York City; Hosp St Anna, Geldrop, the Netherlands; New York Hosp/ Cornell Med Ctr)

Physician Sportsmed 24:87–92, 98, 1996   1–28

Introduction.—Neuropsychological testing is the most sensitive method for detecting neurologic dysfunction associated with boxing. Appropriate controls matched for age, socioeconomic, sociocultural, and education variables must be used before test results can be considered meaningful. Correlations were made between the neuropsychological test results of 42 New York State boxers and their age, boxing records, and exposure variables. References were not made to the general-population norms.

Methods.—Boxers underwent neuropsychological testing and were interviewed regarding neurologic symptoms and boxing history. Computed tomography scans are required for licensure for boxers in New York State. Each boxer's most recent CT scan was reviewed by a neuroradiologist blinded to other data. Scans were rated as normal, borderline, or abnormal.

Results.—The average boxer age was 25.6 years and the mean career duration was 9.5 years. The average number of professional fights per boxer was 10. Sparring practices varied widely from 1–7 days per week (mean, 3.6 days). Two boxers had borderline brain atrophy on CT scan and 2 others had frankly abnormal CT scans. Findings of 1 scan were consistent with posttraumatic encephalomalacia, and the other showed cerebellar atrophy with an enlarged fourth ventricle. Cavum septum pellicidum (CSP) was observed in 6 boxers. There were no significant correlations between the boxers' performance on the neuropsychological tests and age, amateur boxing record, professional boxing record, duration of career, or history of technical knockout/knockout. Increased sparring exposure and the number of rounds per session were inversely correlated with test scores, particularly in the areas of attention, concentration, and memory. Boxers with CSP performed significantly poorer on immediate recall and 1 measure of attention and concentration, compared with other boxers. Boxers with CSP sparred significantly more rounds per week and were significantly heavier than boxers without CSP.

Conclusion.—Sparring involves repetitive blows to the head and may be correlated with significant reductions in cognitive performance. In the absence of a correlation between competition and declining cognitive function, perhaps sparring bouts should be supervised, and boxers may want to decrease the amount and intensity of sparring workouts.

▶ Prior research suggests that although the rate of injury in boxing is higher during matches than during sparring, most injuries occur during the latter because more time is spent sparring. This study of professional boxers relates time spent sparring to subtle deficits in some neuropsychological tests, including impairments in attention, concentration, and memory. A prior study found subtle abnormalities in electroencephalographic patterns and impaired finger-tapping in amateur boxers.[1] More graphic are the 645 deaths in boxing between 1918 and 1983[1] and 5 recent deaths in boxers from the second impact syndrome.[2]

E.R. Eichner, M.D.

References

1. 1994 YEAR BOOK OF SPORTS MEDICINE, pp 27–28.
2. Cantu RC, Voy R: Second impact syndrome: A risk in any contact sport. *Physician Sportsmed* 23:27–34, 1995.

Fatal Cycling Injuries
Noakes TD (Univ of Cape Town, South Africa)
Sports Med 20:348–362, 1995   1–29

Objective.—Bicycle riders have a significant number of injuries, and 1 in every 100 to 400 accidents results in death.

Epidemiologic Factors.—Men have a higher injury rate, boys aged 6 to 12 years have the highest injury rate, and boys aged 10 to 14 years have the highest fatality rates. Most bicycle–motor vehicle accidents are the fault of the cyclist who disobeys traffic laws. Many involve the use of alcohol or prescription drugs such as tranquilizers, antihistamines, and benzodiazepines. Still others result from bicycle malfunction, poor road surface, stunts, going too fast, and riding two on a bike. Children from divorced or emotionally disturbed families are more likely to have accidents. Almost half of accidents occur at intersections.

Site and Nature of Injuries.—Between 13% and 34% of injuries are fractures, 35% are contusions, 26% are lacerations, and 20% are abrasions. The head and face are injured 31% to 81% of the time. The head is injured in approximately 50% of bicycle accidents.

Head Injuries.—Head and neck injuries are responsible for 75% of all deaths after a collision with a car. Most of these bicycle riders were not wearing a helmet. Few cyclists wear helmets in countries that do not promote or legislate wearing of helmets. A well-designed helmet has 3 layers—a firm outer shell, a shock-absorbing middle layer, and a comfort layer—and a chin strap.

Evaluation of Safety Characteristics.—The American National Standards Institute (ANSI) and the Snell Memorial Foundation rate helmet safety.

Preventing Injuries.—Promote helmet use, wear bright cycling clothing, use bicycle lights, separate cyclists from motor vehicles, educate cyclists about traffic laws, maintain roads, maintain bicycles, and ride responsibly. Parents have to play a responsible role in teaching children about safe bicycle riding. Medical professionals need to educate parents about the dangers of cycling. School- and community-based education programs have a small impact. Legislation mandating helmet wear with appropriate penalties and follow-through would be valuable.

Conclusion.—Understanding the factors that result in cycling accidents and ensuring the wearing of helmets that are known to reduce the risk of head injury and death are the primary goals.

▶ This article is a comprehensive review of the subject matter containing 104 references. Clearly, the most important observation is that the few cyclists who either sustained or died of head injuries were wearing adequate helmets at the time of the accident. Helmet use was associated with a reduced incidence of both serious and nonfatal injuries, including concussion, skull fracture, and soft tissue injuries of the face, and shorter hospitalization time.

J.S. Torg, M.D.

Pediatric Head Injuries and Deaths From Bicycling in the United States
Sosin DM, Sacks JJ, Webb KW (Natl Ctr for Injury Prevention and Control, Atlanta, Ga)
Pediatrics 98:868–870, 1996   1–30

Background.—The wearing of bicycle helmets has been found to reduce head injuries by 74% to 85%, which has sparked community efforts to increase helmet use through education, marketing, and legislation. Despite this, only 15% of children in the United States younger than 15 years of age routinely wore helmets in 1991. Among teenagers, rates of helmet use were even lower. Data for the years 1989 through 1993 were analyzed to provide estimates of the potential benefits from increasing bicycle helmet use.

Methods.—Data on all bicycle-related deaths and injuries among children and adolescents treated in emergency departments were obtained to determine traumatic brain injury–related death and head injury rates per 1 million United States residents. Preventable injuries and deaths were estimated by calculating population-attributable risk of head injury from helmet nonuse.

Findings.—A mean of 247 deaths from traumatic brain injury and 140,000 head injuries are related to bicycle crashes annually. If these riders had been wearing helmets, as many as 184 deaths and 116,000 head injuries might have been prevented each year. There were also 19,000 mouth and chin injuries treated annually, especially among the youngest age groups.

Conclusion.—The use of bicycle helmets needs to be increased, especially among young children. Current helmet designs apparently do not prevent injury to the mouth and chin, indicating the need to consider design changes.

▶ Of the more than 1,000 bicycling deaths in the United States each year, three fourths are caused by head injuries and half are in school-age children. Despite evidence that helmets can reduce head injury by up to 85%, in 1991, only 15% of United States children under the age of 15 years routinely wore helmets while cycling. Helmet use rates are even lower in adolescents. This study shows that helmet use by all bicyclists younger than 20 years of age could prevent as many as 184 deaths a year in the United States. We have covered this problem repeatedly in the YEAR BOOK.[1-4] This study also recommends that helmets be improved to prevent mouth and chin injury. See also the next abstract.

E.R. Eichner, M.D.

References

1. 1995 YEAR BOOK OF SPORTS MEDICINE, pp 18–20.
2. 1994 YEAR BOOK OF SPORTS MEDICINE, pp 8–10.
3. 1992 YEAR BOOK OF SPORTS MEDICINE, pp 266–268.
4. 1990 YEAR BOOK OF SPORTS MEDICINE, pp 283–284.

Acute Subdural Hematoma in a High School Football Player
Litt DW (Columbus State Community College, Ohio)
J Athletic Train 29:69–71, 1994   1–31

Introduction.—Head injury is the most common cause of death in football and other sports. The leading cause of death from head trauma is subdural hematoma. The incidence of head injuries may be as high as 40%. In head injuries, there are few objective signs. Postconcussive symptoms may last from 3 to 9 months and include headache and inability to concentrate and maintain work or social relationships. It may be difficult to distinguish these symptoms from normal teenage behavior. Problems with processing information and permanent brain damage have been reported in patients with multiple minor head injuries. A teenage athlete with an apparently minor head injury sustained a second head injury with near catastrophic results.

Case Report.—Boy, 16 years, complained of headache after a collision while playing football. Results of physical examination were normal. The headache persisted during the following week. Findings from a CT scan taken 7 days after injury were normal. The patient continued to report headache pain, but 17 days after the injury, he reported that the headache had disappeared. Testing to re-create the symptoms failed, and the patient was allowed to return to practice. During another football game, he was blindsided by a blow to the right temple. A substitute player was sent into the game. When the patient arrived on the sidelines, he denied any focal neurologic symptoms but then reported dizziness and headache. Shortly thereafter, he began to projectile vomit and became pale and unresponsive. The patient's left pupil was slightly dilated, he had no verbal response, his eyes opened to painful stimulation, and he displayed decerebrate posture. He was rated a Glasgow Coma Scale score of 5. A CT scan at the hospital showed an acute right-sided subdural hematoma with a midline shift. A subdural clot was removed, and at that time, an area of chronic membrane formation indicating subdural trauma in the past was noted. This lesion had not been detected on either CT scan. The patient was discharged and continued to improve. He joined the track team at his high school, and the following spring he was conference champion in various track and field events.

Discussion.—Four months postoperatively, the patient admitted that he had almost constant headaches, diminished concentration, and disrupted sleep between his first and second injuries. The tradition of finding faster ways to return an athlete to competition after a head injury should be reviewed. It can be difficult to determine the extent of minor head injury with traditional physical examination and even CT. Athletic trainers may not be aware of changes in academic performance in athletes who have had a head injury. In this patient, neurologic testing might have detected the effect of the constant headache had the patient been honest about his symptoms, although there was no pretest available for comparison. Mild injuries seen in individuals who participate in contact sports may be ticking time bombs or may result in decreased mental function. The long-term management of mild head injury needs to be improved.

▶ A troubling feature of this case is that a CT scan 1 week after the first injury failed to show the area of subdural trauma later diagnosed by the neurosurgeon, who found an area of chronic membrane formation. Also troubling is that the athlete denied the symptoms he had between day 17 and day 30, the day when full play was again allowed. These 2 features show how tough it can be for the physician to decide when to let the "concussed" player return to play. Athletes who experience a single minor head injury have a fourfold greater risk for sustaining another. This player's second injury caused an acute subdural hematoma. Sometimes—1 or 2 cases a year in U.S. football—the second injury can be rapidly fatal, from the "second impact syndrome." This dreaded complication—as seen in 1 ice hockey player and 5 boxers—has been reviewed, and guidelines for return to play in football were offered.[1] See also the next 3 abstracts.

E.R. Eichner, M.D.

Reference

1. Cantu RC, Voy R: Second impact syndrome: A risk in any contact sport. *Phys Sportsmed* 23:27–34, 1995.

2 Arm

Biomechanics of Overhand Throwing With Implications for Injuries
Fleisig GS, Barrentine SW, Escamilla RF, et al (American Sports Medicine Inst, Birmingham, Ala)
Sports Med 21:421–437, 1996

2–1

Introduction.—Success in overhand throwing often puts the thrower at risk for injury. The biomechanics of the overhand throw (baseball pitch, football pass, and javelin throw) were described, and the implications relative to injury potential were examined.

The Kinetic Chain.—A kinetic chain is used to generate and transfer energy from the larger body parts to the smaller and more injury-prone upper extremity in the throwing motion. Without overloading the shoulder and elbow, the thrower can achieve optimal performance using the kinetic chain. The 6 phases of the overhand throw are wind-up, stride, arm cocking, arm acceleration, arm deceleration, and follow-through. The sequence of motions in the overhand throw are stride, pelvis rotation, upper torso rotation, elbow extension, shoulder internal rotation, and wrist flexion. During overhand throwing, each joint rotates forward and the subsequent joint achieves its rotation back into a cocked position. This allows the connecting segments and musculature to be stretched and eccentrically loaded. With the elbow flexed at about 90 degrees, the shoulder is externally rotated between 150 degrees and 180 degrees at the end of the arm-cocking phase as a result of true glenohumeral rotation, trunk hyperextension, and scapulothoracic motion.

Pathomechanics of Elbow and Shoulder Injuries.—Close to the time of maximum shoulder external rotation, the shoulder and elbow musculature eccentrically contract. This produces shoulder internal rotation torque and elbow varus torque. These arm acceleration motions put the shoulder and elbow at risk for injury. At the end of arm cocking, the ulnar collateral ligament (UCL) is susceptible to injury because tension is put on it that is near its ultimate tensile strength. At the ulna, repetitive tension of the UCL and joint capsule can cause spur formation, which can compress the ulnar nerve. Injuries caused by arm cocking can cause avascular necrosis, osteochondritis dissecans, or osteochondral chip fractures in the lateral shoulder. The shoulder and elbow are at risk for injury during deceleration. The shoulder and elbow muscles produce large compressive forces to resist joint distraction after the ball is released. The posterior elbow can be injured in the arm acceleration phase because of the significant varus torque produced. Wedging of the olecranon into the olecranon fossa can cause impingement. This, in combination with rapid elbow extension during acceleration, can cause osteophytes at the posteromedial olecranon tip, chondromalacia, or the formation of loose bodies. During arm deceleration, the rotator cuff muscles resist distraction, horizontal adduction, and internal rotation while the posterior shoulder muscles are very active in producing compressive force, posterior force, and horizontal adduction torque. This can cause forceful entrapment of the labrum between the humeral head and the glenoid rim that can result in labral tearing. Joint stability can be further compromised with capsular laxity, muscle weakness, or fatigue. A large shoulder inferior force and adduction torque are generated during arm deceleration that can lead to superior translation of the humerus; impingement of the greater tuberosity; tendinitis of the supraspinatus, infraspinatus, or biceps; or abrasive wear. Tear of the superior labrum anterior and posterior could occur with repetitive throwing.

Rehabilitation.—Musculature of both the upper and lower body must be conditioned to maximize performance and minimize the risk of injury because of full body involvement during the throwing motion. Weakness in any segment may result in a deficiency in performance. Injury can result with deficiency in any section of the kinetic chain because compensation increases the demand on other segments. Improper mechanics must be addressed to prevent injuries. Use of high-speed, multijoint, multidirectional exercises (i.e., rubber tubing and plyometric exercises) should be emphasized. Throwers need exercises that emphasize eccentric contraction with appropriate range of motions and speeds of movement. The optimal exercise for throwing is some form of throwing.

Conclusion.—Most throwing injuries of the elbow and shoulder occur during arm cocking and arm deceleration. Exercises that duplicate the motions and loads in throwing can help prevent and rehabilitate throwing injuries.

▶ The authors have included an excellent review of the pathomechanics of elbow and shoulder injuries of throwing athletes and the implications for rehabilitation. They state, "The best exercise for throwing is some form of throwing." They also stress the importance of eccentric muscle contractions when throwing. Eccentric exercises within the appropriate range of motion and at the appropriate speed should be included in throwing exercise and rehabilitation program. Long ball throwing exercises should be included in every pitcher's exercise and warm-up program.

F.J. George, A.T.C., P.T.

Use of Vertebral Levels to Measure Presumed Internal Rotation at the Shoulder: A Radiographic Analysis

Mallon WJ, Herring CL, Sallay PI, et al (Triangle Orthopaedic Associates, Durham, NC; Duke Univ, Durham, NC; Methodist Sports Medicine Ctr, Indianapolis, Ind et al)

J Shoulder Elbow Surg 5:299–306, 1996   2–2

Objective.—Shoulder internal rotation is not easy to measure. The motion was analyzed radiographically to determine the contribution of the glenohumeral and scapulothoracic joints, shoulder extension, and elbow flexion to the motion involved when the arm is placed behind the back.

Methods.—Scapular lateral radiographs, posteroanterior radiographs, and CT scans in 5 positions were obtained of shoulders in 8 normal participants (Fig 1).

Results.—At the maximum internal rotation of 92 degrees, the glenohumeral joint accounted for 65% of the motion and the scapulothoracic joint accounted for 35%. Internal rotation across the chest and hip primarily involved glenohumeral internal rotation, whereas putting the arm behind the back used primarily scapulothoracic joint rotation and in-

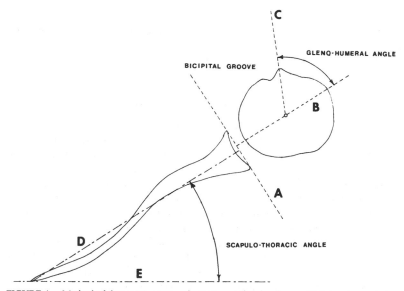

FIGURE 1.—Method of determining internal rotation at the glenohumeral joint and scapulothoracic angle. *Line A* is drawn first, along the glenoid face, connecting the anterior and posterior lips. Next, the center of the humeral head is determined, and perpendicular to *line A* through this center is drawn *line B.* From the center of the humeral head, *line C* is drawn through the lateral ridge of the bicipital groove. The angle of glenohumeral rotation is defined as the angle between *lines B* and *C. Line D* is drawn through the center of the glenoid fossa and exits at the most medial edge of the scapular blade. *Line E* consists of the lower border of the image window or parallel to it. The scapulothoracic angle of internal rotation is defined as the angle between *lines D* and *E.* (Courtesy of Mallon WJ, Herring CL, Sallay PI, et al: Use of vertebral levels to measure presumed internal rotation at the shoulder: A radiographic analysis. *J Shoulder Elbow Surg* 5:299–306, 1996).

volved both extension and internal rotation of the scapula on the thorax. Maximal proximal vertebral reach was provided by elbow flexion.

Conclusion.—Reaching the arm behind the back to the highest vertebral level may not be a good measure of internal rotation because the motion involves more than the internal rotation of the glenohumeral joint.

▶ Shoulder internal rotation is often measured with the arm behind the back, using the highest vertebral level reached by the thumb as the range of motion. This study examined the contribution of the glenohumeral joint, the scapulothoracic articulation, and the elbow joint to producing this range of motion. The authors describe the motion of placing the hand behind the back and reaching upward as 3 motions: maximal internal rotation at the shoulder joint, scapulothoracic extension and internal rotation with the arm behind the back, and elbow flexion to move the thumb superiorly.

Because of the large range of motion produced in associated joints, the authors suggest that reaching the arm behind the back to the highest vertebral level may not be an accurate measure of shoulder medial rotation. Lowered scores in this movement may be the result of restrictions in the associated joints rather than in the glenohumeral joint.

M.J.L. Alexander, Ph.D.

Activation of the Rotator Cuff in Generating Isometric Shoulder Rotation Torque
Jenp Y-N, Malanga GA, Growney ES, et al (Mayo Clinic and Mayo Found, Rochester, Minn)
Am J Sports Med 24:477–485, 1996   2–3

Introduction.—Functions of the rotator cuff have been examined in numerous settings, including various sports activities and exercises. The actual torque output of the shoulder, however, has not been evaluated. Twenty healthy volunteers were recruited for a study designed to examine the electromyographic (EMG) activity of 8 shoulder muscles and to determine the optimal position for generating maximal EMG activity of the rotator muscles in isometric internal and external shoulder rotation.

Methods.—Study participants were 10 men and 10 women ranging in age from 23 to 36 years. All were right handed, and only the right shoulder was tested. Intramuscular wire electrodes were placed to sample the EMG activity of the rotator cuff muscles. A modified Cybex II isokinetic dynamometer was used to measure the isometric shoulder torque in different positions. Axial rotations of the shoulder were included to ensure equal testing throughout the entire range of motion.

Results.—The greatest external rotation isometric force was found to be generated in the frontal and scapular planes in the neutral or full internal rotation positions. The greatest torques for internal rotation isometric force were achieved in the sagittal, dependent, and scapular plane with 45 degrees of elevation in rotational positions of either full or half external rotation. The most active muscles in these positions were the pectoralis major, anterior deltoid, and subscapularis. Rotator cuff muscles generated the greatest EMG activity in neutral to midrotational positions. The subscapularis muscle was best isolated in the scapular plane with 90 degrees of shoulder elevation in neutral rotation. A sagittal plane with 90 degrees of elevation in a half externally rotated position was optimal for isolating the infraspinatus and teres minor muscles. The supraspinatus muscle could not be isolated in any of the tested positions.

Discussion.—Optimal positions for activating the rotator cuff muscles were found to differ from those generating maximal isometric torque. Because the positions recommended for isolating the strength of the subscapularis, teres minor, and infraspinatus muscles did not produce maximal and isolated EMG activity in the supraspinatus muscle, isometric rotation is not a good test for supraspinatus muscle activation.

▶ This paper describes an exhaustive and in-depth analysis of the role of the rotator cuff muscles and the development of shoulder rotation force in various positions of the shoulder. With the use of both fine wire and surface electrodes, the surface muscles of the shoulder and the 4 rotator cuff muscles were examined in 3 planes and in 4 positions of rotation. Several important conclusions were stated: that the rotator cuff is not the primary generator of force in shoulder rotation; that the supraspinatus could not be isolated in any of the positions tested; and that the infraspinatus, teres minor, and subscapularis are best isolated in the scapular plane at 90 degrees of shoulder flexion. This study provides the physician with simple clinical tests for assessing each of these muscles on physical examination after operative repair or nonoperative rehabilitation.

M.J.L. Alexander, Ph.D.

Glenohumeral Translation in the Asymptomatic Athlete's Shoulder and Its Relationship to Other Clinically Measurable Anthropometric Variables
Lintner SA, Levy A, Kenter K, et al (Duke Univ, Durham, NC)
Am J Sports Med 24:716–720, 1996   2–4

Introduction.—Determining the amount of glenohumeral laxity can aid in the examination of patients with suspected shoulder instability. A comparison can then be made between the symptomatic and uninvolved shoulders. The shoulders of 76 Division I collegiate athletes were examined to determine the occurrence of high degrees of translation and the relationship between glenohumeral laxity and other clinically measurable anthropometric variables in asymptomatic athletes.

Methods.—The study group included 44 women and 32 men with an average age of 19 years. Varsity sports represented—tennis, swimming, volleyball, lacrosse, and field hockey—involved both overhead and nonoverhead movement. Both shoulders of participants were examined for passive range of motion: glenohumeral elevation and internal and external rotation at 0 degrees and 90 degrees of abduction. Each athlete was assessed for generalized joint laxity and for the presence of hyperextension of the knees and elbows. Glenohumeral laxity was graded on a scale of 0 (no translation) to 3+ (when the humeral head remains dislocated over the glenoid rim even after removal of the applied force).

Results.—Anterior translation was graded as 0 in 46 shoulders, 1+ in 75 (the humeral head rides up the slope of the glenoid with an applied force, but not over the rim), and 2+ in 31 (the glenoid translates over the edge of the glenoid rim with applied force, but spontaneously reduces when force is removed). Posterior translation was 0 in 13 shoulders, 1+ in 56, and 2+ in 83. There were 38 shoulders with 0 inferior translation, 105 with 1+, and 9 with 2+. No shoulder had translation of 3+ in any direction, and none were asymmetric in all 3 directions (12 men and 12 women exhibited translation asymmetry of at least 1 grade in at least 1 direction). A significant correlation was observed between the dominant hand and increased translation. Translation was not related to range of motion, knee or elbow hyperextension, thumb-to-forearm distance, or duration of sports participation.

Conclusions.—Normal, asymptomatic shoulders can vary considerably in stability values, and up to 2+ translation in any direction is not necessarily abnormal. The normal shoulder may also exhibit asymmetry, with the nondominant shoulder likely to have the greater amount of laxity.

▶ There is a wide range of normal shoulder stability values among the general population, which can be subjectively evaluated by passive range-of-motion testing performed by a qualified physician. Glenohumeral laxity can be graded from 0 to 3+, in which a grade of 0 is essentially no translation; 1+ and 2+ are increasing grades of instability; and a grade of 3+ is when the humeral head remains dislocated over the glenoid rim after removal of force. In this group of athletes, there was a greater degree of external rotation and a lesser degree of internal rotation in the dominant shoulder compared with the nondominant. Comparison of laxity values from side to side revealed a 32% incidence of asymmetry, with the nondominant shoulder having a greater amount of laxity in those with asymmetry. This study reveals that shoulder laxity up to a value of 2+ is common and may not be accompanied by any other shoulder abnormality. Athletes can have lax shoulder joints that are still functional for high-speed athletic activities.

M.J.L. Alexander, Ph.D.

Primary Anterior Dislocation of the Shoulder in Young Patients
Hovelius L, Augustini GBG, Fredin ÖH, et al (Gävle Hosp, Sweden; Region-sjukhuset, Örebro, Sweden; Malmö Allmänna sjukhus, Sweden; et al)
J Bone Joint Surg Am 78A:1677–1684, 1996   2–5

Objective.—Ten-year results after treatment of primary anterior dislocation in 257 shoulders of 255 patients are reported for 247 shoulders in 245 patients.

Methods.—A prospective multicenter study at 27 Swedish hospitals of 257 dislocations (52 female joints) of the glenohumeral joint treated by mobilization for 3 to 4 weeks (Group 1), in a sling until comfortable (Group 2), or varied treatment (Group 3). At 10 years, patients were interviewed, examined, and their shoulders assessed radiographically. Comparisons were analyzed statistically.

Results.—There were no recurrent dislocations in 129 shoulders, although 8 were considered by the patients to be unstable, 11 had 1 recurrent dislocation, 58 with recurrent dislocations were operated, and 49 with recurrent dislocations were not treated operatively. Arthropathy was mild in 23 shoulders, moderate in 16, and severe in 2. There was articular incongruity in 32 shoulders, 23 of which also had arthropathy ($p < 0.0001$) and at least 1 recurrent dislocation compared with 79 of the 176 with a congruent joint ($p = 0.01$). Of 189 patients with bilateral radiographs, 24 had dislocation or subluxation of the contralateral shoulder. Four of these shoulders showed evidence of moderate or severe arthropathy compared with 3 of 165 stable contralateral shoulders ($p < 0.001$). A significant number of patients over age 25 needed surgery. When dislocation recurred within 2 to 5 years after initial injury, operative intervention was not necessary in 24 (22%) of shoulders. Dislocation of the contralateral shoulder occurred in 16% of 12- to 22-year-olds, 21% of shoulders in 23- to 29-year-olds and 3% of shoulders in 30- to 40-year-olds. A Hermodsson lesion present on the initial radiograph in 99 of 185 shoulders, was significantly associated with a worse prognosis at 10 years that shoulders with no lesion.

Conclusion.—At 10-year follow-up, 23 shoulders showed mild arthropathy, 16 had moderate arthropathy, and 2 had severe arthropathy. Some of these shoulders had not had recurrent dislocations. Most recurrent dislocations occurred between years 2 and 5. Patients older than age 25 had a higher operation rate.

▶ The authors' ability to perform a ten year follow-up interview and physical examination on 211 of the 245 patients is most impressive. However, it is important to note that many physicians were involved in the follow-up process and the data was not consistent and, consequently, was not reported. Also, the indications for the surgery varied, having been made by the discretion of the many surgeons involved. In addition to the 58 shoulders that had an operative procedure for recurrent dislocation, at 10 year follow-up an additional 60 shoulders were classified as having had a recurrent dislocation, or were considered by the patient to be unstable.

J.S. Torg, M.D.

Rehabilitation of Injuries in Competitive Swimmers

Kenal KAF, Knapp LD (Greenwood Med Ctr, Midvale, Utah; Univ of Utah, Salt Lake City)
Sports Med 22:337–347, 1996   2–6

Objective.—In swimmers, certain overuse injuries of the shoulder, back, and knee may develop. Understanding the mechanisms of these injuries, along with accurate diagnosis and appropriate treatment, will permit a timely return to competition. The rehabilitation of common injuries in competitive swimmers was reviewed.

Swimmer's Shoulder.—Swimmers need normal function of the scapulothoracic stabilizers for synchronous scapulohumeral motion. Both dynamic and static components contribute to glenohumeral joint stability during shoulder motion. Swimmers generally have hypermobility of the shoulder, except for tightness of the posterior capsule. This can lead to increased anterior humeral translation. With training, there is repetitive microtrauma to the static stabilizers of the glenohumeral joint and to the inferior glenohumeral ligament. The shoulder stretches out, leading to anterior instability. Fatigue often develops in the subscapularis and serratus anterior muscles, leading to asynchronous scapulohumeral motion.

Rehabilitation of swimmer's shoulder may include special strength and stabilization exercises, such as the use of reciprocal pulleys and drawing the alphabet with a handheld weight while in the supine position. These exercises are measured by time, not repetitions, to meet the goal of increased endurance. Swimmers with painful shoulders may recruit the rhomboid muscles during the propulsive phase, sometimes causing tenderness and spasm of these muscles. They may passively adduct the arm across the chest in an attempt to decrease this pain, which serves to stretch the muscles further. Special exercises are needed to train the rhomboids to contract in a more shortened position (Fig 4). To achieve the necessary stretching of the posterior capsule without further stretching the midscapular muscles, the scapula must be stabilized. This can be done by anchoring the scapula with a strap around the chest and over the scapula and stretch by horizontal adduction of the shoulder. Swimmers need education regarding the effects of a forward-shouldered posture on shoulder pain. For swimmers with weak lower trapezius muscles, trapezius strengthening may be achieved by the use of pulleys or by lying down or standing with the elbows bent 90 degrees and externally rotated and the lumbar and cervical spine held flat. Although dips and other exercises for lower trapezius strengthening can be done, care is needed to avoid impinging the tissues under the acromion. For patients with biceps tendinitis, transverse friction massage may be helpful if tolerated. All swimmers with shoulder problems should have their swimming mechanics reviewed.

Back Pain.—For swimmers with back pain, an elastic brace may add stability. The athlete may use a lumbar roll or pillow while sitting or driving and should avoid using a flotation device between the legs while pulling.

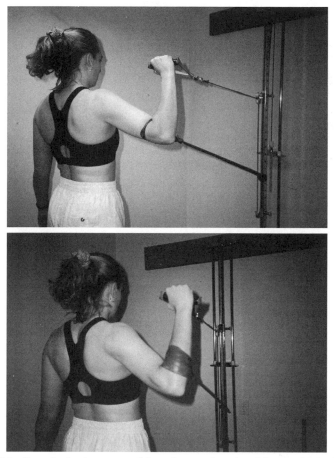

FIGURE 4.—Strengthening the rotator cuff. Isotonic external rotation while strengthening the scapular retractors isometrically (top): elastic tubing is attached from the arm to a stable object in front of the patient so that the scapula is retracted while external rotation is done isotonically with the same upper extremity. Isometric external rotation (bottom): the patient must isometrically hold the arm in external rotation while the scapula is retracted isotonically with the same upper extremity. (Courtesy of Kenal KAF, Knapp LD: Rehabilitation of injuries in competitive swimmers. *Sports Med* 22:337–347, 1996.)

Discussion.—Swimmer's shoulder results from the combined effects of hypovascularity, fatigue, poor stroke mechanics, and abnormal glenohumeral translation. Rehabilitation should focus on regaining functional range of motion and strengthening of the dynamic stabilizers of the glenohumeral joint and scapula. The rehabilitation of back and knee pain in swimmers is reviewed as well.

▶ The authors have described an excellent rehabilitation program for swimmers with shoulder injuries. Their program consists of exercises to stretch the anterior chest muscles and tight posterior shoulder capsule. Strengthening and endurance exercises of the rotator cuff muscles and scapula stabilizers are quantified by time rather than repetitions. Correct stroke and breathing mechanics are reviewed, to prevent shoulder injuries. The authors also recommend avoiding bench presses, dips, pushing off a wall with a kickboard, and other activities that may promote shoulder impingement.

F.J. George, A.T.C., P.T.

Kinematics of the Glenohumeral Joint: Influences of Muscle Forces, Ligamentous Constraints, and Articular Geometry

Karduna AR, Williams GR, Williams JL, et al (Univ of Pennsylvania, Philadelphia; Allegheny Univ, Philadelphia; Univ of Missouri-Kansas City)
J Orthop Res 14:986–993, 1996   2–7

Background.—The glenohumeral articulation's capacity for a great range of motion derives in part from the shallowness of the glenoid cavity. This architecture allows translations of the humeral head with respect to the glenoid, but large translations ultimately lead to joint instability. Because previous studies of glenohumeral translations during normal motions have yielded conflicting results, investigators sought to better understand joint function by examining key factors that control shoulder motions.

Methods.—Cadaver models were used so that devices could be attached directly to bones, providing accurate measurement of 3-dimensional translations. Discrepancies in previous reports of translational patterns may be traced to the use of different types of models. Thus these experiments used both active and passive models on the same human cadaver joints to determine effects of muscle forces. Patterns of translation and rotation were examined in fresh-frozen glenohumeral joints of human cadavers with a 6-degrees-of-freedom magnetic tracking device. Shoulders were positioned from maximal internal to external rotation at several arm positions, reflecting various elevations and planes of motion. Measurements were also made of articular surface geometry and ligament origin-insertion wrap length to assess their influences on joint kinematics.

Results.—For all experiments, the mean net anterior-posterior translation was approximately four-fold larger for the passive model (8.2 mm) than for the active model (2.1 mm). The mean net superior-inferior translation for all experiments was nearly 2.5 times larger during passive (4.2 mm) than during active (1.7 mm) motions. There was also a significant difference between the mean internal-external rotational range of motion during passive positioning (144 degrees) and active positioning (103 degrees). Thus, when joints were positioned passively, large translations were noted at the extremes of motion. But with active positioning there was a tendency for muscle forces to limit humeral head translations, largely by restriction of rotational ranges of motion. The 2 models showed no significant differences in translation, however, when data from the passive model were reanalyzed by considering only the rotational ranges of motion seen actively. Glenohumeral ligament wrap lengths correlated with translations only when the joints were positioned passively.

Conclusion.—By directly comparing the kinematics of active and passive in vitro cadaver models for the same natural glenohumeral joints, several opposite views of the glenohumeral joint can be reconciled. Muscle forces keep the humeral head centered in the glenoid, limiting the rotational ranges of motion and translations in comparison with passive positioning of the joint. Large translations require the increases in rotational ranges of motion associated with the removal of muscle force.

▶ This is an excellent study that "confirms and reconciles several opposing views of the glenohumeral joint noted in the literature." However, the clinical relevance of the observations is not specified.

J.S. Torg, M.D.

Traumatic Tears of the Subscapularis Tendon: Clinical Diagnosis, Magnetic Resonance Imaging Findings, and Operative Treatment
Deutsch A, Altchek DW, Veltri DM, et al (Hosp for Special Surgery, New York)
Am J Sports Med 25:13–22, 1997   2–8

Objective.—Rotator cuff tears rarely involve the subscapularis tendon. The symptoms, diagnoses, magnetic resonance imaging (MRI) evaluations, and operative treatment of 13 patients with 14 rotator cuff tears involving the scapularis tendon are reported.

Methods.—Charts of 13 male patients, aged 18 to 64, seen between 1991 and 1993, were retrospectively reviewed. All patients had had traumatic injury an average of 3 weeks before the initial visit. Two shoulders were diagnosed with a rotator cuff tear isolated to the subscapularis tendon. The remaining 12 shoulders were treated nonoperatively and did not improve in strength and function. Correct diagnoses were delayed for 4 to 24 months. Ultimately arthroscopic surgery was performed on 1 shoulder and arthrotomies on the remaining 13. All shoulders were evaluated by MRI.

Results.—Seven shoulders were injured during sports, and 11 injuries were the result of traumatic hyperextension or external rotation of the abducted arms. All patients reported pain and weakness. Plain radiographs revealed bony abnormalities in 6 shoulders. MRI revealed 13 full-thickness tears and 1 partial-thickness tear. MRI and arthroscopic findings showed 6 shoulders with a medial subluxation of the biceps tendon and 1 shoulder with a biceps rupture (Fig 5). Surgery revealed subscapularis injury in 7 of 13 shoulders only after scar tissue was removed. After surgical repair of the subscapularis tendon 6 shoulders still had biceps tendon instability and required tenodesis of the biceps tendon to the intertubercular groove for stabilization. Shoulders were placed in slings for 5 to 6 weeks with range of motion exercises beginning at week 1, elevation and passive rotation exercises at 4 weeks, deltoid and rotator

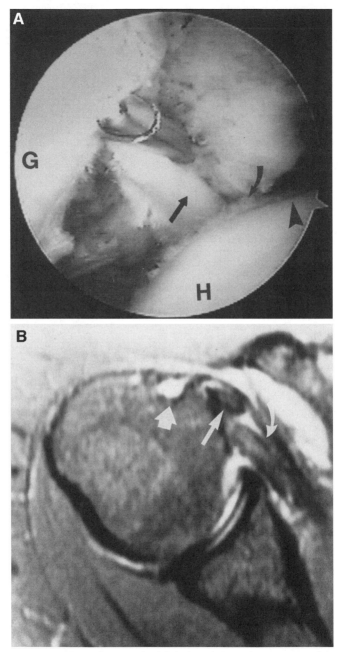

FIGURE 5.—A, An arthroscopic view of a full-thickness subscapularis tear (*curved arrow*) with an associated biceps tendon dislocation (*straight arrow*). The *arrowhead* points to the normal anatomic position of the long head of the biceps tendon. B, T2-weighted axial gradient recalled image demonstrating medial dislocation of the biceps tendon (*straight arrow*) with an empty sheath noted laterally (*arrowhead*). The subscapularis tendon is thinned and irregular (*curved arrow*). *Abbreviations: H,* humeral head; *G,* glenoid. (Courtesy of Deutsch A, Altcheck DW, Veltri DM, et al: Traumatic tears of the subscapularis tendon: clinical diagnosis, magnetic resonance imaging findings, and operative treatment. *Am J Sports Med* 25:13–22, 1997).

cuff muscle isometric exercises at 8 weeks and resistance exercises at 3 months. Return to sports was not allowed for at least 6 months. At an average follow up of 2 years, pain and weakness was completely relieved in 10 shoulders, strength was normal in all shoulders, and external motion was somewhat decreased in 5 shoulders. All patients have returned to work and 12 have returned to their sports activities.

Conclusion.—Proper diagnosis and early surgical repair of tears of the subscapularis tendon result in less pain and improved shoulder function.

▶ This is an excellent paper that clearly defines a somewhat unusual injury. Several important points should be emphasized. The injuries of all the patients in this study were the result of violent, traumatic events such as falls, direct blows, or forceful boxing punches in the absence of antecedent symptoms. The diagnosis of the injury is difficult and often nonspecific, requiring a high index of suspicion. The paper points out that the axial magnetic resonance image provides the most advantageous view of the subscapularis and biceps tendon. Also, arthroscopic examination should be the first step in surgical treatment. However, open repair can be difficult, particularly with larger chronic retracted tears of the subscapularis tendon.

J.S. Torg, M.D.

A Prospective Evaluation of a New Physical Examination in Predicting Glenoid Labral Tears
Liu SH, Henry MH, Nuccion SL (UCLA School of Medicine, Los Angeles)
Am J Sports Med 24:721–725, 1996   2–9

Introduction.—Glenoid labral tears have been identified more easily with improvements in arthroscopic techniques. The ability of clinical evaluation to predict the presence of labral tears preoperatively is poor. Diagnosis is improved with magnetic resonance imaging but is expensive. Reported are results of the "crank test," a highly sensitive and specific examination capable of independently predicting the presence of a glenoid labral tear.

The Crank Test.—With the patient in upright position and the arm elevated 160 degrees into the scapular plane, joint load is applied along the axis of the humerus with one hand. The other hand performs humeral rotation. Pain during the maneuver (usually during external rotation) with or without a click or reproduction of the symptoms (usually during work or athletic activities) is indicative of a positive test result. The crank test should be repeated in the supine position (Fig 2).

Methods.—The crank test was performed in 62 patients with failed conservative treatment for shoulder pain. Average patient age was 28 years.

Results.—Thirty-one of 62 patients had positive crank test results and the other 31 had signs of impingement on physical examination. Glenoid labral tears were observed in 32 patients by arthroscopy. The superior

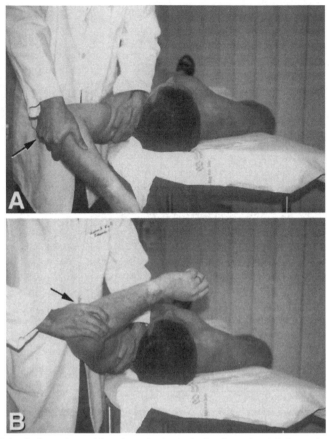

FIGURE 2.—In the supine position, the patient's arm is also elevated to 160 degrees in the scapular plane, applying joint load along the axis of the humerus with one hand (*arrow*) while externally (**A**) and internally (**B**) rotating the humerus with the other hand. (Courtesy of Liu SH, Henry MH, Nuccion SL: A prospective evaluation of a new physical examination in predicting glenoid labral tears. *Am J Sports Med* 24:721–725, 1996.)

labrum was involved in all tears. Two patients with positive crank test results did not have glenoid labral tears; they had partial-thickness, articular-side rotator cuff tears. Sensitivity, specificity, positive predictive value, and negative predictive value of the crank test was 91%, 93%, 94%, and 90%, respectively.

Conclusion.—The crank test was highly accurate in the preoperative diagnosis of glenoid labral tears. Use of the crank test may help decrease the need for expensive imaging techniques.

▶ Of course the beauty of the "crank" test is that it is noninvasive, economical, and reliable.

J.S. Torg, M.D.

Rotator Cuff Injury in Contact Athletes

Blevins FT, Hayes WM, Warren RF (Sports Medicine and Shoulder Service, Hosp for Special Surgery, New York)
Am J Sports Med 24:263–267, 1996   2–10

Introduction.—Rotator cuff injuries usually appear in patients older than 40 years, but some younger individuals who engage in repetitive overhead activities may also experience rotator cuff tears after a traumatic event. In the young patients reviewed here, rotator cuff injuries were the result of direct trauma to the shoulder while playing football.

Methods.—The 10 male football players ranged in age from 24 to 36 years; 9 played at the professional level. In 8 cases the dominant extremity was involved. The patients were interviewed preoperatively to determine details of the injury, symptoms, previous shoulder injuries, and level of

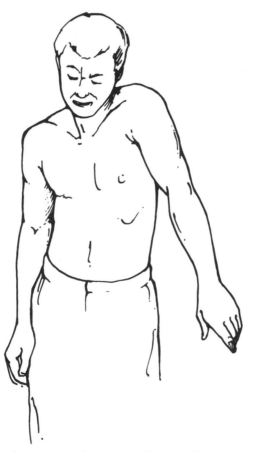

FIGURE 1.—In the shrug sign, scapular rotation with attempted glenohumeral elevation indicates rotator cuff injury. (Courtesy of Blevins FT, Hayes WM, Warren RF: Rotator cuff injury in contact athletes. *Am J Sports Med* 24:263–267, 1996.)

play. Their charts were reviewed for findings of the initial physical examination; data from the operative record were also obtained. Average follow-up was 21 months (range 4 to 88 months). Physical examination at follow-up emphasized muscle strength, active range of motion, and external and internal rotation. The presence or absence of a "shrug sign" (Fig 1) was noted.

Results.—In each case, a specific event—a direct blow to the shoulder—led to pain and weakness in the affected shoulder. All patients did not improve with conservative treatment, and surgery was performed at an average of 9 weeks after the injury. Three partial thickness tears were arthroscopically debrided. The arthroscopically assisted miniarthrotomy technique was used to repair 1 full-thickness tear and 2 partial-thickness tears. Two patients underwent open repair. In the 2 remaining cases, isolated rotator cuff contusions were arthroscopically debrided. Statistically significant improvements in pain and function were recorded postoperatively. The shrug sign, which was positive in 8 patients preoperatively, was negative in all 10 after surgery. Nine of 10 athletes could return to active participation in football, 7 at their preinjury levels.

Discussion.—Young athletes who engage in contact sports may have a rotator cuff injury if shoulder pain is persistent and impingement signs, weakness, and a positive shrug sign are present. Arthroscopic evaluation should be considered if there is no improvement after a rotator cuff rehabilitation program. Diagnoses based on magnetic resonance imaging scans were verified in 4 of 9 patients at surgery. Specificity was 83% for full-thickness tears, but MRI could not distinguish between partial-thickness tears and cuff contusions.

▶ The value of this paper is that it calls attention to the fact that athletes in the 24 to 36 year age group can sustain partial and full-thickness tears of their rotator cuff mechanisms. Certainly, the diagnosis of a rotator cuff injury should be considered in the contact athlete who has a history of having sustained a direct blow to the shoulder associated with persistent pain, impingement signs, weakness and a positive shrug sign. Although all the patients reported significant improvement in both function and decreased pain, 5 did exhibit residual weakness, especially in external rotation.

J.S. Torg, M.D.

An Arthroscopic Technique for Anterior Stabilization of the Shoulder With a Bioabsorbable Tack
Speer KP, Warren RF, Pagnani M, et al (Hosp for Special Surgery, New York City)
J Bone Joint Surg Am 78A:1801–1807, 1996   2–11

Background.—Arthroscopy can be used to reestablish a functional inferior glenohumeral ligament and stabilize the shoulder after injury. This

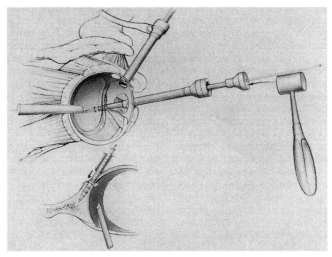

FIGURE 2-B.—The apposition of soft tissue to bone is confirmed by arthroscopic visualization. The upper extremity is generally in neutral rotation and full adduction during the insertion of the implant. (Courtesy of Speer KP, Warren RF, Pagnani M et al: An Arthroscopic Technique for Anterior Stabilization of the Shoulder With a Bioabsorbable Tack. *J Bone Joint Surg Am* 78A:1808–1807, 1996.)

report describes a technique for arthroscopic stabilization of the shoulder using a bioabsorbable tack was described.

Study Group.—The records of the first 52 patients who were managed arthroscopically for the anterior stabilization of the glenohumeral joint with a bioabsorbable tack were reviewed. The study group consisted of 47 male and 5 female patients. The average age of these patients was 28 and the dominant shoulder was affected in 29 of the 52 participants. The injury mechanism was traumatic dislocation in 36 patients, 25 of whom sustained the injury playing contact sports.

Surgical Technique.—A complete glenohumeral arthroscopic examination was performed before surgery. A Bankart lesion was present in 50 patients and a chondral Hill-Sachs lesion in 44 of the 52 patients in this series. The osseous glenoid rim was abraded. A grasper was inserted and used to reduce the labrum and shift it 0.5 to 1.0 cm superiorly on the glenoid rim. A cannulated drill was inserted, and the bioabsorbable tack was impacted over the drill wire (Fig 2b) and inserted under arthroscopic visualization. Two or three tacks were used for each procedure. A sling was employed by the patient for four weeks with pendulum, range-of-motion and isometric forearm exercises. After four weeks, patients were permitted passive forward flexion and elevation of the shoulder and external rotation. At 6 weeks, progression to full range of motion was permitted. Participation in contact sports was not allowed for five months. Follow-up of 49 patients occurred at 24 to 64 months, with the remaining 3 patients interviewed by telephone.

Results.—Among this group of 52 patients 79% were asymptomatic and participated in sports at follow-up. The repair was considered a failure in 21% of the patient group. In four cases, the failure was due to traumatic reinjury during a contact sport, but the remaining seven failures were atraumatic. Due to recurrent instability, eight patients had an open glenoid-based capsulorrhaphy. There was no evidence of tacks in these patients and the Bankart lesions were completely healed.

Conclusion.—This retrospective study of 52 patients who underwent arthroscopic repair for anterior stabilization of the glenohumeral joint with a bioabsorbable tack, indicates that this technique is useful for patients with a traumatic injury and a thick mobile Bankart lesion for repair of the detachment of the labrum. This procedure will not be successful if anatomical reattachment of a displaced Bankart lesion will not restore shoulder stability, and such patients should be treated with open capsulorrhaphy or a capsular shift-type procedure.

▶ The rate of recurrent instability after stabilization with the bioabsorbable tack of 21% is in keeping with that reported for other arthroscopic techniques. To emphasize: this greatly exceeds the rates of recurrence of 0 to 5.5% that have been reported for open capsulorrhaphy.

J.S. Torg, M.D.

Long-term Results of Conservative Treatment for Acromioclavicular Dislocation

Rawes ML, Dias JJ (Leicester Royal Infirmary, England)
J Bone Joint Surg Br 78B:410–412, 1996   2–12

Introduction.—Numerous operative procedures have been developed for the treatment of acromioclavicular dislocation, but none has achieved results superior to those of conservative management. In addition, surgery carries a significant risk of complications and the internal fixation may have to be removed. A review of 30 patients with acromioclavicular dislocation confirms the favorable long-term results of conservative treatment.

Methods.—All patients were treated at the study institution between 1979 and 1982. The group included 25 men and 5 women; their average age was 43. Causes of dislocation were contact sports in 15 cases, road-traffic accidents in 9, and falls in 6. Injuries were all initially classified as Allman grade II. Conservative treatment consisted of wearing a broad arm sling for 3 to 5 weeks, followed by mobilization. Follow-up averaged 12.5 years. Factors considered in assessing outcome were clinical deformity, tenderness of the joint, shoulder range of movement, and pain on resisted abduction and distraction. Standard anteroposterior radiographs were also examined. An additional 5 patients were interviewed by telephone.

Results.—None of the patients sought further medical advice after conservative management of the dislocation. Fourteen reported no discomfort at the area of injury, 15 experienced mild symptoms, and 1 had moderate symptoms. No patient had to give up athletic activities or change jobs because of the injury. Only 2 of the 5 patients interviewed by telephone had mild discomfort. Some deformity was present in 24 cases, but this was obvious in only 8. Radiographs showed that the acromioclavicular joint remained dislocated in 17 patients and was subluxed in 13. Twenty-one patients had ossification around the distal clavicle. The radiologic appearances of the joint had not changed significantly since these patients' 5-year review.

Conclusion.—Despite deformity of the acromioclavicular joints after conservative treatment for dislocation, there was no clinical deterioration at long-term follow-up and adequate functional adaptation was achieved. Surgery to restore the anatomy of the joint is not required for a good outcome.

▶ It is important to note that the conclusion regarding the efficacy of conservative treatment for acromioclavicular dislocation applies to grades I to III. None of the injuries reported were of the Grades IV, V, or VI type. Also to be noted is the fact that there was no randomized control group for comparison of results. Albeit, however, I agree with the conclusions of the authors.

J.S. Torg, M.D.

Posterior Instability of the Glenohumeral Joint
Hawkins RJ, Janda DH (Steadman-Hawkins Clinic, Vail, Colo; Inst for Preventative Sports Medicine, Ann Arbor, Mich)
Am J Sports Med 24:275–278, 1996   2–13

Background.—Posterior instability of the glenohumeral joint remains a difficult condition to treat. Although the majority of patients will respond to a nonoperative rehabilitation regimen, for those patients who do not respond, surgical treatment remains an option. Various surgical procedures have been tried with little success for these patients. This paper describes a posterior capsulotendinous tensioning procedure for patients with posterior instability of the glenohumeral joint who do not respond to nonoperative treatment.

Study Group.—The study group consisted of 17 patients with recurrent posterior glenohumeral instability who underwent posterior capsulotendinous tensioning procedures from June 1986 to July 1990. These patients were unable to perform activities of daily living. Preoperatively, the average pain rating score was 5 out of 10 at rest and 9 out of 10 with activity. Six of these patients had previous anterior reconstructions. The average patient age was 27 years at operation. Fourteen patients were available for an average of 44 months of follow-up, which consisted of patient interviews and a physical examination.

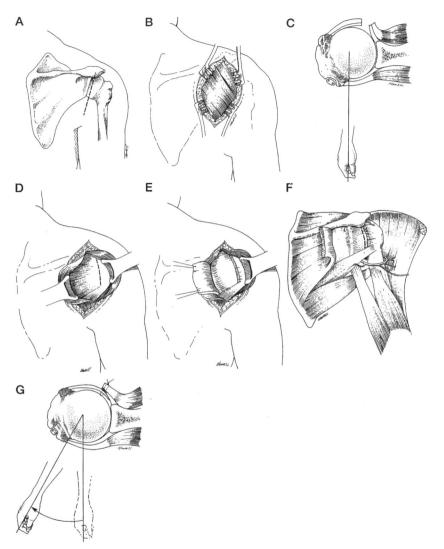

FIGURE 1.—The posterior capsular tensioning procedure for posterior glenohumeral instability. (Courtesy of Hawkins RJ, Janda DH: Posterior instability of the glenohumeral joint. *Am J Sports Med* 24:275–278, 1996.)

Operative Technique.—The patient was placed in the lateral decubitus position. A longitudinal incision was made from 2 cm medial to the posterolateral corner of the acromion to the posterior axilla (Fig 1). The underlying deltoid muscle was split to reveal the infraspinatus and teres minor muscles. A deltoid muscle retractor was placed over the humeral head and under the acromion and the arm was placed in neutral rotation. A vertical incision was made through the infraspinatus tendon and the capsule. When the capsulotomy was complete, the joint was visualized and the arm was externally rotated so that the lateral stump of the capsule could be sutured into the intact posterior labrum. The medial portion of the capsule and infraspinatus muscle were sutured laterally over the repair. The arm was capable of 20 degrees of internal rotation at this point. A routine wound closure was performed. The arm was placed in about 20 degrees of abduction and 20 degrees of external rotation with the upper arm slightly posterior to the coronal plane, and an orthosis or shoulder spica cast was put in place. The patient's shoulder was immobilized for 4 to 6 weeks. After removal of the orthosis, a 3-stage rehabilitation program was initiated. The first stage consisted of passive range of motion exercises for 2 weeks. This was followed by active range of motion and terminal stretching for 4 weeks. The final stage consisted of rotational and scapular strengthening, with continued terminal stretching. Six months of aggressive postoperative rehabilitation were necessary before a return to sports activities or occupational tasks.

Results.—After surgery, the average range of motion was 174 degrees forward elevation and 69 degrees external rotation. Posterior instability did not recur. The average pain rating score was 2 out of 10 at rest and 4 out of 10 with activity. All patients were improved after surgery. Four patients remained minimally disabled in activities of daily living, 6 patients had shoulder fatigue at work and 4 patients were unable to return to full athletic activities. Thirteen of the 14 patients available at follow-up were satisfied with the outcome of this procedure.

Conclusions.—A posterior capsulotendinous tensioning procedure was performed for patients with posterior instability of the glenohumeral joint who did not respond to conservative management. Although this procedure was more successful than others that have been used to treat this condition, it was not ideal because patients continued to have some shoulder discomfort. Posterior capsulotendinous tensioning should be considered for the management of patients with posterior instability of the glenohumeral joint who do not respond to conservative management.

▶ The authors emphasize that in their experience the majority of patients with posterior instability of the glenohumeral joint respond to a nonoperative program. All patients in this study, however, were unable to perform activities of daily living, occupational activities, and athletic activities. Although all but one were satisfied with their surgical outcomes, it is concluded that "the procedure described is an imperfect aberration in that not all patients return to aggressive labor and work and several patients were unable to return to recreational sports activity."

J.S. Torg, M.D.

Arthroscopic Anterior Labral Reconstruction Using a Transglenoid Suture Technique

Mologne TS, Lapoint JM, Morin WD, et al (Naval Med Ctr, San Diego, Calif)
Am J Sports Med 24:268–274, 1996   2–14

Background.—Ideally, surgical treatment of traumatic anterior glenohumeral instability would repair the torn or detached labrum and reestablish the integrity of the inferior glenohumeral ligament. Historically, the open Bankart procedure has been the gold standard in surgical management of these lesions. However, arthroscopic stabilization of the glenohumeral joint is now possible. A 3-year experience with arthroscopic transglenoid suture reconstruction of the anteroinferior glenoid labrum in athletic patients in the military was reviewed in a retrospective study.

Operative Technique.—A diagnostic arthroscopic examination was performed with standard anterior and posterior shoulder arthroscopic portals. The frayed labral or rotator cuff muscular tissue was debrided and the scapular neck abraded to bleeding bone in the area of labral attachment. Polydioxanone sutures were placed in the labrum. One or two 2-mm Beath pins were placed through the glenoid, drilled across the scapular neck, and placed through the infraspinatus muscle. Then, 0-PDS labral sutures were delivered through the holes with the Beath pins and tied posteriorly over the infraspinatus fascia. Postoperatively, the shoulder was immobilized for 6 weeks before passive motion is begun. Active motion was begun at 8 weeks, and resistive exercises were begun after full motion was achieved.

Methods.—The inpatient and outpatient records of 48 patients undergoing 49 arthroscopic procedures were reviewed. The patients had 3 types of injuries: a history of traumatic glenohumeral dislocation (29 patients), traumatic recurrent glenohumeral subluxation (12 patients), and shoulder pain and apprehension on testing, but no subjective instability (7 patients). Follow-up data included the occurrence of recurrent instability, functional outcome, and return to athletic participation. Predictors of recurrent instability were analyzed.

Results.—Recurrent instability was reported during follow-up in 45% of the patients with a history of glenohumeral dislocations and 33% of the patients with a history of glenohumeral subluxations. In the dislocation group, the functional results were good or excellent in 52%, fair in 14%, and poor in 34%. Functional results in the subluxation group were good or excellent in 50%, fair in 25%, and poor in 25%. In the shoulder pain group, functional results were good or excellent in 63% and poor in 37%. Full athletic participation was achieved in 48% of the dislocation group, 33% of the subluxation group, and 71% of the shoulder pain group. Compliance with postoperative immobilization for 6 weeks was the only significant predictor of outcome. There was a complication rate of

14%, with 7 complications in 5 patients. The complications included suprascapular nerve palsy in 3 patients and traction-induced musculocutaneous nerve palsy, septic shoulder, portal abscess, and adhesive capsulitis in 1 patient each.

Conclusions.—Arthroscopic transglenoid suture for anterior labral reconstruction was associated with a high rate of recurrent instability in athletic patients in the military, although the risk of recurrent instability was reduced in patients with immobilized shoulders for a full 6 weeks postoperatively. Suprascapular nerve palsy emerged as a significant potential complication of the procedure. Therefore, this arthroscopic technique is not recommended for the management of glenohumeral instability in young athletic patients.

▶ The 41% overall postoperative recurrent instability rate in this study is both unacceptable and unexplainably high. In view of the fact that the shoulders were immobilized for 6 weeks and did not return to full unlimited activity until 6 months, this procedure clearly has no advantage over the open Bankart procedure.

J.S. Torg, M.D.

Complications of Type I Coronoid Fractures in Competitive Athletes: Report of Two Cases and Review of the Literature

Liu SH, Henry M, Bowen R (UCLA School of Medicine, Los Angeles)
J Shoulder Elbow Surg 5:223–227, 1996   2–15

Purpose.—There are 3 types of coronoid fracture: type I, tip avulsion; type II, fractures involving less than 50% of the coronoid; and type III, fractures involving more than 50% of the coronoid. Treatment varies by type of fracture. Whereas elbow instability is a known complication of type III and sometimes type II fractures, type I fractures are generally thought to heal uneventfully. This report describes 2 athletes with type I elbow fractures that did not respond to conservative treatment.

Patients.—The patients were both young adults, one injured while waterskiing and the other during a judo tournament. Radiographs demonstrated type I coronoid fractures, and both patients were treated with an elbow brace and active and passive range of motion. Though elbow motion improved, both patients continued to have pain. In the waterskiier, arthroscopic evaluation was performed 3 months after the injury. This patient was found to have a displaced and hypertrophic coronoid process. This process was attached to the coronoid base by fibrotic scar tissue, and was interfering with flexion and extension. These tissues were arthroscopically debrided, and the patient was able to return to recreational sports after 6 weeks of bracing and physical therapy. The judoist underwent arthroscopic removal of 2 loose fracture fragments after 2 months of unsuccessful physical therapy. She was able to return to her sport after 2 months.

Discussion.—Not all type I coronoid fractures in athletes will heal with conservative treatment. Patients who continue to have pain or restricted motion after 3 months of conservative therapy should be considered for surgery. Those with intraarticular loose bodies should undergo early arthroscopy.

▶ As is pointed out, type I fractures of the coronoid really present a problem. There are potential complications, and the authors suggest that in the competitive athlete, this fracture should be recognized and treated early. This, of course, deals with the complication in that no change in the conservative management of the initial fracture is suggested.

J.S. Torg, M.D.

The Results of Operative Resection of the Lateral End of the Clavicle
Eskola A, Santavirta S, Viljakka T, et al (Orthopaedic Hosp of the Invalid Found, Helsinki; Tampere Univ, Finland; Central Hosp of Middle-Finland, Jyväskylä)
J Bone Joint Surg (Am) 78A:584–587, 1996   2–16

Introduction.—Although most patients undergoing operative resection of the lateral end of the clavicle for painful conditions of the acromioclavicular joint are reported to have a good outcome, 1 series found results to be poor in more than 20% of cases. To assess long-term results of the procedure, 73 patients were examined an average of 9 years after operation.

Methods.—The procedures were done at 3 hospitals in Finland between 1973 and 1985. Patients had an average age of 43 years; 52 were men and 21 were women. The painful condition of the acromioclavicular joint was caused by a traumatic event in 40 patients, 32 of whom had a complete separation of the joint and radiographic signs of osteoarthrosis. Eight patients had a fracture of the lateral end of the clavicle, and 33 had primary acromioclavicular osteoarthrosis. An average of 16 mm was resected, and the amount of resection was similar in the 3 patient groups.

Results.—At follow-up evaluation, outcome was considered good in 21 patients, satisfactory in 29, and poor in 23. Only 1 of 8 patients who had a fracture of the lateral end of the clavicle had a good result; 4 had a poor result. Forty-six patients reported pain in the shoulder with exertion, and 16 had limited glenohumeral motion. Strength was reduced in the involved upper extremity of 18 patients. Forty-five patients were able to return to their previous work, but 11 of 21 whose work involved strenuous manual labor retired because of disability or had to transfer to different work. There was a significant association between pain at follow-up and a greater extent (greater than 10 mm) of resection.

Discussion.—Operative resection of the lateral end of the clavicle for treatment of painful conditions of the acromioclavicular joint yields results that are unpredictable and often poor at long-term follow-up. Resection is not advised for patients hoping to return to strenuous manual work or athletic activities. When operative treatment is undertaken, resection of the lateral end of the clavicle should not exceed 10 mm.

▶ A common cause of acromioclavicular joint pain seen in a sports medicine practice is osteolysis of the distal end of the clavicle. Unfortunately, it does not appear that this problem occurred in the patients in this study. The significance of this is that in my experience, better results occur when there is adequate resection of the distal end of the clavicle in those patients with osteolysis.

J.S. Torg, M.D.

Direct Injury to the Axillary Neve in Athletes Playing Contact Sports
Perlmutter GS, Leffert RD, Zarins B (Harvard Med School, Boston)
Am J Sports Med 25:65–68, 1997   2–17

Background.—Nerve injury, frequently associated with a burning pain (a "burner" or "stinger"), is one of the most serious complications of contact sports. This injury can result from a direct blow to the shoulder, neck or head, causing shoulder depression and contralateral neck flexion. This report describes axillary nerve injuries associated with a direct blow to the anterior lateral deltoid muscle in athletes playing contact sports.

Study Group.—The study group consisted of 11 male athletes, identified from a retrospective review of medical records, who had clinical and electrocardiographic evidence of injury to the axillary nerve and who were studied for more than 2 years. Nine of these injuries were sustained during football tackles and 2 were sustained during hockey collisions. The average age of these patients was 19 years. Nine athletes had "burners" at the time of injury. The mechanism of injury was a direct blow to the anterior lateral deltoid muscle in 7, with a concurrent shoulder depression and contralateral neck flexion in 4.

Treatment.—All athletes participated in a rehabilitation program. Four underwent axillary nerve exploration an average of 5.5 months after injury. All the patients had extensive scarring of the posterior branch of the axillary nerve at operation. Neurolysis was performed in all cases.

Results.—The average time from injury to correct diagnosis was 6.5 weeks. At 31- to 276-month follow-up, all patients had residual defects of axillary sensory and motor nerve function. There was no deltoid muscle improvement in 3 patients, some improvement in 2 patients and major improvement in 6 patients. Shoulder function remained excellent, with all participants maintaining full range of motion and good motor strength. Axillary nerve exploration and neurolysis had no effect on outcome. Although there was no case of full recovery of axillary nerve function, 10 of 11 athletes returned to their previous level of sports activity, including professional athletics.

Conclusions.—This report describes a series of patients with direct injury to the axillary nerve. Although neurologic recovery was incomplete in all study participants, functional recovery was excellent. It is recommended that athletes with axillary nerve injuries return to contact sports only when they have full range of motion in the shoulder and muscle strength is good. Nerve exploration should be reserved for patients with suspected nerve rupture. A thorough cervical spine and neurologic examination should be performed on every athlete who sustains a "burner" injury to ensure proper diagnosis of axillary nerve injury.

▶ This paper represents the first comprehensive and well-documented report dealing with direct blow injuries to the axillary nerve resulting from contact sports. Clearly, this is an unusual injury and I can't recall having encountered the problem myself. As noted, most axillary nerve injuries occurring in athletic activities are caused by glenohumeral dislocation. It is interesting to note that of the 4 patients who came to surgery, all were found to have extensive scarring of the posterior branch of the axillary nerve. However, of note, the authors "do not believe axillary nerve exploration is warranted in a patient who sustains a direct injury and should be reserved for a patient in whom one suspects a rupture of the axillary nerve, such as that seen after traumatic shoulder dislocation."

J.S. Torg, M.D.

The Pathomechanics of Chronic, Recurrent Cervical Nerve Root Neurapraxia

Levitz CL, Reilly PJ, Torg JS (Univ of Pennsylvania, Philadelphia; Allegheny Univ, Philadelphia)
Am J Sports Med 25:73–76, 1997   2–18

Introduction.—The proposed injury mechanisms for chronic, recurrent cervical nerve root neurapraxia, or the chronic burner syndrome, are: brachial plexus stretch or traction injury, nerve root compression in the neural foramina, or injury from a direct blow to the brachial plexus. These injuries occur most often in football and other collision sports. The pathomechanics of chronic burner syndrome are described, and its clinical findings are characterized.

Methods.—Of 55 football players evaluated, 11 were professional, 37 were intercollegiate, and 7 were scholastic players. Patients were evaluated by physical examination and magnetic resonance imaging, and the mechanism for injury was classified for each patient.

Results.—The mechanism of injury was extension combined with ipsilateral-lateral deviation in 46 patients (83%) and axial compression in 9 patients (17%). Physical examination revealed 39 patients (70%) with positive Spurling's sign and 40 patients (72%) with persistent weakness of the deltoid and spinatus muscle groups. Twenty-nine patients (53%) had developmentally narrowed cervical stenosis. Degenerative disk disease was noted on magnetic resonance imaging in 47 patients (85%). Of these, 19 patients had bulging of the intervertebral disk, 15 had protrusion of the disk, and 12 had herniation of the disk (Fig 1). Narrowing of the neural foramina from bony hypertrophy (Fig 2) was observed in 3 of 7 patients with no evidence of disk disease. Of 47 patients (94%) with disk disease,

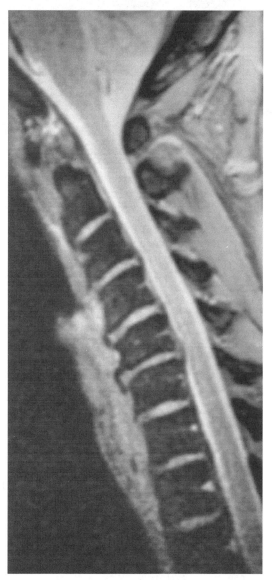

FIGURE 1.—Magnetic resonance scan of a player with chronic burner syndrome with a disk bulge at C3-4 and C4-5 and a disk herniation at C5-6 that indents the cord. (Courtesy of Levitz CL, Reilly PJ, Torg JS: The pathomechanics of chronic, recurrent cervical root neurapraxia. *Amer J Sports Med* 25:73–76, 1997.)

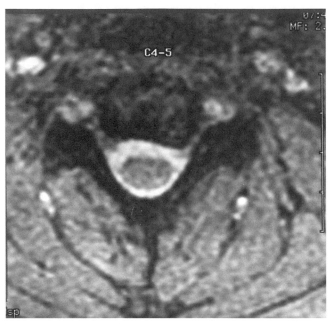

FIGURE 2.—Magnetic resonance scan of a player with chronic burner syndrome with narrowing of the intervertebral foramina with decreased space for the nerve root. (Courtesy of Levitz CL, Reilly PJ, Torg JS: The pathomechanics of chronic, recurrent cervical root neuraprazia. *Am J Sports Med* 25:73–76, 1997.)

involvement of the C4-5, C5-6, or C6-7 levels was observed. Sixteen patients had involvement of multiple levels. Ten of 11 professional football players (91%) had disk disease related to other abnormalities on radiographs.

Conclusion.—Cervical stenosis was observed in most football players seen for recurrent burner syndrome. Athletes with combined disk disease and cervical spinal canal stenosis may have alterations in cervical spine mechanics that could make them more prone to chronic burner syndromes.

▶ Noteworthy is the fact that this is the first published study in which magnetic resonance imaging analysis was correlated with the clinical findings and presumed pathomechanics of the chronic burner syndrome.

J.S. Torg, M.D.

Upper Limb Nerve Entrapments in Elite Wheelchair Racers
Boninger ML, Robertson RN, Wolff M, et al (Univ of Pittsburgh, Pa; Ohio State Univ, Columbus)
Am J Phys Med Rehabil 75:170–176, 1996   2–19

Background.—Peripheral nerve entrapments are common manual wheelchair users (MWUs). If these injuries are caused by repetitive stress during wheelchair propulsion, then wheelchair athletes who participate in activities that increase the time spent pushing a wheelchair would be at increased risk for development of carpal tunnel syndrome. To determine whether peripheral nerve entrapments among MWUs are caused by the pushing of the wheelchair, the prevalence of upper limb nerve injuries was assessed in a group of elite wheelchair racers and compared with the prevalence reported in the literature for all MWUs.

Study Design.—All 12 wheelchair racers participating in the United States Olympic Committee Wheelchair USA training camp in 1994 were recruited into this study group. Each racer completed a questionnaire that included sex, age, dominant hand, type of disability, disability duration, training schedule, years of competition, hours per week spent in the wheelchair, history of upper limb injury and type of treatment received. A focused physical examination, included bilateral upper limb nerve conduction studies, was performed.

Findings.—The study group consisted of 11 men and 1 woman. Their average age was 33 years. These racers pushed their chairs an average of 56 miles per week for training. Of the 12 racers in the study group, 6 had evidence of median mononeuropathy. Of these 6, 5 had evidence of bilateral mononeuropathy. Ulnar mononeuropathy at the wrist was present in 25% and ulnar mononeuropathy at the elbow was present in 25% of the study group. Radial nerve injury was detected in 17%. The duration of disability accounted for a significant amount of the variance in the median sensory amplitude and the mean ulnar palmar amplitude. None of the other variables was associated with the results of nerve conduction studies.

Conclusions.—This study of a population of elite wheelchair racers revealed a 50% prevalence of median mononeuropathy, similar to that reported for the general population of wheelchair users. Nerve conduction abnormalities were not related to amount of training or years in competition but were associated with disability duration. This finding suggests that neuropathy is not primarily caused by the pushing of the wheelchair but may be caused by the forces on the wrist during chair transfer. Further research is required to assess potentially modifiable risk factors associated with the development of neuropathy among wheelchair users.

▶ As pointed out by the authors, the reason that this group of elite racers was not predisposed to neuropathy at a greater rate that the general wheelchair-using population may be because neuropathy in all wheelchair users has little to do with pushing the wheelchair. Rather, it is proposed that the neuropathy may be solely attributable to forces during transfers to and from the wheelchair.

J.S. Torg, M.D.

Radiologic Measurement of Superior Displacement of the Humeral Head in the Impingement Syndrome

Deutsch A, Altchek DW, Schwartz E, et al (Hosp for Special Surgery, New York; Catholic Med Ctr of Brooklyn and Queens, Elmhurst, NY; Case Western Reserve Univ, Cleveland, Ohio)

J Shoulder Elbow Surg 5:186–193, 1996   2–20

Background.—The impingement syndrome is common. In cases of rotator cuff injury, even without a full-thickness tear, there may be a relative imbalance of forces across the glenohumeral joint, and as the rotator cuff weakens, the deltoid would generate a relative increase in upward shear force. The superior displacement of the humeral head during abduction

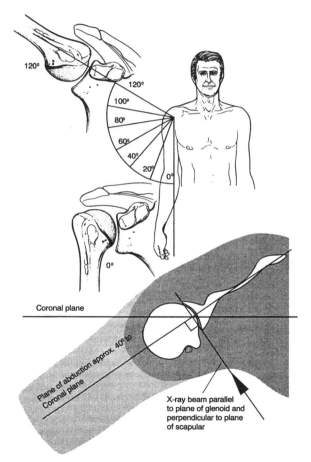

FIGURE 2.—Sequential radiographs. The study consisted of a series of anteroposterior roentgenograms in the plane of the scapula with the arm in neutral rotation. Roentgenograms were obtained at 20-degree intervals as the arm was elevated in the plane of the scapula from 0 to 120 degrees. (Courtesy of Deutsch A, Altcheck DW, Schwartz E, et al: Radiologic measurement of superior displacement of the humeral head in the impingement syndrome. *J Shoulder Elbow Surg* 5:186–193, 1996.)

then functionally narrows the subacromial space, resulting in an impingement phenomenon. Measurements of the excursion of the humeral head on the face of the glenoid, arm angle, scapulothoracic angle, and glenohumeral angle with the arm elevated in the plane of the scapula were obtained to compare the motion of the normal shoulder with that of shoulders with stage II and stage III impingement syndrome.

Methods.—Twelve patients with normal shoulders (group 1), 15 with stage II impingement syndrome (group 2), and 20 with rotator cuff tears or stage III impingement (group 3) participated in the study. A series of anteroposterior radiographs were obtained in the plane of the scapula with the arm in neutral rotation. Radiographs were obtained at 20-degree intervals as the arm was elevated from 0 to 120 degrees, while the subjects held in their hand a weight that was 2.5% of their body weight.

Findings.—No significant change was noted in the position of the humeral head with arm elevation in group 1. Group 2 patients had significant superior displacement of the center of the humeral head with arm elevation. Group 3 patients had a significant rise during the first 40 degrees of abduction. The mean position of the humeral head in groups 2 and 3 was superior to the mean head position in group 1. Group 2 and 3 patients did not differ significantly in head position (Fig 2).

Conclusion.—These data support a biomechanical theory for the development of impingement syndrome. In patients with excessive cuff deficiency caused by a massive tear or disease, surgical repair may be unable to achieve the goal of restoring the centering ability of the rotator cuff. In patients with minor injury, proper strength training should restore the normal deltoid-rotator cuff force couple and decrease the likelihood of superior displacement of the humeral head and impingement.

▶ Rotator cuff injury is a common precursor to more serious pathology of the shoulder joint, including impingement syndrome. Supraspinatus and infraspinatus act to hold the humeral head in the glenoid fossa during abduction of the arm from deltoid action, which also tends to lift the humerus superiorly. Impingement syndromes are often accompanied by upward movement of the humeral head on the glenoid fossa during arm elevation, caused by weakness or injury to the rotator cuff muscles.

The movement of the humeral head during arm elevation was examined in a group of normal patients, a group with stage II impingement, and a group with rotator cuff tears. The analysis of the roentgenograms indicated that there was distinct upward displacement of the humeral head for both the impingement group and the group with rotator cuff tears. The upward motion of the humeral head further increases the impingement as compression occurs below the coracoacromial arch. This impingement produces acromial and greater tuberosity osteophyte formation, which produces greater degeneration of the supraspinatus muscle. The study suggests that early rehabilitation and strengthening of rotator cuff strains is important for preventing the later stages of impingement and loss of range of motion.

M.J.L. Alexander, Ph.D.

Parsonage-Turner Syndrome (Acute Brachial Neuritis)

Misamore GW, Lehman DE (Methodist Sports Med Ctr, Indianapolis, Ind)
J Bone Joint Surg (Am) 78A:1405–1408, 1996   2–21

Introduction.—Brachial neuritis (Parsonage-Turner syndrome) usually has a sudden onset, with severe pain in the shoulder girdle area followed by muscle weakness in the shoulder. Diagnosis can be difficult because the symptoms of brachial neuritis are similar to those of a number of disorders. A retrospective review of 7 cases discussed the onset, treatment, and resolution of brachial neuritis.

Methods.—Between 1985 and 1992, 14 of more than 6,500 patients seen by the senior author for shoulder-related problems received a diagnosis of brachial neuritis. Seven of the 14 were excluded because of incomplete workup or follow-up. The other 7 patients, all men, had a mean age of 35 years when first seen for shoulder complaints. None had antecedent trauma or a systemic disorder that might affect the musculoskeletal system; all had electromyographic studies consistent with brachial neuritis and experienced a spontaneous decrease in pain and weakness. Treatment consisted of analgesics, physical therapy, and rehabilitation exercises. The minimum follow-up was 2 years.

Results.—The patients' intense pain continued for 3 to 21 days before spontaneous resolution. A dull ache, usually not related to activity, was experienced after the period of pain. The onset of subjective weakness occurred at a mean of approximately 4 weeks after initial onset of the disorder. All 7 patients showed a consistent pattern of electromyographic changes, with fibrillation potentials and positive waves seen 3 to 4 weeks after pain onset. All reported pain to be relatively minor after 3 months. Six patients had no residual pain at 1-year follow-up, and 1 had minor activity-related aching. The outcome was unchanged at long-term follow-up (mean, 6 years). Shoulder weakness was slower to resolve than pain, and 3 patients have continued to experience mild, persistent weakness.

Conclusions.—Parsonage-Turner syndrome typically has a large male-to-female ratio. The exact cause of the disorder remains uncertain, but trauma generally is not considered to be a factor. Diagnosis, made primarily by exclusion, becomes more obvious when pain decreases spontaneously and weakness develops.

▶ This is an important article. Although low on the list, acute brachial neuritis should be considered in the differential diagnosis of patients with shoulder pain without a history of antecedent trauma. This is particularly true of those who are seen with bilateral complaints. Although the prognosis is "reasonably good," complete restoration of strength does not always occur. More importantly, although recovery can be quite protracted, there is no place for surgery in the management of the disorder.

J.S. Torg, M.D.

Burner Syndrome: Recognition and Rehabilitation

Nissen SJ, Laskowski ER, Rizzo TD Jr (MeritCare Med Group, Fargo, ND; Mayo Clinic, Rochester, Minn; Mayo Clinic, Jacksonville, Fla)
Physician Sportsmed 24:57–64, 1996   2–22

Background.—Brachial plexus injury, referred to as burner syndrome, occurs commonly in contact sports, especially football. This injury is not always benign. An adolescent football player with burner symptoms that resolved quickly but resulted in later shoulder weakness and neck pain was described.

Case Report.—Boy, 15 years, was initially seen with left neck and shoulder pain and left shoulder weakness that had persisted for 1 week. His medical history included 2 neck injuries while playing football. The first injury occurred during a tackle. The opponent's leg hit the left side of the patient's neck, causing his head to snap back and to the right. His left arm immediately felt "paralyzed and numb," and severe pain occurred in his left shoulder and neck. These symptoms resolved in 5 minutes, and he did not seek medical evaluation. One week later, the patient was injured again when butting helmets with an opponent. This caused severe shooting pain in the left side of his neck and arm, together with weakness in the left upper extremity. One week after this incident, the boy sought medical attention.

Physical assessment demonstrated antigravity strength of the left supraspinatus muscle with an inability to accept any resistance, mild weakness of the deltoid and biceps with an inability to accept full resistance, and reduced left biceps and brachioradialis deep tendon reflexes. The patient also had a positive drop arm test and an equivocal Neer impingement test. Diagnostic imaging results were normal. Overall, the findings were most consistent with a grade 2 burner. Treatment consisted of ice applied to the left upper trapezius muscle and supine active assisted range-of-motion exercises of the left shoulder, seated active assisted range-of-motion exercises with a pulley, shoulder shrugs, and active range-of-motion exercises of the elbow and neck without neck extension. The patient was told not to participate in football or physical education activities.

One month later, weakness on manual muscle testing of the external rotators and deltoid was minimal. He still had occasional paraspinal neck pain, but his neck range of motion was full and painless. At 2 months, strength and deep tendon reflexes were normal, and he had no arm or neck pain. Although the patient refrained from playing football for the rest of the season, he was able to play competitive basketball 4 months after the initial injury.

Conclusion.—Proper classification of burner injuries relies on detailed serial clinical examinations. Conditions to exclude are cervical root lesions, shoulder injuries, and other plexus or nerve involvement. Rehabilitation consists of physical modalities and range of motion, stretching, and strengthening exercises for the cervical, shoulder, and elbow muscles. Preseason strengthening exercises and protective devices help prevent burner injuries.

▶ In football, burners are very common, greatly underreported, and tend to recur, with ever less force required to produce the lesion. It is widely agreed—but not always followed in practice—that the athlete who experiences a burner should not be allowed to compete until he is pain free and symptom free, with full range of neck motion and complete arm and shoulder strength.[1] This practical article covers causation, recognition, grading, treatment, rehabilitation, and return-to-play criteria; it offers useful tips on preventing burners via exercise, equipment, and proper technique of play.

A recent study covers the pros and cons of 3 different cervical orthoses (the neck roll, the "Cowboy Collar," and a customized orthosis used by the Vanderbilt University football team) used to limit neck motion and help prevent burners. Burners should not be taken lightly; complete recovery from a grade 2 or 3 injury may take 6 months or more.

E.R. Eichner, M.D.

References

1. 1993 Year Book of Sports Medicine, pp 32–34.
2. Hovis WD, Limbird TJ: An evaluation of cervical orthoses in limiting hyperextension and lateral flexion in football. *Med Sci Sports Exerc* 26:872–876, 1994.

Compression of the Lateral Antebrachial Cutaneous Nerve by the Biceps Tendon
Gillingham BL, Mack GR (Naval Med Ctr, San Diego, Calif)
J Shoulder Elbow Surg 5:330–332, 1996   2–23

Introduction.—In the case presented, an active duty marine experienced pain and paresthesias in the lateral antebrachial cutaneous nerve (LACN) distribution of his left arm after slam-dunking a basketball. Surgery was undertaken when conservative treatment failed to relieve symptoms. The literature relating to this uncommon entity, compression of the LACN by the biceps tendon, is reviewed.

Case Report.—A 21-year-old man was medically evacuated from duty in Saudi Arabia because of persistent pain and paresthesias extending from the elbow flexion crease to the base of the thumb. He traced his symptoms to an event 10 months earlier, but also reported a 2-year history of a grating sensation and left elbow pain during push-ups. Removal of a loose body (1 × 2 cm), which appeared to have originated from the articular surface of the olecranon, relieved elbow symptoms. Two months after this procedure, physical examination revealed normal range of motion in the left arm and good grip strength. Sensory examination confirmed decreased sensation in the distribution of the LACN.

When exploratory surgery was performed at the elbow, the lateral edge of the biceps tendon was found to be compressing the LACN when it emerged from between the biceps and brachialis muscle bellies (Fig 1). Compression of the nerve was accentuated by elbow extension and forearm pronation. The nerve was decompressed by means of an oblique incision in the lateral edge of the biceps tendon, creating a triangular flap (Fig 2) that was sutured to the remaining tendon. There was no further compression, and the patient experienced immediate and complete pain relief after sur-

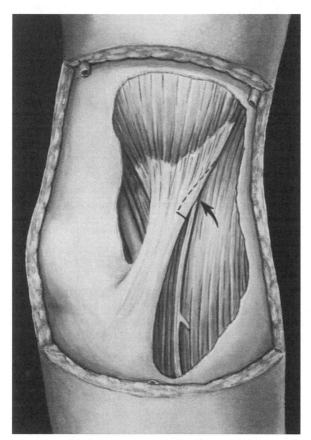

FIGURE 1.—Intraoperative findings. Focal compression of LACN by biceps aponeurosis is present *(arrow). Solid transverse line* represents location of relaxing incision. *Dashed line* represents line along which proximal triangular flap was folded. *Abbreviation: LACN,* lateral antebrachial cutaneous nerve. (Courtesy of Gillingham BL, Mack GR: Compression of the lateral antebrachial cutaneous nerve by the biceps tendon. *J Shoulder Elbow Surg* 5:330–332.)

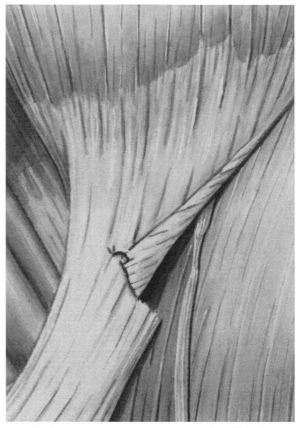

FIGURE 2.—Completed procedure. Compression on LACN relieved by reflecting triangular flap of aponeurosis and tendon medially and suturing to remaining tendon. Focal hyperemia and narrowing of LACN was present. *Abbreviation: LACN,* lateral antebrachial cutaneous nerve. (Courtesy of Gillingham BL, Mack GR: Compression of the lateral antebrachial cutaneous nerve by the biceps tendon. *J Shoulder Elbow Surg* 5:330–332.)

gery. At 3-month follow-up, results of the sensory examination were normal, as were the results of manual muscle testing of supination and elbow flexion. The patient remains asymptomatic 4 years later.

Discussion.—Compression of the LACN at the elbow by the lateral edge of the biceps tendon is a rarely recognized entrapment neuropathy, with only 19 cases reported to date. Symptoms include sensory loss pain over the anterolateral aspect of the elbow, aggravated by elbow extension and forearm pronation. Physical examination may reveal a positive Tinel's sign just lateral to the biceps tendon. Patients often have a history of injury or overuse of the elbow. Surgical decompression can usually relieve symptoms when conservative therapy is ineffective.

▶ Although it is stated that late rupture of the biceps tendon has not been observed in patients treated with surgical decompression, this potential complication is certainly a consideration. As this article points out, another surgical technique described involves freeing the nerve between the brachialis and biceps tendon without cutting the biceps.

J.S. Torg, M.D.

Internal Fixation of Acute Stable Scaphoid Fractures in the Athlete
Rettig AC, Kollias SC (Methodist Sports Medicine Ctr, Indianapolis, Ind)
Am J Sports Med 24:182–186, 1996   2–24

Introduction.—Scaphoid fractures are commonly treated with casts and usually require 9 to 12 weeks for healing. Although playing casts may be appropriate for athletes desiring to return to play, open reduction and internal fixation can offer an early return to sports requiring maximal dexterity. The 12 athletes described were treated with Herbert screw fixation for acute midthird scaphoid fractures.

Methods.—Patients ranged in age from 17 to 31 years; 8 participated in basketball, 2 in baseball, and 2 in archery. All were treated within 4 weeks of the injury. The fractures were nondisplaced in 10 cases and minimally displaced in 2. Most surgical procedures were performed through a volar Russe-type approach. Patients wore a short arm-thumb spica splint for 7 to 10 days, followed by a resting splint and a program of stretching and strengthening at home. Return to sport was approved when the patient could participate without pain or use of a supportive device. During the healing period patients were regularly examined for grip strength, range of motion, and point tenderness.

Results.—With an average follow-up of 2.9 years, 11 of the 12 athletes had radiographic union of the fracture. Average time to union was 9.8 weeks. Range of motion of the wrist was symmetric in 9 of 12 patients, and 10 had grip strength equal to or greater than the injured side. Archers returned to their sport at an average of 3.5 weeks after surgery; basketball players required 6 weeks and baseball players 5.8 weeks. Except for the patient with nonunion, (a basketball player with insulin-dependent diabetes) patients were pleased with surgical results.

Conclusion.—For athletes who desire an early return to sports and accept the risks of surgery, internal fixation of an acute midthird scaphoid fracture is a viable alternative to cast treatment. The procedure was safe and outcome excellent in this small series of patients, but longer follow-up is advisable before internal fixation is widely recommended in such cases.

▶ It is interesting to note that the senior author has previously reported on the management of midthird scaphoid fractures in the athlete.[1] His conclusions were that "in season athletes with stable mid-third scaphoid fractures can safely achieve early return to sport with a playing cast or rigid internal fixation with a Herbert screw." These two methods of treatment yielded comparable union rates with other series, and it appears that the athletes are not at increased risk of union failure or nonunion as a result of participation in sports. In that study, clinical and radiographic healing averaged 10.8 and 11.2 weeks, respectively, for those treated surgically and 13.7 and 14.2 weeks for those treated nonoperatively. Also, return to sports averaged 8 weeks in the surgical group and 4.3 weeks in the nonoperative group. However, in the more recent study, athletes whose activities precluded the use of a playing cast and were treated with internal fixation returned on an average of 5.8 weeks. So for this group, those precluded from use of a playing cast, surgery appears to delay a return to activity for 2 weeks. It would appear that this is an important fact in the athlete's decision-making process.

J.S. Torg, M.D.

Reference

1. Rettig AC, Weidenbener EJ, Gloyeske R: Alternative management of midthird scaphoid fractures in the athlete. *Am J Sports Med* 22:711–714, 1994.

Magnetic Resonance Imaging Versus Bone Scintigraphy in Suspected Scaphoid Fracture
Tiel-van Buul MMC, Roolker W, Verbeeten BWB Jr, et al (Univ of Amsterdam, The Netherlands)
Eur J Nucl Med 23:971–975, 1996   2–25

Background.—Fractures of the scaphoid account for up to 80% of wrist injuries and are an important cause of wrist disability. Nonunion is a frequent occurrence, particularly when the fracture line is proximal to the entry of the blood supply of the scaphoid. The ideal diagnostic procedure would have the same favorable characteristics as a bone scan, which is noninvasive and highly sensitive, but without a radiation burden to the patient. By using the bone scan as a reference method, magnetic resonance imaging (MRI) was evaluated for its suitability in the acute phase after carpal injury.

Methods.—Twenty-seven patients with clinically suspected scaphoid fracture were seen during the study period. Eight initially had positive results on a radiographic series, and 19 were included in the comparison of MRI and scintigraphy. Three patients could not undergo MRI because of claustrophobia, leaving 16 patients available for analysis. All patients were initially immobilized in a plaster cast. Three-phase radionuclide bone scintigraphy was obtained at least 72 hours after the injury with 200 MBq technetium-99m methylene diphosphonate. Bone scans were considered positive if both dynamic and static images showed focally increased activity in the scaphoid region. The carpal radiographs, MR images, and bone scans were reviewed by a panel of radiologists and a nuclear physician.

Results.—In all 16 patients the bone scan and MRI were obtained on the same day (a mean of 10 days after the trauma). Three-phase bone scintigraphy was positive for scaphoid fracture in 7 patients; MRI was positive in 5. Both modalities were negative in 6 patients. Two patients with negative MRI results appeared to have interosseal fluid in the carpus and were treated as if they had a scaphoid fracture; initial radiographs were retrospectively found to be positive for scaphoid fracture in 1 of these cases. In another case, surgery confirmed a fracture after MRI showed a perilunar luxation without a fracture. The 2 remaining patients had a hot spot in the region of MCP I with a negative MRI; therapy was adjusted in both.

Conclusion.—This is the first report of the use of MRI in the acute phase after carpal injury and when initial radiographs were negative. Although MRI shows promise in this setting, it is costly and not superior to 3-phase scintigraphy.

▶ In this the era of cost containment, in addition to the superior reliability of bone scintigraphy in the diagnostic management of patients with suspected scaphoid fractures, the excessive cost of MRI may well be the most important determinant in not using this modality.

J.S. Torg, M.D.

Non-union of the Scaphoid
Trumble TW, Clarke T, Kreder HJ (Univ of Washington, Seattle)
J Bone Joint Surg Am 78A:1829–1837, 1996   2–26

Background.—Treating scaphoid non-union is challenging. Several screws have been developed to provide stabilization for long periods and to reduce the duration of postoperative immobilization. The outcomes of bone grafting and internal fixation with 1 of 2 types of screws and temporary placement of Kirschner wires parallel to the screw to prevent rotation were reviewed.

Methods.—Thirty-four patients had been treated. Sixteen patients (Group 1) received a Herbert screw between 1986 and 1989, and 18 (Group 2) received a 3.5 mm cannulated AO/ASIF screw between 1990 and 1992. The 2 groups did not differ clinically or radiographically.

Findings.—Tomographically confirmed time to union was a mean 7.6 months in Group 1 and 3.6 months in Group 2, a significant difference. Both treatments significantly improved the alignment of the scaphoid and reduced carpal collapse. Time to union was significantly shorter when screw placement was in the central third of the scaphoid, regardless of the screw type used. Seventeen of the 18 cannulated screws and 7 of the 16 Herbert screws had been placed centrally.

Conclusions.—Time to union after fixation with the AO/ASIF cannulated screw was shorter than that after Herbert screw use, though the rate of central placement in the proximal pole of the scaphoid was higher for the cannulated screw than for the Herbert screw. Improved lateral intra-scaphoid angle alignment was associated with an overall improvement in the range of motion.

▶ It is important that the 94% union rate was most likely related to the strict inclusion criteria. Excluded were patients who had severe avascular necrosis, fracture of the proximal pole, or osteoarthritis, all being associated with a decreased rate of union.

J.S. Torg, M.D.

Wrist Pain in a Young Gymnast: Unusual Radiographic Findings and MRI Evidence of Growth Plate Injury
DiFiori JP, Mandelbaum BR (Univ of California, Los Angeles; Santa Monica Orthopaedic and Sports Medicine Group, Calif)
Med Sci Sports Exerc 28:1453–1458, 1996   2–27

Introduction.—Chronic wrist pain has a prevalence of 46% to 79% in elite and nonelite gymnasts. The criteria for diagnosing this injury in skeletally immature gymnasts are difficult to establish because of anatomical variants of the normal physis. Unusual radiographic findings and MRI evidence of growth plate injury in a young gymnasts were reported.

Case Report.—Girl, 10 years, was seen for a 3-week history of bilateral dorsal wrist pain after averaging 8 hr/wk of training for 1 year. Symptoms were most noticeable when she was performing handstands, handsprings, and round-offs. She did not miss practice sessions, but the quality of her performance was affected by pain. Icing and range-of-motion exercises did not ease the discomfort. Pain was elicited on radial deviation of the left wrist and during axial compression with the wrist in extension. The right wrist was not tender on palpation.

Radiographs showed rare cleft radial and ulnar epiphyses and epiphyseal spur formation. Metaphyseal and epiphyseal ischemia of the growth plate was observed on MRI. Gradient echo imaging of the left wrist showed widening of the growth plate and an inhomogeneous signal within the physis (Fig 2). Physeal cartilage extension into the metaphysis was observed in the left wrist. The diagnosis was bilateral distal radial stress injuries with cleft epiphyses. All gymnastic participation was stopped. The patient responded well to conservative treatment of ice, splinting, and activity modification. She was able to return gradually to gymnastics by a 7-month follow-up visit. Radiographs at follow-up revealed improvement in growth plate appearance, and an epiphyseal spur was observed. Two months later, the girl quit gymnastics because of lack of interest.

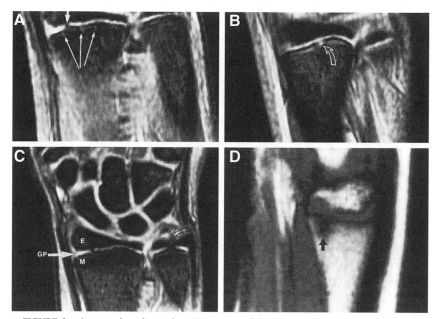

FIGURE 2.—**A,** coronal gradient echo (GRE) image of the left wrist shows a region of low signal within the distal radial growth plate extending from the epiphysis to the metaphysis, corresponding to the linear striation seen on the plain films (*short arrow*). Three linear high signal areas are seen in the distal metaphysis, consistent with vertical fractures as described by Shih (23) (*long arrows*). **B,** coronal GRE image of left wrist showing region of high signal intensity emanating from the growth plate and extending into the metaphysis, indicative of physeal cartilage extension (*arrow*). (The linear area of high signal in the radial epiphysis is an artifact.) **C,** coronal GRE image of the right wrist shows widening of the distal radial growth plate and inhomogeneity of the signal intensity within the growth plate. The cleft ulnar epiphysis appears as an area of high signal within the epiphysis (*arrow*). The cleft radial epiphysis is not seen on this view. *Abbreviations: E,* epiphysis; *M,* metaphysis; *GP,* growth plate. **D,** Sagittal view of right wrist using a short TR sequence demonstrates area of low signal within the distal radial metaphysis suggestive of a bone bruise (*arrow*). (Courtesy of DiFiori JP, Mandelbaum BR: Wrist pain in a young gymnast: Unusual radiographic findings and MRI evidence of growth plate injury. *Med Sci Sports Med* 28(12):1453–1458, 1996.)

Conclusion.—The patient had several confusing radiographic abnormalities. Magnetic resonance imaging has an important role in evaluating wrist pain in young gymnasts. Increased awareness of this injury is needed.

▶ This report emphasizes the fact that the risk of stress injury of the distal radial growth plates in young, skeletally immature females is not limited to elite gymnasts and can best be diagnosed by MRI, which outperforms the radiograph in distinguishing signs of injury from anatomical variants. Controversy arose recently regarding the toll that training takes on female gymnasts,[1] including the possibility that the "female athlete triad" (disordered eating, amenorrhea, and osteopenia) predisposes to stress fractures. Actually, research, so far, suggests that among female gymnasts, athough disordered eating and menstrual problems are common, bone mineral density tends to be high, not low, perhaps from the high-impact loading of the sport.[2–4]

E.R. Eichner, M.D.

References

1. Tofler IR, Stryer BK, Micheli LJ, et al: Physical and emotional problems of elite female gymnasts. *N Engl J Med* 335:281–283, 1996.
2. Robinson TL, Snow-Harter C, Taaffee DR, et al: Gymnasts exhibit higher bone mass than runners despite similar prevalence of amenorrhea and oligomenorrhea. *J Bone Miner Res* 10:26–35, 1995.
3. Kirchner EM, Lewis RD, O'Connor PJ: Bone mineral density and dietary intake of female college gymnasts. *Med Sci Sports Exerc* 27:543–549, 1995.
4. Dyson KD, Blimkie CJR, Davison KS, et al: Gymnastic training and bone density in preadolescent females. *Med Sci Sports Exerc* 29:443–450, 1997.

3 Chest, Spine, and Hip

The Effect of Protective Football Equipment on Alignment of the Injured Cervical Spine: Radiographic Analysis in a Cadaveric Model
Palumbo MA, Hulstyn MJ, Fadale PD, et al (Brown Univ, Providence, RI)
Am J Sports Med 24:446–453, 1996   3–1

Background.—The protective helmet and shoulder pads worn by football players complicate the standard immobilization process in the event of a neck injury. Emergency medical personnel often follow a protocol that requires helmet removal in cases of presumed cervical spine injury, whereas sports medicine professionals almost universally recommend leaving the helmet in place to prevent neurologic injury. The effect of protective football equipment on the alignment of the intact lower cervical spine and on the partially destabilized C5–C6 motion segment was determined in a cadaveric study.

Methods.—Testing procedures were performed with the use of 15 human cadavers (9 men and 6 women with an average age of 75 years). In all specimens, the lower cervical spine was tested in an intact condition. In an 8-member subset of specimens, selected because few degenerative changes were present at the C5–C6 intervertebral space, the C5–C6 motion segment was tested in both an intact and a 2-column, partially destabilized condition. Cadavers were placed supine on a backboard, and lateral cervical radiographs were obtained in 4 conditions: no protective equipment, helmet only, helmet and shoulder pads, and shoulder pads only. In the 8-member subset, a second set of radiographs was obtained after a distractive-flexion stage 3 injury was simulated.

Results.—Radiographs of the intact cervical spine specimens showed that wearing both helmet and shoulder pads did not result in a significant change in cervical lordosis when compared with the no-equipment condition. Cervical lordosis was significantly decreased (mean, 9.6 degrees) in the helmet-only setting and significantly increased (mean, 13.6 degrees) in the shoulder pads–only condition. Destabilized specimens under the helmet-only test situation exhibited significant increases in C5–C6 forward angulation (mean, 16.5 degrees), posterior disk space height (mean, 3.8 mm), and dorsal element distraction (mean, 8.3 mm) (Fig 3).

Discussion.—Improper handling of a football player who has a compromised spinal column can lead to significant neurologic injury. These experimental results indicate that immobilization with the helmet only or

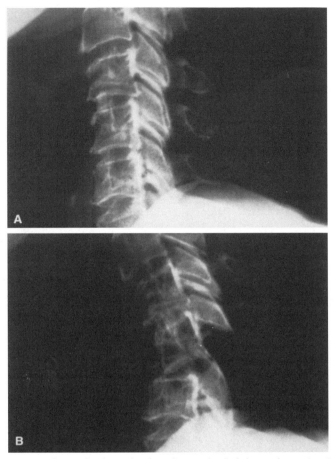

FIGURE 3.—Lateral cervical radiographs of a cadaver under the helmet-only test situation. A, intact condition; B, partially destabilized condition. (Courtesy of Palumbo MA, Hulstyn MJ, Fadale PD, et al: The effect of protective football equipment on alignment of the injured cervical spine: Radiographic analysis in a cadaveric model. *Am J Sports Med* 24:446–453, 1996.)

the shoulder pads only violates the principle of splinting the cervical spine in neutral alignment. With certain exceptions, both protective devices should remain in place during immobilization. The face mask should be removed if rescue breathing must be initiated, and both pads and helmet should be removed when CPR is required.

▶ This study should put an end to any controversy that may still exist regarding emergency removal of football helmets.[1, 2] In emergency situations, the helmet and shoulder pads should be thought of as a single unit if a cervical injury is suspected. Either leave them both in place or remove them both very carefully, with the neck stabilized according to established protocol.[3] Removal may or may not be necessary for CPR.

F.J. George, A.T.C., P.T.

References

1. 1994 Year Book of Sports Medicine, pp 30–32.
2. 1995 Year Book of Sports Medicine, pp 221–222.
3. Feld F: Management of the critically injured football player. *J Athletic Train* 28:206–212, 1993.

Electromyographic Activity of the Cervical Musculature During Dynamic Lateral Bending

Lu WW, Bishop PJ (Univ of Hong Kong; Univ of Waterloo, Ont, Canada)
Spine 21:2443–2449, 1996   3–2

Objective.—The myoelectric activity of selected cervical muscles was studied in 5 young, healthy men during dynamic loading. Although there have been numerous biomechanical investigations of the cervical spine, few studies have focused on the muscular activities of the neck.

Methods.—Study participants ranged in age from 25 to 34 years; none had a history of neck problems. All were tested with the head and neck in the neutral and prebent positions. A light cord from the right side of a helmet ran over a pulley and was connected to a force transducer (Fig 1). Dynamic loads were applied laterally to create peak dynamic loads ranging from about 40 to 100 N. Four pairs of surface electromyographic (EMG) electrodes were applied to each side of the lateral cervical triangle area. Three trials for each loading level and each head position were applied to each participant. Force and EMG data were recorded, and cross-correlations from linear envelope (LE) EMG were calculated.

Results.—Applied loads ranged from 70 to 96 N for the 2-kg mass and from 31 to 52 N for the 0.9-kg mass. There were time delays of 75–165 msec between the peak applied force and the peak electromyogram. In one

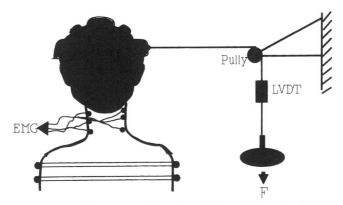

FIGURE 1.—Rear view of test setup with cord attached to pull the subject's head to the right. *Abbreviations: EMG,* electromyography; *LVDT,* Linear Variable Differential Transducer. (Courtesy of Lu WW, Bishop PJ: Electromyographic activity of the cervical musculature during dynamic lateral bending. *Spine* 21:2443–2449, 1996.)

participant, higher EMG activity was recorded from the levator scapulae and splenius group muscles; another showed higher activity from the scalenus group and the trapezius and semispinalis. Overall, muscles on the left side, which functioned as agonists to resist the applied loads, demonstrated higher LE-EMG amplitude than did those in the right side. Within study subjects, the LE-EMG profiles were consistent under the same trial conditions.

Conclusions.—Knowledge of the muscular activity of the neck can help to determine the mechanism of neck injury and to guide injury prevention strategies. In this study of healthy volunteers, EMG profiles and the cross-correlation coefficients for cervical muscles showed highly reproducible intrasubject muscle synergies that were not sensitive to the magnitude of applied load or to the posture of the head before loading. There were variations, however, in intersubject muscle activity patterns.

▶ Few studies have been conducted that have examined the role of the neck muscles in dynamic loading of the head. This study examined the responses of 3 of the major neck muscles to dynamic loading produced by free-falling masses attached to a head collar. As seen in many EMG studies, there was considerable variation in the muscle activity between individuals. As might be expected, the muscle activity was greater on the contralateral side than the side on which the load was dropped. The patterns of muscle activity within each individual did not change much with an increase in external load or with postures of the head, but they were different between individuals. These interindividual variations may explain why, under the same impact conditions, some people may sustain tissue injuries and others may not. These muscles are important in sharing loads on the cervical spine under direct impact or in whiplash conditions; but the lack of consistency in muscle activity reveals little about their individual role in neck injury prevention.

M.J.L. Alexander, Ph.D.

Dynamic Electromyographic Analysis of Trunk Musculature in Professional Golfers

Watkins RG, Uppal GS, Perry J, et al (Kerlan Jobe Orthopaedic Clinic, Los Angeles; Inland Empire Spine Inst, Riverside, Calif; Rancho Los Amigos Hosp, Downey, Calif; et al)

Am J Sports Med 24:535–538, 1996   3–3

Background.—Although back pain among golfers is prevalent, the importance of trunk muscle testing in golfers has not been fully investigated. Which trunk muscles are active during the different phases of the professional golfer's swing was investigated.

Methods and Findings.—Muscle activity was studied in 13 professional male golfers during their swing. Surface electrodes were placed to record the level of muscle activity in the right and left abdominal oblique, right and left gluteus maximus, right and left erector spinae, and upper and lower rectus abdominis muscles. The signals were synchronized electronically with photographic images of the various phases of the golf swing. Images were recorded in slow motion by motion picture photography. Five phases of the swing were identified: take away, forward swing, acceleration, early follow-through, and late follow-through. Although the golfers' swings had individual differences, reproducible patterns of trunk muscle activity were noted throughout all phases of the swing.

Conclusion.—The trunk muscles play an important role in stabilizing and controlling the loading response for maximal power and accuracy in the golfer's swing. These data can be used in the development of a golfers' rehabilitation program that emphasizes trunk muscle strengthening and coordination exercises.

▶ Golf is the fastest growing sport of the 1990s and is played by golfers of all ages and abilities. Golfers do not usually engage in a preplay flexibility and warm-up regimen, thus producing a high rate of injury among golfers who may lack adequate trunk strength, coordination, and flexibility. The key role played by the trunk musculature of a skilled golfer is unquestioned, and this timely examination of trunk muscle activity reinforces its importance in developing speed in the club head.

The abdominal oblique muscles are active in all phases of the swing, as might be expected, as is the erector spinae group; however, their greatest activity occurs during the downswing phase. The gluteus maximus muscles show their greatest activity during the downswing phase, with greater activity in the gluteus maximus on the left side than on the right side during the downswing phase. In the follow-through phase, the trunk is decelerating while trunk muscle activity continues to decrease. One useful application of these results would be to compare them with the trunk muscle activity of less skilled golfers, to examine differences in these patterns, and to relate this muscle activity to the incidence of low back pain in golfers.

M.J.L. Alexander, Ph.D.

The Incidence of Spearing During a High School's 1975 and 1990 Football Seasons
Heck JF (Richard Stockton College, Pomona, NJ)
J Athletic Train 31:31–37, 1996   3–4

Objective.—Spearing and head-first injuries in football can result in spine injury and concussion. Since a rule outlawing spearing was made in 1976, the incidence of these injuries has declined. The incidence of spearing in 2 football seasons, 1 before and 1 after the rule change, were compared.

Methods.—Videotapes of 9 high school football games each season (1975 and 1990) played by a skilled team were reviewed to determine the incidence of all types of spearing. The incidence of spearing and position spearing during the 2 seasons were compared using the independent t test.

Results.—The cumulative incidence of spearing during the 1990 season was 1/2.4 plays and during the 1975 season was 1/2.5 plays. During the 1990 season the incidence of spearing by running backs increased. Running backs had the highest number of spears in both seasons. The incidence of spearing among ball carriers was similar in both seasons. During the 1990 season, tacklers were almost 4 times more likely to spear when the ball carrier speared. The incidence of concurrent tackler spearing increased by 21% during the 1990 season, whereas the incidence of independent tacker spearing decline.

Conclusion.—It does not appear that the rule banning spearing had much impact.

▶ Twenty years ago, in 1976, the National Collegiate Athletic Association and the National Federation of State High School Associations recognized the role of axial loading as the causative factor in catastrophic cervical spine injuries and implemented rules to preclude at-risk playing techniques. A subsequent dramatic reduction in football-incurred quadriplegia has been well documented.[1] These two articles (Abstracts 3–4 and 3–5) that certain members of the coaching community have either not learned, forgotten, or have been in violation of the principle learned from this experience. I trust that we will not have to "invent the wheel all over again" as the article by Lawrence et al. indicates is happening in Louisiana.

J.S. Torg, M.D.

Reference

1. Torg JS, Vegso JJ, O'Neil MJ, et al: The epidemiologic, pathologic, biomechanical, and cinematographic analysis of football-induced cervical spine trauma. *Am J Sports Med* 18:50–57, 1990.

High School Football-related Cervical Spinal Cord Injuries in Louisiana: The Athlete's Perspective

Lawrence DW, Stewart GW, Christy DM, et al (Louisiana State Office of Public Health, New Orleans; Tulane Univ, La)

J La State Med Soc 149:27–31, 1997   3–5

Introduction.—Among organized team sports, football is associated with a high incidence of serious injuries. The rate of cervical spinal cord injuries sustained by high school football players is particularly high in Louisiana. Instead of 1 catastrophic neck injury every 14 years, as would be expected given the national rate of 0.4 per 100,000 players per year, Louisiana has averaged 2.3 per year for the past 7 football seasons. A 1994 survey of 596 Louisiana high school football players assessed their safe tackling knowledge, attitudes, and practices.

Methods.—The players represented 13 public and 3 private high schools in southeastern Louisiana. Questionnaires, which were completed during preparticipation physical examinations, sought data on player demographics, attitudes about the game, behavior during practice and competition, and knowledge of injury prevention. Coaches were contacted to determine if they were showing a training video on proper tackling. The video demonstrates proper technique and emphasizes the risk involved in using the top of the helmet to tackle, block, or strike opponents.

Results.—Respondents had a mean age of 16.2 years. Approximately one-third incorrectly answered "yes" when asked if it was within the rules to tackle by using the top of their helmet (29%) and reported that they had tackled someone in this manner (33%). Although 23% said they had been warned by an official not to tackle with the head down, 28% said they had been taught to use this unsafe method; 83% reported that a coach had trained them in this dangerous and illegal tactic. Many felt that their equipment would prevent potentially paralyzing injuries. All 11 coaches knew of the Louisiana Safe Tackling video, but 5 said they lacked time to show it and 6 thought that it might cause the players to play less aggressively.

Discussion.—Catastrophic football injuries continue to be a problem in Louisiana, 2 decades after national organizations made the deliberate use of the helmet against an opponent illegal. Coaches and team physicians must teach proper tackling technique and its importance for the prevention of catastrophic neck injuries, and football officials must use the spearing penalty as a deterrent to head-first contact. Also recommended are supervised neck muscle strengthening exercises.

Athletes With Cervical Spine Injury
Maroon JC, Bailes JE (Allegheny Gen Hosp, Pittsburgh, Pa; Hahnemann Univ, Pittsburgh, Pa)
Spine 21:2294–2299, 1996   3–6

Background.—Though athletic injuries to the cervical spine are uncommon, they can be different to diagnose and treat. A simple classification system consisting of 3 broad types of injuries was presented to facilitate management decisions.

Classification of Athletic Injuries to the Cervical Spine.—Type I injuries cause permanent damage to the spinal cord. This type of injury includes paralysis, anterior cord syndrome, Brown-Sequard syndrome, central cord syndrome, and mixed incomplete syndrome. Type II injuries are transient after athletic trauma. Spinal concussion, neurapraxia, and burning hands syndrome are examples. Type III injuries consist of radiographic abnormalities only. This type includes congenital spinal stenosis, acquired spinal stenosis, herniated cervical disk, unstable fracture or fracture and dislocation, stable spinal fracture, ligamentous injury, and Spear Tackler's spine.

Management.—Initial management of athletic injuries to the spine consists of cervical immobilization. Patients are withdrawn from sports participation until the exact nature of their injury and degree of risk are established. Athletes with permanent neurologic injury are not allowed to return to competition.

Conclusions.—The classification system described should provide a general framework within which clinicians can make rational decisions about management and return to sports participation. Such injury may be prevented by instruction in proper athletic techniques.

▶ This is basically a review article dealing with cervical spine injuries in the athlete from a neurosurgical perspective. The admission of the authors that "temporary spinal cord dysfunction, including transient quadriplegia, is not completely understood on a pathophysiologic basis" clearly indicates both their lack of experience in dealing with this problem clinically as well as a lack of familiarity with the subject as presented in the orthopedic literature.[1] This fact, of course, can present a patient management problem with those dealing with cervical cord neurapraxia in the field.

J.S. Torg, M.D.

Reference

1. Torg JS, et al: The pathomechanics and pathophysiology of cervical spinal cord injury. *Clin Orthop Rel Res* 321:259–269, 1995.

Experimental Impact Injury to the Cervical Spine: Relating Motion of the Head and the Mechanism of Injury

Nightingale RW, McElhaney JH, Richardson WJ, et al (Duke Univ, Durham, NC)
J Bone Joint Surg 78A:412–421, 1996   3–7

Introduction.—There is a lack of consensus in the orthopedic community of the classifications of injury to the neck. In the past, reviews of radiographs and magnetic resonance images, studies of patient histories, and reconstruction accidents have been the basis for classifying mechanism of injury to the cervical spine. The actual motions of the cervical spine should be known to understand the mechanism of cervical injury rather than just displacements seen on radiographs. The head and neck of a human cadaver were used in an impact model to study the traumatic deformations and forces to the cervical spine. The clinical relevance of the injuries that were produced was also evaluated.

Methods.—With the head and neck in an anatomically neutral position, 11 human cadaver heads were dropped in an inverted posture (Fig 1). Recordings were taken of the forces, moments, and accelerations at 1000 frames per second. At the time of impact, the velocity was 3.2 m/sec.

Results.—The mechanism of injury to the spine did not correspond to the observable motion of the head. After impact, injury occurred at 2.2 to 18.8 milliseconds and before there was a noticeable motion of the head. The local deformations of the cervical spine at the time of the injury described the classification of the mechanism of the injuries. In describing the local mechanism of injury, the classification is a useful tool. Observations were made of buckling of the cervical spine, involving extension

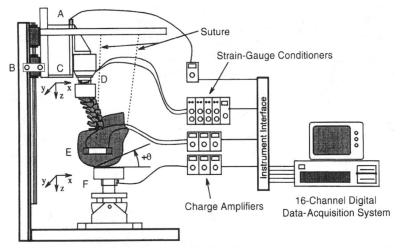

FIGURE 1.—Diagram of the test apparatus, showing the accelerometer on the torso mass (*A*), the optical velocity sensor (*B*), the carriage and torso mass (*C*), the 6-axis load-cell at the first thoracic level (*D*), the accelerometers on the head (*E*), and the impact surface and 3-axis load-cell (*F*). The angle of the impact surface was varied according to the sign convention shown. (Courtesy of Nightingale RW, McElhaney JH, Richardson WJ, et al: Experimental Impact Injury to the Cervical Spine: Relating Motion of the Head and the Mechanism of Injury. *J Bone Joint Surg* 78A:412–421, 1996.

between the third and sixth cervical vertebrae and flexion between the seventh and eighth cervical vertebrae (Fig 5). Deformations are so complex that they can give rise to many mechanisms of injury.

Conclusion.—After a vertical impact of the head, classic concepts of flexion and extension of the head as a mechanism of injury do not apply. The mechanism of injury is not reliably indicated by the motions of the head, which often are used to classify the injury. Concomitant flexion and extension in different regions of the cervical spine may be caused by the complex buckling of the cervical spine. The local mechanism should be the basis for treatment.

▶ The results of this study confirm what we have been saying for 20 years regarding the pathomechanics of athletically incurred cervical spine injury.[1] That is, "biomechanical analysis of those injuries resulting in cervical spine fracture-dislocation has disclosed the previously unrecognized mechanism: non-accidental loading of the straight and cervical spine reacting to maximum axial compressive deformation of a segmented column."

J.S. Torg, M.D.

Reference

1. Torg JS, Truex R Jr, Quedenfeld TC, The National Football Head and Neck Injury Registry. Report and conclusions, 1978. *JAMA* 241:1477–1479, 1979.

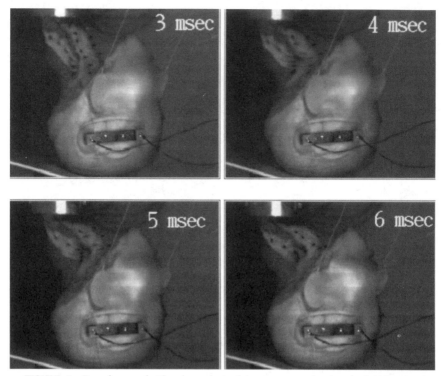

FIGURE 5.—Four frames of video data, obtained 1 msec apart, showing the initial serpentine deformation (at 3 msec) followed by a rapid transition to buckling (at 6 msec). Buckling involved flexion of the seventh and eighth cervical motion segments and extension of the third through sixth cervical motion segments. (Courtesy of Nightingale RW, McElhaney JH, Richardson WJ, et al: Experimental impact injury to the cervical spine: Relating motion of the head and the mechanism of Injury. *J Bone Joint Surg* 78A:412–421, 1996.)

Factors Related to Quadriplegia in Football and the Implications for Intervention Strategies

Bishop PJ (Univ of Waterloo, Ontario, Canada)
Am J Sports Med 24:235–239, 1996   3–8

Background.—Serious cervical spine injuries have long been associated with American football. The biomechanical and epidemiologic factors associated with cervical quadriplegia were reviewed.

Factors Related to Quadriplegia in Football.—The main cause of spinal cord quadriplegia in American football is axial compressive loading. This occurs when a player is struck forcibly on the crown of the helmet, subjecting the small cervical vertebrae to a large compressive force that can produce stress exceeding the failure limit of the spine. Several factors influence the outcome in axial collisions. These include the available kinetic energy, displacement needed to dissipate the energy, and end conditions of a collision.

To develop effective preventive strategies, both biomechanical and epidemiologic findings must be considered. Neck loading needs to be kept at a level less than the failure limit of the cervical spine. Because cervical quadriplegia is rare among football players, however, protective devices intended to reduce the forces on the cervical spine may not markedly decrease the incidence of this injury. In fact, the introduction of new protective equipment may result in the occurrence of other injuries.

Conclusions.—The biomechanical and epidemiologic factors associated with cervical quadriplegia among American football players were reviewed in this article. Such factors must be considered in attempts to design preventive strategies.

▶ This excellent review emphasizes the principle that the occurrence of cervical quadriplegia resulting from football injuries is not a function of equipment. That is, neither the football helmet nor other protective devices cause or will prevent these injuries. Specifically, axial loading, a function of technique, is responsible for cervical spinal injuries resulting in quadriplegia. Thus, as this article concludes, to be considered are modifications of behavior so that crown-first contact with the head was not only discouraged, but eliminated.

J.S. Torg, M.D.

A Retrospective Study of Cervical Spine Injuries in American Rugby, 1970 to 1994

Wetzler MJ, Akpata T, Albert T, et al (American Orthopaedic Rugby Football Assoc, Washington Crossing, Pennsylvania; Rugby Magazine, New York, NY; Thomas Jefferson Univ, Philadelphia; et al)
Am J Sports Med 24:454–458, 1996   3–9

Objective.—As the popularity of rugby increases in the United States, so does the incidence of cervical spine injuries. Results of a retrospective study of the occurrence of cervical spine injuries in U.S. rugby players between 1970 and 1994 were presented.

Methods.—Data from medical reports and the American Orthopaedic Rugby Football Association of 59 cervical spine fractures or significant ligamentous injuries were collected.

Results.—Of the injured players, 30 were junior level, 28 were men's club players, and 1 was a woman. There were 2.36 injuries per year during the study period. Forwards were injured significantly more often than backs. Hookers were injured significantly more often than other players. Most (57) injuries occurred during games; 34 of those occurred during scrimmaging, and 21 of those during the scrum. Most injuries (72%) occurred during tackles outside the scrum; 18 players were injured during tackles, and 7 happened during rucks and mauls. Whereas junior level teams outside the U.S. have a 30% to 40% incidence of cervical spine injuries, U.S. players at the junior level experience a 50.8% incidence. U.S.

players are more prone to injury because they are bigger, stronger, and less experienced than their foreign counterparts. Furthermore, in the United States, rugby is an amateur sport with minimal coaching where players learn the sport while playing it.

Conclusion.—The high cervical spine injury rate, particularly among junior-level rugby players in the United States, argues for rugby law and regulation changes and increased coaching and playing experience that would decrease the incidence of injuries, particularly cervical spine injuries, among the players.

▶ This is an important paper if for no other reason that it is the first study that examines cervical spine injuries in the United States from rugby. It should be noted that these injuries have been recognized as a major problem by physicians in the British Commonwealth nations. Specifically, the incidence of cervical spine injuries, excluding those occurring in the United States, is approximately 3 per 100,000 athletes. A review of the recent literature reveals that, unfortunately, rule changes have not been successful in reducing this number. It is pointed out that "the situation in the U.S. is complicated because many athletes are former football players who have been taught to use their heads as 'weapons' during a tackle and deliver a blow to the ball carrier."

J.S. Torg, M.D.

Cervical Spinal Stenosis With Cord Neurapraxia and Transient Quadriplegia

Torg JS (Hahnemann Univ, Philadelphia)
Sports Med 20:429–434, 1995   3–10

Background.—The syndrome of neurapraxia of the cervical spinal cord with transient quadriplegia occurs as a result of compressive deformation of the spinal cord. Patients have sensory changes, including burning pain, tingling, and numbness, and motor changes ranging from weakness to paralysis. The episodes may be quite brief, with recovery in 10 to 15 minutes, or last for as long as 36 hours. The occurrence of transient quadriplegia in athletes and its relation to further injury is discussed.

Findings.—The literature contains few reports of transient quadriplegia in athletes, yet the prevalence of this problem is relatively high. Several published studies describe the syndrome in football players, some of whom had transient quadriplegia after neck hyperflexion or hyperextension. One player was found to have developmental cervical stenosis. There appears to be no relation between cord neurapraxia and permanent quadriplegia. None of the 117 known quadriplegics in the National Football Head and Neck Injuries Registry had a history of cord neurapraxia, and none of the 45 patients in the transient cohort has become quadriplegic.

Discussion.—With the ratio method for determining the sagittal spinal canal diameter, the standard measurement of the canal is compared with the anteroposterior width of the vertebral body at the midpoint of the corresponding vertebral body. A spinal canal vertebral body ratio of <0.8 at one or more levels has an extremely high sensitivity, supporting the concept of cord neurapraxia resulting from the transient, reversible compression deformation of the spinal cord. Athletes with uncomplicated developmental narrowing of the cervical canal do not have a predisposition for permanent neurologic injury. Continued participation in contact activities is contraindicated, however, for those who have had an episode of cervical cord neurapraxia associated with ligamentous instability, intervertebral disk disease with cord compression, significant degenerative changes, magnetic resonance imaging evidence of cord defects or swelling, neurologic symptoms of >36 hours' duration, or when there is more than 1 recurrence of the neurapraxia.

The Relationship of Developmental Narrowing of the Cervical Spinal Canal to Reversible and Irreversible Injury of the Cervical Spinal Cord in Football Players
Torg JS, Naranja RJ Jr, Pavlov H, et al (Hahnemann Univ, Philadelphia; Univ of Pennsylvania, Philadelphia; Hosp for Special Surgery, New York City)
J Bone Joint Surg Am 78A:1308–1314, 1996   3–11

Introduction.—Developmental narrowing of the cervical spinal canal is a consistent finding in athletes who have experienced an episode of neurapraxia of the cervical spinal cord with transient quadriplegia. This syndrome is associated with sensory or motor changes or both, that usually resolve in 10 to 15 minutes. An epidemiologic study was conducted to determine whether a relationship exists between a developmentally narrowed cervical canal and reversible and irreversible injury of the cervical cord.

Methods.—Study subjects were 4 groups of football players and a control group of 105 nonathletes. The 5 cohorts included: 227 asymptomatic college football players with no known history of transient neurapraxia of the cervical spinal cord (cohort I); 97 professional football players who were asymptomatic and had no known history of transient neurapraxia of the cervical cord (cohort II); 45 high school, college, and professional football players who had experienced at least 1 episode of transient neurapraxia of the cervical spinal cord (cohort III); 77 former athletes who were permanently quadriplegic after a football injury in high school or college (cohort IV); and 109 men aged 15 to 38 who had been evaluated for neck symptoms (cohort V).

For each cohort, the mean and standard deviation of the diameter of the spinal canal, the diameter of the vertebral body, and the ratio of the diameter of the spinal canal to that of the vertebral body were determined for the third through sixth cervical levels. The criterion for developmental narrowing is a ratio of the diameter of the spinal canal to that of the vertebral body of 0.80 or less. Thus, the sensitivity, specificity, and positive

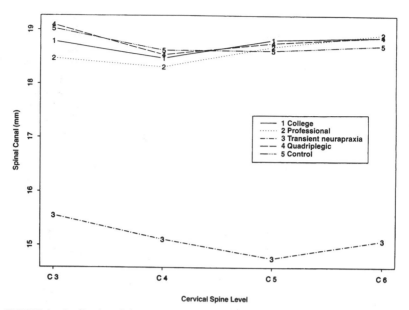

FIGURE 1.—Profile plot of the mean diameters of the spinal canal, demonstrating a significantly smaller value in cohort III compared with that in all of the other cohorts (P <0.05). With the numbers available, no significant difference was found among cohorts I, II, IV, or V. (Courtesy of Torg JS, Naranja RJ Jr, Pavlov H, et al: The relationship of developmental narrowing of the cervical spinal canal to reversible and irreversible injury of the cervical spinal cord in football players. *J Bone Joint Surg Am* 78A:1308–1314, 1996.)

predictive value of this ratio in relation to transient neurapraxia was evaluated. Participants in cohorts III and IV were surveyed to determine the relationship between transient neurapraxia and permanent neurologic injury.

Results.—The cohorts differed in mean diameter of the spinal canal, mean diameter of the vertebral body, and the mean ratio of these diameters. Cohort III had a significantly smaller mean diameter of the cervical spinal canal and mean ratio than the other 4 cohorts (Fig 1). None of the 77 former football players who were quadriplegic reported an episode of transient quadriplegia before the major injury, and none of the 45 athletes who had symptoms of transient quadriplegia had a subsequent injury that led to a permanent neurological deficit. A ratio of ≤0.80 or less had a high sensitivity (93%) for transient neurapraxia, but a low positive predictive value (0.2%).

Conclusion.—Most individuals who have had an episode of transient neurapraxia of the cervical cord have a spinal canal and vertebral body ratio ≤0.80 at 1 or more levels of the cervical spine. Among those with a stable spine, however, developmental narrowing of the cervical canal does not appear to predispose to permanent, catastrophic neurologic injury. Such a finding should not prevent an athlete from participation in contact sports.

▶ The data presented clearly indicate that developmental narrowing of the cervical canal without associated instability does not predispose an individual to permanent neurologic injury and therefore should not preclude an athlete from participation in contact sports.

J.S. Torg, M.D.

Pathogenesis of Sports-related Spondylolisthesis in Adolescents: Radiographic and Magnetic Resonance Imaging Study
Ikata T, Miyake R, Katoh S, et al (Univ of Tokushima, Japan)
Am J Sports Med 24:94–96, 1996   3–12

Introduction.—To clarify the pathogenesis of spondylolisthesis in individuals with this condition, 165 young athletes were studied; 77 with spondylolysis and spondylolisthesis (the slip group) were compared with 88 with spondylolysis only (the nonslip group). Although various factors are thought to be involved, there is no clear evidence on what causes slippage to develop.

Methods.—Those in the slip group were aged 9 to 18 years and were seen at a sports clinic from 1987 through 1993. Spondylolisthesis was defined as a vertebral slippage of more than 5%. Radiographic studies showed pars defects ranging from early stage (ill-circumscribed radiolucent defects) to the terminal stage (a wide defect with reactive sclerosis and hypertrophy). Results of MRI studies were classified as grade 0 (normal), grade I (concave, irregularity, or thinning), or grade 2 (separation, detaching, or both). Disk degeneration was graded as normal, mild, moderate, or marked. Findings in the slip group were compared with those of similar studies in the age-matched nonslip group.

Results.—End-plate lesions at the lower surface of L5, the upper surface of S1, or both were seen on T1-weighted MRI scans of 68% of the nonslip group and 100% of the slip group. All patients in the slip group, but only 2% of the nonslip group, had a grade 2 lesion. In the slip group, end plate lesions showed characteristic changes of slippage between the cartilaginous and osseous end plates. Five different types of slippage were identified according to the location of end plate lesions. Most common was a partial slip of L5 or S1 (40%). Disk degeneration was apparent in 51% of the slip group but in only 19% of the nonslip group. Twenty-two of 51 patients who were followed up radiographically for more than 1 year showed an average slippage development of 9.8%. The development and progression of slippage occurred most often in patients whose skeletal age was in the cartilaginous stage. Wedging of the L5 vertebral body and rounding of the sacrum progressed as slippage developed.

Conclusions.—Because no slippage was associated with the early stage of a pars interarticularis defect, the advanced stage of this defect in an immature spine is a risk factor for spondylolisthesis. The L5 wedging and

S1 rounding alterations are considered sequelae of end plate lesions, rather than the cause of spondylolisthesis.

▶ This is an interesting study detailing the deformities that occur in the lumbosacral spine in youngsters with spondylolisthesis. However, the presumption that a pars defect, that is, spondylolysis, results in a mechanical weakness in the neural arch and necessarily leads to spondylolysis is incorrect. As the article points out, the results show that the more mature spine has a lower risk of slippage development or progression. I believe that the presence of a pars defect without elongation in adolescents does not constitute a contraindication to participation in vigorous physical activity.

J.S. Torg, M.D.

Cervical and Lumbar MRI in Asymptomatic Older Male Lifelong Athletes: Frequency of Degenerative Findings
Healy JF, Healy BB, Wong WHM, et al (Univ of California, San Diego)
J Comput Assist Tomogr 20:107–112, 1996   3–13

Objective.—To determine the incidence of asymptomatic abnormalities seen in cervical and lumbar spine imaging.

Background.—The cervical and lumbar spine are among the first areas to show evidence of degenerative joint disease on imaging studies. On MRI scans of the aging spine, various abnormalities can be seen that produce no symptoms. These abnormalities may confuse the evaluation of spinal symptoms.

Methods.—MRI of the spine was performed in 19 male athletes between 41 and 69 years old who were highly active. Subjects were asymptomatic and at their normal athletic activity. Spine, athletic, and sports injury histories were taken.

Results.—The incidence of asymptomatic degenerative findings on MRI scans was similar to that seen in other populations. Degenerative changes included disk protrusion and herniation, spondylosis, and spinal stenosis. The incidence of these changes increased with older age. The most dramatic-appearing cervical disk protrusion was seen in a 45-year-old triathlete. This subject had excellent strength and flexibility, but reported experiencing a mildly stiff neck after riding a bicycle more than 80 miles or hang-gliding more than 3 hours. He had raced more than 700,000 miles with his head in extreme extension. In these subjects, all imaging findings were asymptomatic and did not interfere with athletic activity.

Discussion.—The findings seen in this study group were similar to those seen in other populations. These subjects are asymptomatic and very active. MRI findings must be evaluated with a clinical history and results of a physical examination. MRI of the spine can show many abnormalities that do not produce signs or symptoms. These findings may be given undeserved importance by personal injury litigators, worker's compensation authorities, and others.

▶ Although this study did not involve a detailed analysis of the significance of cervical MRI changes, the observations presented support our position that cervical spondylolysis in the younger athlete need not necessarily be an absolute contraindication to participation in collision activities. Clearly, a detailed study of the significance of degenerative changes in the older male athlete would be most helpful and informative.

J.S. Torg, M.D.

Time-dependent Changes in the Lumbar Spine's Resistance to Bending
Adams MA, Dolan P (Univ of Bristol, England)
Clin Biomech 11:194–200, 1996   3–14

Introduction.—Frequent bending and lifting are associated with low back pain, and such movement is the highest known risk factor for acute disk prolapse. A cadaveric study was conducted to determine how bending moment is affected by the speed of movement and by repeated and sustained loading.

Methods.—Thirty-one lumbar spines were collected at routine necropsy from individuals ranging in age from 19 to 87 years. None had a history of spinal injury or prolonged bed rest. The spines were dissected into motion segments consisting of 2 vertebrae and the intervening disk and ligaments. Motion segments were subjected to compressive and bending loads on a hydraulic materials testing machine. The effect of loading rate on resistance to bending was evaluated in 25 specimens. Also examined were the effects of repeated flexion movements on a motion segment's resistance to bending (8 specimens), the effects of sustained flexion (12 specimens), and the effect of sustained compressive loading on a motion segment's resistance to bending (20 specimens).

Results.—Compared with slow movements, rapid flexion movements increased the peak bending moment by 10% to 15%. Repeated flexion during a period of 5 minutes reduced the peak bending moment by an average of 17%. The average reduction in peak bending moment by 5 minutes of sustained flexion was 42%. Repeated flexion led to a small and steady fall, whereas sustained flexion caused a large and rapid fall (Fig 3). Results of 2 hours of compressive creep loading included a 1.1-mm reduction in height of the intervertebral disks, a 12% increase in the range of flexion, and a 41% reduction in peak bending moment.

Discussion.—When applied to movements and postures in living people, the scale of the changes observed in this experimental study suggests that the risk of bending injury to the lumbar disks and ligaments depends on the loading rate and loading history, as well as on the loads applied to the spine. Reduced resistance to bending after creep loading increases with age, probably because old disks creep faster.

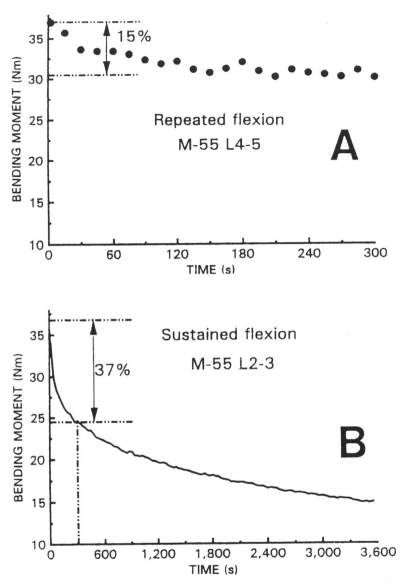

FIGURE 3.—**A**, repeated flexion movements reduced this specimen's resistance to bending by 15% over 300 seconds. *Circles* indicate the peak bending moment in every fifth loading cycle. **B**, sustained bending has a much larger effect on the bending moment. After 1 hour, the specimen appears to be approaching equilibrium. (Courtesy of Adams MA, Dolan P: Time-dependent changes in the lumbar spine's resistance to bending. *Clin Biomech* 11:194–200, copyright 1996, with kind permission from Elsevier Science Ltd., The Boulevard, Langford Lane, Kidlington 0X5 1GB, UK)

▶ This study is an excellent attempt to relate the authors' work with cadaveric vertebral specimens to the stresses on the spine during daily activities. Their studies suggest that the risk of back injury increases as the speed of movement increases, as the compressive forces on the disk are higher because of muscle contraction. Also, repetitive lifting may lead to muscle fatigue, which may produce fatigue damage to the annulus layers of the disk. Activities such as gardening may cause the spine to undergo viscoelastic creep, and this prolonged stretching of the ligaments and disks may be responsible for the backache associated with prolonged stooping. The study suggests that patients with back pain need to consider the size of a load being lifted, but also the speed of lifting, the number of repetitions, and the length of time in the forward flexed position.

M.J.L. Alexander, Ph.D.

Role of Muscles in Lumbar Spine Stability in Maximum Extension Efforts
Gardner-Morse M, Stokes IAF, Laible JP (Univ of Vermont, Burlington)
J Orthop Res 13:802–808, 1995   3–15

Objective.—The lumbar spine can withstand in vivo compression loads that exceed 2,600 N, approximately 30 times the force leading to instability during in vitro measurements. Stabilization is thought to come from activated muscles that behave like force generators and springs. Results of a study investigating whether muscle stiffness alone is adequate to stabilize the spine in response to small perturbations were presented.

Methods.—Distribution of muscle force was determined by linear programming with equilibrium and physiologic constraints and used to calculate the maximum extension effort, muscle forces, and motion segment. These values were then used to perform an eigenvalue buckling analysis of spinal stability using a lumbar spinal model (Fig 1). Axial muscle stiffness k_m (Newton-meters) was calculated using the formula $k_m = q(T/l_m)$, where T is the active muscle force determined by muscle force distribution calculations, l_m is the muscle length in millimeters, and q is a multiplier assumed to be the same for all muscles.

Results.—Eigenvalues (buckling load multipliers) greater than 1 indicated stability. Spinal stability increased nonlinearly as active muscle stiffness parameter q increased. Below a critical q value, the spine became unstable. A flexed and extended spine was metastable. Muscle stiffness values were less sensitive to changes in posture than to changes in spinal stiffness, indicating that degenerative changes that reduced stiffness also increased instability. Small perturbations could cause the spine to buckle without active muscle stiffness, demonstrating that the muscles had to act like springs in addition to behaving as force generators. For stability, q had to be greater than 3.7.

Conclusion.—Changes in spinal equilibrium, spinal stiffness, or muscle stiffness can result in spinal instability and lead to self-injury.

▶ Modeling the lumbar spine is difficult because of the complex motion of the segments and the differing stiffness characteristics of the spinal structures. This model determined the importance of the lumbar spine muscula-

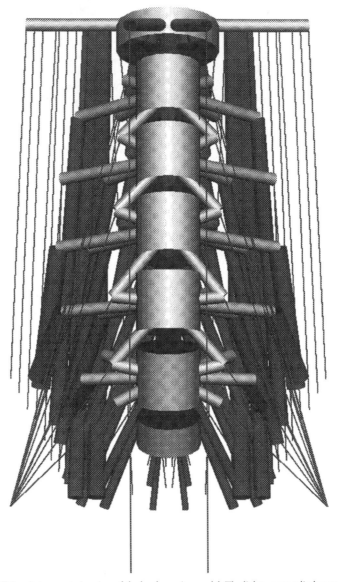

FIGURE 1.—Anteroposterior view of the lumbar spine model. The lighter gray cylinders represent the lumbar vertebrae, with rigid connections supporting muscle attachments. The thorax is a rigid body to which all thoracic muscles attach. The position of S1 is indicated by a simple cylinder. The rest of the sacrum and the pelvis (which were fixed) are not shown. Active muscles (activity corresponding to the maximum, extension effort) are shown as *cylinders* with diameters proportional to their physiologic cross-sectional areas, and inactive muscles are shown as *thin lines*. (Courtesy of Gardner-Morse M, Stokes IAF, Laible JP: Role of muscles in lumbar spine stability in maximum extension efforts. *J Orthop Res* 13:802–808, 1995).

ture in stabilizing the spine when maximally activated but not to the point at which spine buckling would occur. The important role of feedback from muscles and resulting changes in length and stiffness are critical in maintaining trunk stability and spinal control. Poor muscular control or altered vertebral segment stiffness could produce spinal instability and lower back injury. This study emphasized the importance of inherent muscle stiffness in stabilizing the lumbar spine and noted that alterations in this stiffness could lead to damage in the lower back.

M.J.L. Alexander, Ph.D.

Spine and Spinal Cord Injuries in Downhill Skiers
Prall JA, Winston KR, Brennan R (Univ of Colorado, Denver; Provenant St Anthony Central Hosp, Denver)
J Trauma: Injury Infect Crit Care 39:1115–1118, 1995   3–16

Objective.—Spine and spinal cord injuries (S/SCIs) are the most serious injuries had by skiers and often result in lifetime costs of $500,000 or more. To improve the effectiveness of triage of injured skiers and increase awareness of clinicians for S/SCIs in skiers, the incidence, patterns, and injuries associated with S/SCIs were described.

Methods.—Between 1982 and 1993, of 636 consecutive injured skiers, 126 (53 men), aged 13 to 75 years, with S/SCIs were treated at a level I trauma center in Denver, Colo. Demographic data, injury scoring, associated injuries, level and severity of S/SCIs, and duration of hospital care were recorded and statistically compared with similar patients with other types of skiing injuries.

Results.—Sixty-nine patients had 1 fracture and 38 had 2 or more fractures. There were 18 patients with SCIs; 11 were complete. There were significantly more cervical- than thoracic- or lumbar-associated SCIs. Spinal fractures most commonly occurred at C6, T12, and L1. The most common type of fracture was compression (38%). Almost one-third of these patients also had head and thoracic, abdominal, and extremity injuries. SCIs were caused by falls in 60% of patients and by collisions in 30%. Cervical injuries generally resulted from collisions with other skiers, whereas thoracolumbar injuries were more likely to result from running into a stationary object. Patients with thoracolumbar injuries were significantly more likely than patients with cervical injuries to have injuries to the torso or extremities. Patients were treated with 32 spinal fusions and received 12 halo traction vests.

Conclusion.—Most SCIs in skiers result from falls. Most cervical spine injuries result from collisions with other skiers. The incidence of SCI in this study was 17%.

▶ In evaluating these data it is important to differentiate between those of the 126 skiers with spine injury as opposed to those with concomitant cord injury. In the latter group there were 20, 11 of whom had permanent lesions and are appropriately described as being "most chronically debilitating." Noteworthy is the fact that it was observed that speed was a preeminent factor in virtually all these accidents and invariably resulted from skier-skier collision.

J.S. Torg, M.D.

Strength, Mobility, Their Changes, and Pain Reduction in Active Functional Restoration for Chronic Low Back Disorders

Taimela S, Härkäpää K (DBC Internatl, Vantaa, Finland; Rehabilitation Found, Helsinki)
J Spinal Disord 9:306–312, 1996   3–17

Objective.—Whereas acute low back pain improves with most treatments, chronic low back pain improvement is modest for most patients, with no treatment being any better than another. Studies have found that patients' psychological symptoms and personal pain control abilities were significantly related to treatment outcome and early retirement. Results of a study analyzing associations between muscular strength and mobility parameters and their changes, and pain reduction were presented.

Methods.—Functional restoration was studied in 143 patients (55 men) with chronic back pain ($n = 46$) or chronic back and neck pain ($n = 97$) who participated in a 12-week multidisciplinary treatment program. Trunk muscle strength and low back mobility were measured at the beginning and end of the study. Sociodemographic variables, health history, and pain history were assessed in a questionnaire.

Results.—Low back pain decreased in 79% of patients and increased or did not change in 21% after the study. Mobility and muscle strength increased in more than 75% of patients. Pain reduction was significantly correlated with changes in both strength and mobility. Patients with reduced back pain and those whose pain was not reduced had similar strength and mobility measurements. Strength and mobility increases were not significantly associated with decreases in pain. Low back pain intensity and duration at baseline and pain reduction were significantly associated. Pain was more likely to decrease in patients who had more pain. Pain regularity and pain reduction were not correlated.

Conclusion.—Pain in patients with low back pain decreased significantly as muscle function and mobility increased. The magnitude of pain reduction was not related to the magnitude of improvement of muscle function and spinal mobility.

▶ Most patients with low back pain will experience some improvements in pain and mobility over time, regardless of the treatment modality. This group of patients attended a 12-week back treatment program that included classes in strength, mobility, and back care. Pain reduction was monitored throughout the treatment program. The findings were interesting in that they found no significant relationship between increases in strength and mobility and decreases in pain. Although there was a reduction of pain in the majority of patients, the improvement in function was not related to the amount of pain decrease. Clinicians should expect that changes in strength and mobility will not always be accompanied by significant changes in low back pain.

M.J.L. Alexander, Ph.D.

Influence of Saddle Type Upon the Incidence of Lower Back Pain in Equestrian Riders
Quinn S, Bird S (Canterbury Christ Church College, UK)
Br J Sports Med 30:140–144, 1996   3–18

Introduction.—Equestrian sports have a high rate of injury, and most injuries result from falls or kicks. Even more common, however, are overuse injuries including lower back pain produced by compressive forces transmitted through the rider's vertebral column during riding. A questionnaire completed by 108 equestrian riders was designed to investigate the potential influence of saddle type on the incidence of lower back pain.

Methods.—Saddle types were categorized into 2 broad classes: the traditional or classic English type and the deep-seated saddle. Within the former category are dressage, general-purpose, jumping, and hunting saddles; the latter includes the Western and long-distance riding saddles. The deep-seated saddle provides the rider with maximum comfort and security during long periods of riding and allows a more upright position to be assumed. A traditional saddle is thought to be more likely to result in lower back pain. Riders eligible to complete the questionnaire were older than age 18 and had been riding for at least 3 years. Sixty-five used the traditional, general-purpose saddle and 43 used the deep-seated Western saddle.

Results.—Lower back pain was reported by 48% of riders, but the incidence was significantly higher in the general purpose saddle group (66%) than in the Western saddle group (23%). This difference was also marked when men and women riders were analyzed separately. Women had a higher incidence of lower back pain than men regardless of saddle type. Neither the age of the rider nor the number of hours spent riding each week appeared to be related to the incidence of lower back pain. In the general-purpose saddle group, however, those who had been riding for more than 15 years had a higher incidence of lower back pain than those who had been riding for shorter periods.

Discussion.—Low back pain is commonly reported by equestrian riders, especially by women and by riders who have used a general-purpose saddle for more than 15 years. The deep-seated, Western style saddle, although not suited to all equestrian activities, provides better support and is far less likely to cause lower back pain than the general-purpose, English style saddle.

▶ The authors have successfully demonstrated a high incidence of low back pain among equestrian riders and demonstrate an association with the use of the general-purpose saddle. Unfortunately, no attempt was made to identify the pathologic diagnosis. That is, was the pain caused by degenerative disk disease, facet arthritis, spondylolysis, muscle strain, and so forth?

J.S. Torg, M.D.

Spinal Manipulation for Low Back Pain: An Updated Systematic Review of Randomized Clinical Trials
Koes BW, Assendelft WJJ, van der Heijden GJMG, et al (Vrije Universiteit Amsterdam, The Netherlands; Maastricht Univ, Limburg The Netherlands)
Spine 21:2860–2873, 1996   3–19

Introduction.—Guidelines of the Agency for Health Care Policy and Research (United States) and the Clinical Standard Advisory Group (United Kingdom) support the use of manipulation for low back pain. A computer-aided search was conducted to evaluate literature on manipulation for low back pain and to determine whether the new guidelines are supported with results from sound randomized clinical trials (RCTs).

Methods.—A MEDLINE search was conducted for the years 1966–1995. Reports were assessed and given scores based on: quality of methods, study population, interventions, measurement of effect, data presentation and analysis, conclusion of authors regarding spinal manipulation, and results based on the main outcome measure.

Results.—Thirty-six RTCs met inclusion criteria. Of a possible score of 100 points, the highest score for a trial was 60 points. Most trials were of poor quality. Nineteen trials (53%) indicated favorable results for spinal manipulation. Five additional trials (14%) reported positive results in 1 or more subgroups only. Of 5 trials with a score of 50–60 points, 3 were positive and 2 were positive only for a subgroup of patients. Inconsistent results were observed for 11 trials that compared manipulation with placebo therapy. There was no definite relationship between the methodologic score and overall outcome. Of 12 trials evaluating only patients with acute low back pain, 5 reported positive results, 4 reported negative results, and 3 reported positive results in a subgroup. Of 8 trials comparing manipulation with other conservative treatment modalities for patients with subacute or chronic low back pain, 5 reported positive results, 2 reported negative results, and no conclusion was reported in 1. Of 16 trials reporting an effect measurement of at least 3 months, 6 reported positive effects of manipulation.

Conclusion.—Evidence for efficacy of manipulation in patients with acute low back pain was not convincingly demonstrated with sound RCTs. Manipulation may be effective in some subgroups of patients with acute or chronic low back pain.

Clinical Significance.—Findings of an updated systematic review of RCTs support additional research efforts on manipulation for low back pain. Hopefully high-quality methodology will be a priority for future investigations.

▶ I agree with the conclusion of the authors that "...the efficacy of manipulation for patients with acute low back pain has not been convincingly demonstrated with sound randomized clinical trials." Also, the efficacy of manipulation has not been established for chronic conditions. However, spinal manipulation is a modality somewhat unfamiliar to most physicians and probably lies more within the realms of the "art of medicine." The subjective nature of the therapeutic response is such that "a methodologic quality may be difficult to obtain." Note that the authors do conclude that there certainly are indications that manipulation might be effective in some groups of patients with low back pain.

J.S. Torg, M.D.

Can Variations in Intervertebral Disc Height Affect the Mechanical Function of the Disc?
Lu YM, Hutton WC, Gharpuray VM (Clemson Univ, South Carolina; Emory Univ, Atlanta, Ga)
Spine 21:2208–2217, 1996   3–20

Background.—Disk height varies among individuals and with different disk levels, abnormal conditions and clinical treatments. The effect of disk height on the mechanical behavior of a human lumbar spine segment was examined.

Methods.—A 3-dimensional finite element model of L2–L3 disk body unit was used in the parametric studies. Disks of 8 mm, 10 mm, and 12 mm heights were investigated, with disk cross-sectional area, finite element mesh density, and all other parameters kept constant.

Findings.—Disk height variations significantly affected axial displacement, the posterolateral disk bulge, and the tensile strength in the peripheral anulus fibers. However, such variation only minimally affected intradical pressure and the longitudinal stress distribution at the endplate–vertebra interface (Fig 8).

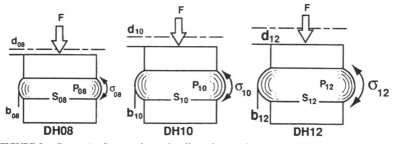

FIGURE 8.—Composite diagram shows the effect of an axial compressive force (F) on axial displacement (d), disk bulge (b), intradiskal pressure (p), longitudinal stress at the inferior end-plate–vertebra interface (S), and tensile stress on the peripheral anulus fibers (s). The magnitude of each parameter for the 3 models is indicated schematically by the size of the letter used (i.e., $d_{08} < d_{10} < d_{12}$; $b_{08} < b_{10} < b_{12}$; $P_{08} \sim P_{10} \sim P_{12}$; $S_{08} \sim S_{10} \sim S_{12}$; $\sigma_{08} < \sigma_{10} < \sigma_{12}$). (Courtesy of Lu YM, Hutton WC, Gharpuray VM: Can variations in intervertebral disk height affect the mechanical function of the Disk? *Spine* 21:2208–2217, 1996.)

Conclusion.—Axial displacement, posterolateral disk bulge, and tensile stress in the peripheral anulus fibers are a function of axial compressive force and disk height. Variations in disk height may compromise the conclusions of experimental and analytic studies that do not consider geometric parameters.

▶ Intervertebral disks have large variations in both disk height and disk cross-sectional area, and these variations may cause differences in response to applied stresses. Because it is difficult to measure these stresses in vivo, the use of finite element models has become a useful technique for evaluating the effects of different types of mechanical stress on structures such as the disk. The finite element model includes all of the mechanical characteristics of the structures that comprise the disk, including the cartilaginous end plates and the layers of the annulus fibrosus.

Generally, it was found that greater disk height was associated with greater deformation of the disk under compressive stress, producing greater impingement of the disk on structures close by. Disks with a higher height-to-area ratio generated higher values of axial displacement, disk bulge, and tensile stress on the annulus fibers. The study suggests that under compression, thinner disks may impinge less on associated structures than thicker disks; however, these are structural differences that cannot be controlled. Under the same compressive force, greater disk bulging and greater impingement on the nerve roots may occur in a disk with greater disk height, suggesting that some lower back pain syndromes are related to disk height.

M.J.L. Alexander, Ph.D.

Validation of Two 3-D Segment Models to Calculate the Net Reaction Forces and Moments at the L_5/S_1 Joint in Lifting

Plamondon A, Gagnon M, Desjardins P (Université Laurentienne, Sudbury, Ont, Canada; Université de Montréal)
Clin Biomech 11:101–110, 1996   3–21

Introduction.—The tasks involved in manual materials handling (MMH) are a major hazard to industrial workers. Various 3-dimensional (3-D) dynamic biomechanical models are designed to estimate stresses from MMH tasks. Two 3-D segment models (free-body diagram models) were evaluated for their validity and sensitivity in estimating the net reaction forces and moments at the L_5/S_1 joint. Because most validation studies have been done on 2-D models, there is little information on 3-D linked-segment models.

Methods.—Two dynamic 3-D multisegment models applied to lifting materials were evaluated: a lower body model and an upper body model. Three healthy young men (mean age, 28 years) took part in the study. Participants had a mean mass of 69 kg and a mean height of 1.74 m. The task performed under experimental conditions consisted of lifting a load of

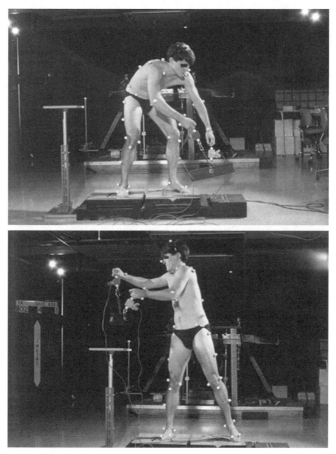

FIGURE 1.—Illustration of the task. (Courtesy of Plamondon A, Gagnon M, Desjardins P: Validation of two 3-D segment models to calculate the net reaction forces and moments at the L_5/S_1 joint in lifting. *Clin Biomech* 11:101–110. Copyright 1996, with kind permission from Elsevier Science Ltd, The Boulevard, Langford Lane, Kidlington OX5 1GB, UK.)

9.6 kg from a low shelf (0.05 m) on the participant's left, turning 180 degrees, and placing the load on a high shelf (0.8 m) to his right (Fig 1). Two speeds of lifting were employed: normal and fast. The mode of lifting was not standardized. Results from the 2 models were compared in terms of joint reaction forces and joint reaction moments at L_5/S_1.

Results.—Comparisons between the lower body model and the upper body model at normal speed yielded very similar curves. Correlations for the data from both models were generally above 0.95. The root mean square (RMS) differences, which varied between 10 and 15 N for the forces with a maximum difference of 59 N, were generally larger in the fast speed condition. The sensitivity analysis yielded similar trends. Errors in the segment accelerations accounted for a proportion of the error, the result of an increase in the RMS differences between models with an increase in lifting speed. The lower body model was thought to have some advantages over the upper body model in this task, which did not require large accelerations from the lower part of the body.

Conclusions.—Correlations between the reaction moments from both the upper body model and the lower body model were generally above 0.95, and RMS differences were generally below 10 Nm (although they could reach 38 Nm). Sensitivity analysis of the models demonstrated similar trends. With the upper body model, hand transducers are recommended to accurately measure characteristics of the load. It is important that trunk anthropometric data be as precise as possible.

▶ There is considerable interest in the field of biomechanics in modeling the lower back, because of the increasing number of injuries to this vulnerable area. Most models attempt to calculate the joint reaction forces and moments at the L_5/S_1 junction, which is the site of a large majority of lower back lesions. Injuries to the lower back often occur because of lifting motions, or a combination of lifting and twisting the trunk. In this study, a lifting task was modeled that consisted of twisting and lifting a load of 9.6 kg, which is well below the maximal lifting load tolerance of 50 kg suggested by the National Institute for Occupational Safety and Health (NIOSH). Two models were examined—one using the segments of the lower body and one using the segments of the upper body—and the forces and moments of each model were compared. The force and torque output of the lower body model was found to be the smoothest and likely the most representative of the task, possibly because of the lower rate of acceleration of the lower body. This paper suggests that upper body models of spinal movements may be subject to some inaccuracy because of the higher accelerations of the upper body segments relative to those of the fixed lower body.

M.J.L. Alexander, Ph.D.

Pulmonary Barotrauma: Diagnosis in American Football Players: Three Cases in Three Years
Levy AS, Bassett F, Lintner S, et al (Duke Univ, Durham, NC)
Am J Sports Med 24:227–229, 1996   3–22

Background.—Many reports have discussed various types of injuries caused by blunt trauma in football players. However, few have looked at pulmonary and thoracic injuries related to this sport. For several reasons, it may be difficult to recognize a small pneumothorax in an athlete. Three cases of pneumothorax occurred in football players.

Case Report 1.—A receiver, 21, was hit in the left axilla by an opponent's helmet. His initial difficulty in breathing resolved within 5 minutes, but he did not return to play. He was resting comfortably after the game, but the next day he complained of trouble catching his breath when climbing stairs. The day after that, a chest radiograph showed 70% pneumothorax without rib fracture. The patient was treated with a chest tube in the emergency department. He returned to play 2 weeks later, with his ribs taped and covered with a flak jacket.

Case Report 2.—A fullback, 22, landed on his left side, on the football, after being tackled. He felt better within a few minutes, but he had increased pain on deep breathing when he was asked to run on the sideline. A radiograph taken in the training room showed 40% pneumothorax with no rib fracture. Again, the patient was treated by chest tube and returned to play 2 weeks later with his ribs protected.

Case Report 3.—A tight end, 22, was tackled on his right side after a pass reception. He returned to play, but complained of being unable to slow his breathing. Although the initial radiograph showed no abnormalities, a repeat radiograph obtained 15 minutes later showed 5% to 10% apical pneumothorax. He was admitted to the hospital, where he was found to have a 20% pneumothorax. Treatment consisted of tube thoracostomy for 4 days. Return to activity was as in the first 2 cases.

Discussion.—These 3 cases of pneumothorax in football players appear to be related to barotrauma, probably occurring when the player is hit at full inspiration with a closed glottis. This diagnosis may be difficult to make in athletes participating in contact sports—sore ribs and temporary windedness are common, well-conditioned athletes probably require a larger ventilatory loss to have dyspnea at rest, and the noise on the field may make it impossible to auscultate the lungs. Winded football players should be required to run on the sidelines before they are allowed to return to play. The return to activity should be gradual and with rib protection when play is resumed.

▶ This report of 3 cases of pneumothorax from football emphasizes how an athlete may be able to tolerate a large unilateral pneumothorax—up to 40% or even 70%—with relatively little breathlessness, at least at rest. Given the noise of the crowd, sideline diagnosis can be difficult; the authors advise a "sideline-running test" before allowing back in the game a player who has been "winded." Despite the need for chest-tube therapy, these football players were back in the game in 2 weeks, with ribs taped and wearing flak jackets. None had rib fractures; the proposed mechanism for pneumothorax here is forced expiration against a closed glottis. Another recent report notes that, even while the athlete is wearing a rib vest protector, rib fracture with pneumothorax can occur during football.[1]

E.R. Eichner, M.D.

Reference

1. Cvengros RD, Lazor JA: Pneumothorax—A medical emergency. *J Athl Training* 31:167–168, 1996.

108 / Sports Medicine

Assessing Acute Abdominal Pain: A Team Physician's Challenge

Bergman RT (Lansing, Mich)
Physician Sportsmed 24:72–76, 81–82, 1996   3–23

Background.—When an athlete reports abdominal pain, the physician must make an evaluation and a working diagnosis, then decide whether the patient may return to training and competition (Fig 1). A review was presented to aid physicians in this decision-making process.

Valuable Historical Information.—Abdominal pain can indicate either serious or minor conditions. In evaluating athletes with such pain, physicians should remember that athletes often tolerate pain better than nonathletes, seeking medical attention later than is typical. History-taking should include a record of mode of onset, progression, character, and severity of pain; the activity during which pain was first noticed; the initial location of the pain and any change in its location; associated symptoms and their temporal relationship to the abdominal pain; factors that aggravate the pain; menstrual history and reproductive status; medications and

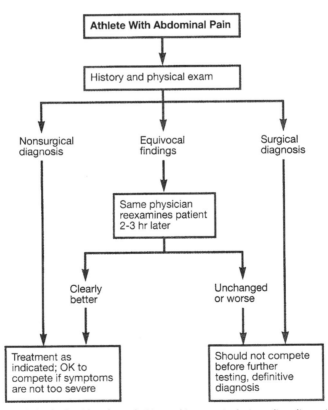

FIGURE 1.—A simple algorithm shows decision-making steps in the immediate diagnosis of abdominal pain. (Courtesy of Bergman RT: Assessing acute abdominal pain. *Physician Sportsmed* 24:72–76, 81–82, copyright 1996, reproduced with the permission of McGraw-Hill, Inc.)

supplements used; and previous episodes, family history of similar problems, peers with similar symptoms, food intolerance, allergies, sudden changes in training or diet, and travel to regions with endemic disease.

Physical Examination.—Physicians should first explain to the patient what the examination will involve, then begin with auscultation, starting in the area farthest from the site of the worst pain. If pain caused by a certain maneuver increases with voluntary guarding, the source of pain is the abdominal wall. The source is visceral if guarding decreases it. If the patient seems to overreact to palpation, the physician should ask questions and have the patient answer during palpation. The patient will stop talking while guarding if the pain is as severe as it seems. Finally, gross tests for rebound tenderness should be avoided; light percussion provides just as much information.

Conclusion.—Diagnosing abdominal pain is challenging, especially for team physicians with restricted access to ancillary tests and specialists. Typically, pain caused by a serious condition arises suddenly; is continuous, progressively worse, and long lasting; begins during inactivity; and is not near the umbilicus.

▶ This article can perhaps best serve as an outline and quick check for the team physician faced with an athlete with acute abdominal pain. It lists nearly 40 causes of such pain and covers telltale clinical features of 7 common causes, together with practical tips on how to examine the abdomen. It also gives general advice on how to proceed after the initial workup and whether a given patient needs further testing or can continue to train or compete. Traumatic splenic rupture was covered last year;[1] splenic rupture in infectious mononucleosis is covered this year (abstract 8–33). Recent articles remind us that acute abdominal pain evoked by exercise can occasionally stem from constipation or adhesions.[2, 3]

E.R. Eichner, M.D.

References

1. 1996 YEAR BOOK OF SPORTS MEDICINE, pp 302–305.
2. Anderson CR: A runner's recurrent abdominal pain: One simple solution. *Physician Sportsmed* 20:81–83, 1992.
3. Lauder TD, Moses FM: Recurrent abdominal pain from abdominal adhesions in an endurance triathlete. *Med Sci Sports Exerc* 27:623–625, 1995.

Comparison of Prediction Models for the Compression Force on the Lumbosacral Disc
Kee D, Chung MK (Keimyung Univ, Taegu, Korea; Univ of Science and Technology, Pohang, Korea)
Ergonomics 39:1419–1429, 1996   3–24

Introduction.—One of the most frequently performed tasks in industrial sites and real-life situations are manual materials handling tasks, such as

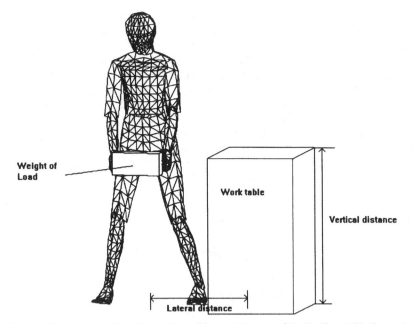

FIGURE 1.—Representation of 3 experimental factors. (Courtesy of Kee D, Chung MK: Comparison of prediction models for the compression force on the lumbosacral disc. *Ergonomics* 39:1419–1429, 1996, Taylor & Francis, publishers.)

lifting, lowering, holding, carrying, pushing, or pulling. These tasks are regarded as the primary source of low back pain and overexertion, and 1 of 4 industrial overexertion injuries are attributed to 1 of these tasks. These tasks should be designed ergonomically and safely. The effect of vertical distance, lateral distance, and weight of load during asymmetric lifting on the L5–S1 compressive forces that are computed from 3 representative prediction models was examined.

Methods.—The prediction models were linear programming–based models, a double linear programming–based model, and electromyographic (EMG)-assisted models. The relationships between the compressive forces obtained from these 3 models were examined along with the 1991 National Institute for Occupational Safety and Health (NIOSH) lifting indices computed for varying asymmetric lifting conditions. The design included 2 volunteers who performed 36 task conditions with vertical distance, lateral distance, and weight of load used as experimental factors (Fig 1). Electromyographic signals from 6 trunk muscles were measured to calculate the L5/S1 compressive forces (Fig 2). The Motion Analysis System was used to record postural data and locations of load.

Results.—All 3 factors were reflected well with the EMG-assisted model. Only weight of load was reflected in the 2 linear programming–based models. From the EMG-assisted model, low lifting index values were observed for relatively high L5–S1 compressive forces, which suggested

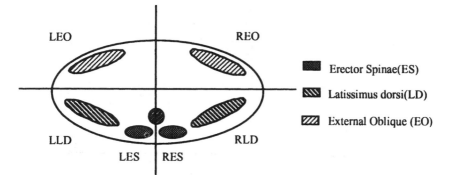

FIGURE 2.—Cross-sectional view of the 6 trunk muscles at the L5–S1 disk. (Courtesy of Kee D, Chung MK: Comparison of prediction models for the compression force on the lumbosacral disc. *Ergonomics* 39:1419–1429, 1996, Taylor & Francis, publishers.)

that the 1991 NIOSH lifting equations may not fully evaluate the risk of dynamic asymmetric lifting tasks.

Conclusion.—The varying conditions of asymmetric lifting tasks were more properly reflecting by the EMG-assisted model in comparison with the linear programming–based models.

▶ Three models that predict compressive forces on the L5–S1 disk of the lumbar spine were examined during an asymmetric lifting task. Two of the models simply calculated muscle forces based on the loads lifted and the position of the loads, whereas the third model used EMG force estimates to determine muscle force magnitudes. It was concluded that the EMG-assisted model better represented the coactivation of muscles that occurred during the lifting task; as well, it more accurately portrayed the forces during a dynamic lift. This paper suggests that forces on the lower back during lifting tasks estimated by computer models may be underestimated because of the lack of consideration of antagonist contraction. Design of lifting tasks must allow for underestimates from static computer models.

M.J.L. Alexander, Ph.D.

Hip Joint Forces During Load Carrying
Bergmann G, Graichen F, Rohlmann A, et al (Free Univ of Berlin)
Clin Orthop 335:190–201, 1997   3–25

Introduction.—Biological factors and mechanical loads affect the course of diseases and other conditions like proximal femur fractures, coxarthrosis, Perthes' disease, and unstable hip implants. Patients with hip disorders on 1 side ask on which side they should carry loads; however, no in vivo data are available. Using a simplified static model, the effects of the load magnitude and the carrying method on the hip joint forces were calculated (Fig 1).

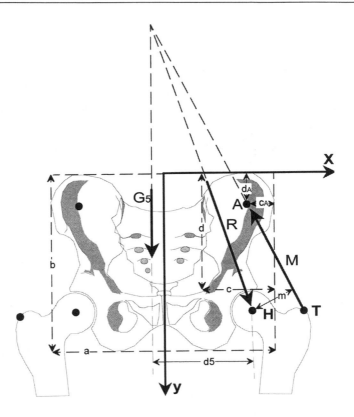

Becken3   30.11.94

FIGURE 1.—Forces and sizes of the hip. Static model in the frontal plane. *H* is the center of the femoral head of the supporting leg. *G5* is the weight of the body minus the stance leg. *M* is the force in the abductor muscles. *M* has to counterbalance *G5*. Because of its shorter lever arm, *M* is much bigger than *G5*. The hip joint force *R*, the sum of *G5* and *M*, is higher than *M*. In anteroposterior radiographs, the hip has the sizes *a* and *b*. The idealized origin point *A* of the abductor muscles at the iliac bone (c_a, d_a) was chosen after Debrunner, and the insertion point *T* at the greater trochanter was chosen after Pauwels. For patients without a radiograph, the *x* position and *y* position of the points *H, A,* and *T* were taken from average data. (Courtesy of Bergmann G, Graichen F, Rohlmann A, et al: Hip joint forces during load carrying. *Clin Orthop* 335:190–201, 1997.)

Methods.—The gait data of 6 volunteers were used to observe the maximum forces during slow walking. The spatial hip joint force could be measured with 1 patient who had 2 instrument hip implants. To check the validity of the calculated results, the forces obtained by both methods for the same steps were compared. To prove that load carrying with abducted arm, as when using a large basket for shopping, may have an additional influence on the hip joint forces, additional force calculations and measurements were performed.

Results.—For the patient who had instrument endoprostheses implanted in both hips, the measured values were slightly higher than the calculated 1; however, overall results were similar. At the ipsilateral hip joint, the force is kept constant or is even slightly lowered by carrying a load on 1 side. On the opposite side, there is a large increase in force. In the contralateral joint, there are two-thirds higher forces when carrying 25% of body weight with 1 hand when compared with the loaded side. Both hip joint forces increase by 25% if this load is evenly distributed between the 2 sides. Additional relief of the ipsilateral joint can be achieved in unilateral load carrying if the upper body is held upright and the load carrying arm is abducted, such as when using a large shopping basket.

Conclusion.—Increased forces at the affected hip joint should be avoided in patients with proximal femur fractures, coxarthrosis, and some other unilateral diseases. Heavy loads should be avoided; however, if this is not possible, the load should be carried on the side to be relieved, and the arm should be held as far away from the body as possible by using a large basket for shipping and by keeping the upper body upright.

▶ Hip joint diseases are very common in the aging population, as well as in individuals of all ages with arthritis. Hip joint reaction forces increase depending on the magnitude of the loads, and the location of the load relative to the affected hip. Patients with unilateral hip disorders often want to know on which side they should carry loads to minimize forces on the hip. A mathematical model was developed to calculate maximal hip joint forces in various load carrying situations, and with the load in either or both hands. Because of the increase in moment arms when the load is carried on the ipsilateral side, the forces on the contralateral side increase in proportion to the increased torque. Individuals with hip joint pathologic conditions should carry the load on the affected side with the arm abducted as far as is comfortable, because this decreases the moment arm for the weight and for the load. However, this will increase the forces on the nonaffected hip, which may eventually lead to problems on this joint. Use of a backpack or carrying the load evenly distributed between both hands may avoid problems caused by unilateral carrying.

M.J.L. Alexander, Ph.D.

A New Pelvic Tilt Detection Device: Roentgenographic Validation and Application to Assessment of Hip Motion in Professional Ice Hockey Players

Tyler T, Zook L, Brittis D, et al (Lenox Hill Hosp, New York; Long Island Univ, Brooklyn, NY; New York Med College, Valhalla)
J Orthop Sports Phys Ther 24:303–308, 1996   3–26

Background.—Playing ice hockey has been hypothesized to shorten the iliopsoas muscles and increase the likelihood of lumbosacral strains and hip injuries. Whether ice hockey players show decreased hip extension range of motion compared with age-matched controls was studied.

Methods.—The Thomas test was used with an electric circuit device to determine pelvic tilt motion. Six subjects were radiographed during the Thomas test to validate the device. Testing of 25 professional hockey players and 25 age-matched controls was then performed. The effect of sport and side were determined with a 2-way analysis of variance.

Results.—Compared to age-matched controls, the ice hockey players showed a reduced mean hip extension range of motion ($p < 0.0001$). No difference was found between right and left side and sport did not interact with side of the body. Decreased extensibility of the iliopsoas muscle in ice hockey players was thus demonstrated.

Discussion.—Specific features of the skating motion that favor shortening of the iliopsoas were identified. Ice hockey players must flex both the knee and hip to compensate for the anterior shift of the center of gravity caused by the skates; the stiffness of the skate does not allow plantar flexion. Stretching the iliopsoas is difficult when wearing skates, and players often sit on the bench in a hip-flexed position. Hip flexor muscles are also important in backward skating. Hip extensibility may be lost by requirement of action through a limited range of motion. Shortening of the iliopsoas muscles with an increase in lumbar lordosis may result. A hockey player's general conditioning should include a specific program of stretching directed at the anterior soft tissues of the hip.

▶ This study indicates that an iliopsoas flexibility and stretching program should be a part of the conditioning and warm-up programs of ice hockey athletes. The authors conjecture, "whether or not a tight iliopsoas predisposes the hockey player to low back pathology." There have been numerous anecdotal reports of low back pain in preseason hockey camps.

F.J. George, A.T.C., P.T.

Nontraumatic Hip Pain in Active Children: A Critical Differential
Gerberg LF, Micheli LJ (Albert Einstein College of Medicine, Bronx, NY; Harvard Med School, Cambridge, Mass)
Physician Sportsmed 24:69–74, 1996   3–27

Background.—When evaluating an active young person seeking care for hip pain, clinicians should consider the many possible nontraumatic entities with similar symptoms, as well as injury. The patient described below, found to have Legg-Calvé-Perthes (LCP) disease, illustrates the importance of a thorough examination and referral when needed.

> *Case Report.*—Boy, 8 years, with a 6-month history of intermittent pain in the left hip was brought for medical care. The boy was a Little League baseball player and reported that the pain was initially most noticeable during baseball practice. He had no history of acute trauma or illness. When crutches and activity restriction were ineffective, the patient was referred to an orthopedics

sports medicine clinic. Physical assessment was notable only for an antalgic limp, marked discomfort on palpation over the entire left hip region, and significant pain on internal rotation and hip abduction. The hip was also found to have a reduced range of motion in abduction, internal rotation, and flexion compared with the contralateral hip.

A full laboratory workup yielded no abnormalities.

Plain radiographs showed a "moth-eaten" radiolucency suggesting osteopenia of the femoral epiphysis and neck. The femoral epiphysis was observed to be shortened. On a bone scan, there was evidence of avascularity of the left femoral epiphysis, consistent with a diagnosis of LCP disease. Treatment with a Petrie cast with the hip in 30-degree abduction and 30-degree internal rotation resulted in containment of the femoral epiphysis in the acetabulum. After 2 weeks in the cast, the boy was free of pain. At 6 weeks, the cast was removed and physical therapy was begun. Nine months after the initial diagnosis, the patient was asymptomatic. Eventually, he resumed sports participation with no difficulty.

Conclusion.—There are many nontraumatic causes of hip pain such as slipped capital femoral epiphysis, septic arthritis, transient synovitis, juvenile rheumatoid arthritis, and bone tumor. In this patient with LCP disease, radiographs and bone scans were useful for documenting and staging the disease and for assessing treatment efficacy. The treatment of choice for LCP is generally nonoperative containment of the femoral epiphysis with a cast or orthosis, although the aggressiveness of treatment depends on disease stage.

▶ This is a useful, practical clinical article for the physician seeing a child with a limp and hip pain. Although trauma must be ruled out, nontraumatic cases of hip pain are also common in children. The cause here—avascular necrosis of the femoral head—is covered in detail. Other common nontraumatic "mimics" are outlined, including slipped capital femoral epiphysis (the most common nontraumatic hip problem in adolescents, calling for immediate non–weight-bearing treatment), septic arthritis (fever is a clue), transient synovitis, rheumatoid arthritis, and tumors. Stress fracture of the femoral neck (in an adult runner) was covered in the 1994 YEAR BOOK.[1]

E.R. Eichner, M.D.

Reference

1. 1994 YEAR BOOK OF SPORTS MEDICINE, pp 97–98.

Labral Lesions: An Elusive Source of Hip Pain. Case Reports and Literature Review

Byrd JWT (Vanderbilt Univ, Nashville, Tenn)
Arthroscopy 12:603–612, 1996   3–28

Introduction.—The labrum is the fibrocartilaginous rim that lines the circumference of the acetabulum (Fig 4). Labral lesions can be a significant source of disabling hip pain. Cause of injury can be major trauma, twisting injuries, and degenerative changes. Diagnosis is difficult because tearing can be undectable on radiographs. Described is the use of arthroscopy in the diagnosis and treatment of 3 patients with labral lesions of the hip.

> *Case Report 1.*—A 35-year-old man had a 14-year history of intermittent pain, catching, and giving way of the right hip after a motorcycle accident. A painful pop within the hip joint could be elicited by flexion combined with rotational motion. Radiographs and CT scan were normal. An extensive complex tearing of the anterior half of the labrum that was displaced into the weight-bearing portion of the joint was viewed on arthroscopy. He had prompt resolution of symptoms after arthroscopic debridement.
>
> *Case Report 2.*—A 26-year-old man was seen 6 weeks after a hyperextension injury of the left hip after rebounding a basketball. He was unable to bear weight and had a painful click in the hip. Radiographs and MRI were normal. A painful click could be elicited with active rotational motion. Arthroscopy showed the lateral labrum to be hypermobile with a hemorrhagic partial sep-

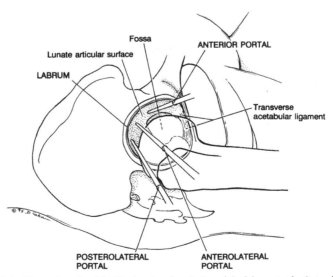

FIGURE 4.—Illustration of a right hip showing the relation of the labrum to the 3 standard portals used in hip arthroscopy. (Courtesy of Byrd JWT: Labral lesions: an elusive source of hip pain. Case reports and literature review. *Arthroscopy* 12:603–612, 1996.)

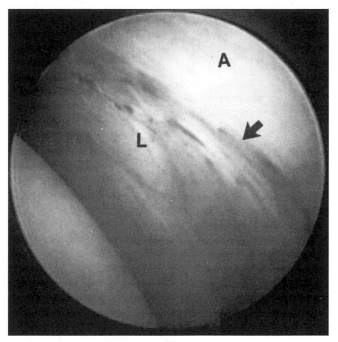

FIGURE 2.—A 26-year-old man with 6-week history of painful clicking in the left hip after an extension injury. Arthroscopic view of the left hip from the anterior portal, viewing laterally. The labrum (*L*) is hemorrhagic and partially separated (*arrow*) from its bony attachment to the lateral acetabulum (*A*). (Courtesy of Byrd JWT: Labral lesions: an elusive source of hip pain. Case reports and literature review. *Arthroscopy* 12:603–612, 1996.)

aration from its bony attachment to the acetabulum (Fig 2). Acute entrapment of the labrum was relieved and symptoms subsided.

Case Report 3.—A 68-year-old man had a 5-month history of intractable mechanical right hip pain after a lengthy car trip. He had a long-standing history of problems with degenerative disk disease. Physical examination showed modest limitation of motion in both hips and radiographs showed osteoarthritis of both hips that was slightly more advanced in the right hip. Arthroscopy showed a large displaced degenerative tear of the labrum posteriorly. The area was debrided and most symptoms subsided for about 15 months. He underwent total hip arthroplasty after symptoms returned.

Conclusion.—Arthroscopic debridement of labral tears can provide significant improvement in select patients. There are many variations in the arthroscopic anatomy of the acetabular labrum. Careful clinical evaluation and diagnostic exclusion are important tools for this elusive problem.

▶ This article calls attention to and documents labral lesions as a contributing source of mechanical hip pain. Interestingly, it concludes that labral tearing can be readily assessed and in many instances successfully treated by arthroscopy. However, it lacks a satisfactory description of arthroscopic technique and does not present data with regard to a long-term follow-up.

J.S. Torg, M.D.

The Superiority of Magnetic Resonance Imaging in Differentiating the Cause of Hip Pain in Endurance Athletes

Shin AY, Morin WD, Gorman JD, et al (Naval Med Ctr, San Diego, Calif; Midelfort Clinic, Eau Claire, Wis; Naval Hosp, Portsmouth, Va)
Am J Sports Med 24:168–176, 1996   3–29

Background.—The consequences of a missed or untreated femoral neck stress fracture can be catastrophic in young, active patients. The diagnostic accuracy of MRI in the assessment of hip pain in military endurance athletes was studied.

Methods.—Nineteen soldiers undergoing endurance training were included. All had hip pain, negative radiographic results, and radionuclide bone scans consistent with femoral neck stress fracture. Bone scan findings were positive for femoral neck stress fracture in 22 hips. MRI was performed in each patient, along with 6-week follow-up plain radiography.

Findings.—On MRI, femoral neck stress fractures were differentiated from a synovial pit, iliopsoas muscle tear, iliopsoas tendinitis, obturator externus tendinitis, avascular necrosis of the femoral head, and a unicameral bone cyst. The diagnosis of stress fracture was confirmed on the follow-up radiographs, which showed healing callus in patients with stress fractures. No changes were observed on the follow-up radiographs of patients with diagnoses other than stress fractures. The accuracy of MRI in determining the cause of hip pain was 100%. By contrast, radionuclide bone scan had an accuracy of 68% for femoral neck stress fractures, with a 32% false-positive rate.

Conclusions.—MRI should be the primary diagnostic modality used to assess endurance athletes with hip pain. It is superior to radionuclide bone scan in differentiating femoral neck stress fractures from other causes of hip pain.

▶ As the authors have pointed out, soft tissue inflammation, synovitis, neoplasm, infections, and stress fracture may all produce positive bone scan results. Thus, considering the potential morbidity that a missed and untreated femoral neck stress fracture presents, the finding that MRI has a 100% diagnostic accuracy is an important observation. I agree with the authors' recommendation that "MRI in this specific patient population be used as a primary diagnostic modality."

J.S. Torg, M.D.

Surgical Management of Refractory Trochanteric Bursitis
Slawski DP, Howard RF (USAF Med Ctr, Scott Air Force Base, Ill)
Am J Sports Med 25:86–89, 1997   3–30

Background.—The most common symptom of trochanteric bursitis is pain in the greater trochanter region radiating down the thigh or buttocks. The majority of these patients respond to nonsteroidal antiinflammatory medication, iliotibial band stretching, ice and warm packs, ultrasound, and local anesthetic/corticosteroid injections. Patients who do not respond to this treatment regimen are treated with a variety of surgeries. One surgeon's experience with the surgical management of refractory trochanteric bursitis was reviewed.

Study Group.—The study group consisted of 4 women with 6 affected hips and 1 man with 1 affected hip. The average age of the participants was 40.3 years. Each participant had pain in the greater trochanter region without a snapping or popping sensation. All patients had undergone the standard conservative treatment regimen for at least 1 year without improvement. The patients were limited by hip pain in all activities. The average preoperative Harris hip score was 51.7 of 100. Preoperative radiographs and technetium-99m scintigraphs were all normal.

> *Surgical Technique.*—The iliotibial band was longitudinally divided over the greater trochanter. There was spontaneous retraction of the fascial edges, resulting in 2 to 4 cm of separation. Deep retractors further retracted the iliotibial band edges to expose the trochanteric bursa, which was excised with needle-tip electrocautery. The iliotibial band gap was not repaired, but the rest of the wound was closed in layers. The average operative time was 30 minutes, and the average blood loss was 28 mL. Full weightbearing was initiated immediately. Range of motion and strengthening were initiated as tolerated under supervision. Return to full activity was encouraged.

Results.—Four patients with 6 affected hips were available at an average of 20 months' follow-up. The average Harris hip score had increased to 95.0. All patients were satisfied with the results of surgery and had returned to unrestricted athletic activities.

Conclusions.—For those patients with trochanteric bursitis that is refractive to conservative treatment, surgical treatment with longitudinal release of the iliotibial band and bursectomy appears to be a safe and effective treatment.

▶ The authors emphasize that nonoperative treatment results in successful clinical outcome in the great majority of patients with trochanteric bursitis. Thus, the importance of patient selection is apparent. The necessity in differentiating between primary greater trochanteric bursitis and the so-called "snapping hip" should be pointed out. The latter may be caused by several poorly defined conditions, one of which is painful snapping of the iliotibial band over the greater trochanter. For this condition, Zoltan et al.[1] described a procedure in which an ellipsoid excision of the iliotibial band over the trochanter and a subgluteal bursectomy is performed.

J.S. Torg, M.D.

Reference

1. Zoltan DJ, Clancy WG Jr, Keene JS: A new operative approach to snapping hip and refractory trochanteric bursitis in athletes. *Am J Sports Med* 14:201–204, 1986.

Stress Fracture of the Pubic Ramus in Female Recruits
Hill PF, Chatterji S, Chambers D, et al (Cambridge Military Hosp, Aldershot, England)
J Bone Joint Surg Br 78B:383–386, 1996   3–31

Background.—Stress injuries in normal bone subjected to repeated cyclic loading are well-documented complications of military training. The occurrence of stress fractures of the pubic ramus in one group of female recruits was reported.

Methods and Findings.—Twelve stress fractures of the inferior pubic ramus occurred in 11 military recruits during basic training in a 4-month period (Fig 2). Eleven of these fractures occurred in women. This was attributed to the introduction of mixed-sex training, in which women had to increase their stride length to march with men. The presenting symptom was chronic groin pain that did not settle with rest. Clinical diagnoses were confirmed by radiographic assessment in all but 1 patient, who underwent ^{99m}Tc bone scanning. No new cases of stress fracture of the pelvis have been reported since the required stride length among military recruits was reduced.

Conclusions.—This cluster of pelvic stress fractures, occurring almost exclusively in women, was found to be caused by the practice of mixed-sex training, which forces female recruits to march with longer strides. The diagnosis of this injury was delayed partly because recruits were penalized for missing training, which discouraged them from taking the time to seek medical attention.

▶ It is important to note that stress fractures of the pubic ramus may be responsible for prolonged symptoms and disability. However, with activity modification, they all eventually heal.

J.S. Torg, M.D.

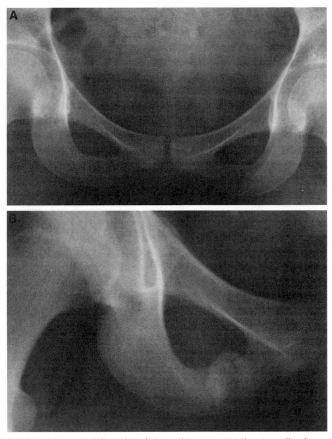

FIGURE 2.—Stress fracture of the right inferior pubic ramus (A) showing callus formation 6 weeks after presentation (B). (Courtesy of Hill PF, Chatterji S, Chambers D, et al: Stress fracture of the pubic ramus in female recruits. *J Bone Joint Surg Br* 78B:383–386, 1996.)

4 Leg

Plyometric Training in Female Athletes: Decreased Impact Forces and Increased Hamstring Torques
Hewett TE, Stroupe AL, Nance TA, et al (Deaconess Hosp, Cincinnati, Ohio)
Am J Sports Med 24:765–773, 1996   4–1

Introduction.—Jump-training programs have been designed to address the higher incidence of serious knee injuries in female athletes in jumping sports, compared to male athletes. The effects of a jump-training program on the mechanics of landing and the strength of lower extremity musculature were evaluated in female athletes involved in jumping sports.

Methods.—Eleven female high school volleyball players and 9 male athletes were matched by height, weight, and age. Female research subjects were compared to male research subjects before and after a training program. Testing included vertical jump height and muscle strength testing. Female athletes underwent 6 weeks of a training program that included jumping and landing techniques and jumping for increased vertical height and increased strength. Participants stretched immediately before jumping and after weight training. Two-hour training sessions were held 3 times weekly.

Results.—Landing forces were decreased 22% after training. Knee adduction and abduction moments decreased by about 50% (Fig 5). These moments were significant predictors of peak landing forces. There was no change in peak landing flexion and extension moments or knee flexion angles. After training, female athletes had lower landing forces and lower adduction and abduction moments, compared to male athletes. There was a 26% and 13% increase in hamstring-to-quadriceps muscle peak torque ratios on the nondominant and dominant sides, respectively. After training, there was a 44% and 21% increase in hamstring muscle power on the dominant and nondominant sides, respectively. The peak torque ratios were significantly higher in male athletes and untrained athletes. After training, these ratios were similar in males and females. Trained females had about a 10% increase in mean vertical jump height.

Conclusion.—Female athletes had a marked imbalance between hamstring and quadriceps muscle strength before undergoing a 6-week training program. These athletes experienced a considerable increase in hamstring muscle peak torque and power after the training program.

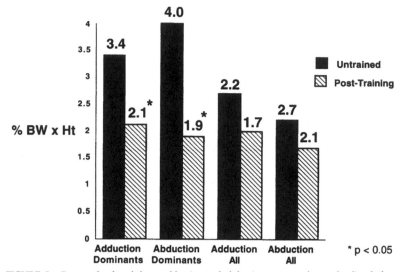

FIGURE 5.—Bar graph of peak knee adduction and abduction moment data at landing before and after training. The female subjects were grouped according to the dominant moment (adduction or abduction) and all the female subjects grouped together (all). (Courtesy of Hewett TE, Stoupe AL, Nance TA: Plyometric training in female athletes: Decreased impact forces and increased hamstring torques. *Am J Sports Med* 24:765–773, 1996.)

▶ If one of the factors underlying the increased risk of anterior cruciate ligament injuries in female athletes is an imbalance between hamstring and quadriceps muscle strength, it is encouraging to know that a relatively short training program can bring the hamstring-to-quadriceps ratio up to that of the male athletes. Although the training program in this study was rather time-consuming and was designed specifically for volleyball players; it could be made more general and more efficient for athletes in other sports.

B.L. Drinkwater, Ph.D.

Hamstring Muscle Injuries Among Water Skiers: Functional Outcome and Prevention
Sallay PI, Friedman RL, Coogan PG, et al (Duke Univ, Durham, NC)
Am J Sports Med 24:130–136, 1996   4–2

Objective.—Hamstring muscle tears are common in water skiers. Results of a study to define the mechanisms of injury, describe the associated pathologic changes, determine the functional limitations, and suggest measures for prevention are presented.

Methods.—Between 1987 and 1993, 12 patients (4 women), aged 18 to 51, with partial or total avulsion of the muscle at or near the ischial tuberosity insertion were examined by an orthopedic surgeon and interviewed about the exact mechanism of injury, recovery, activity limitations, and residual pain. Five patients had an MRI scan and 1 had a CT scan.

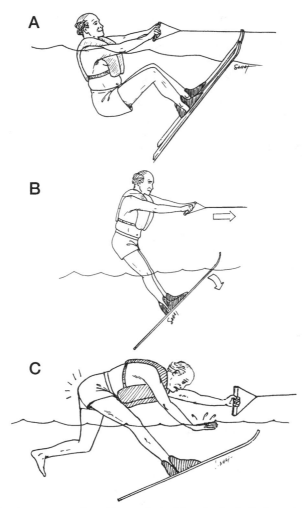

FIGURE 1.—**A**, proper crouch position at the begining of takeoff. **B**, the novice skier tends to straighten the knees prematurely, causing the ski tips to submerge. **C**, the continued forward momentum pulls the skier forward causing extreme flexion at the hip. (Courtesy of Sallay PI, Friedman RL, Coogan PG, et al: Hamstring muscle injuries among water skiers: Functional outcome and prevention. *Am J Sports Med* 24:130–136, 1996).

Results.—Six patients were novice skiers and 6 were experienced. The mechanism of injury was improper body position during takeoff that resulted in forced, severe hip flexion (Fig 1). MRI and CT scans demonstrated 5 complete avulsions and 1 partial tear. Convalescence averaged 7 weeks before patients were able to walk without a limp. It took 3 months to 1.5 years before patients were able to return to vigorous activities. Seven patients returned to their previous sports but at reduced activity levels. Five patients with complete disruptions had pain or cramping when participating in sports requiring running. Isokinetic results in 2 of these patients demonstrated average concentric hamstring and quadriceps muscle deficits of 61% and 23%, respectively, when compared with the contralateral leg. Two patients underwent delayed surgical repair; 1 had an excellent result and 1 had a poor result.

Conclusion.—Proximal avulsion of the hamstring muscle is common in water skiers and results from failure to maintain the proper crouch position during takeoff. Complete recovery is lengthy. Five of 12 patients were unable to return to preinjury activity levels. Two patients needed surgical repair. Surgical repair at the acute stage is recommended for these injuries to avoid problems with chronic scarring, atrophy, and retraction.

▶ This article clearly demonstrates that hamstring muscle injuries resulting from water skiing are an entirely different entity than those commonly seen in relation to other activities. The proximal avulsion of the muscle complex from the ischium results in prolonged convalescence with nonoperative treatment with the patient unable to return to preinjury level of activity. Although the authors currently repair complete hamstring muscle avulsions during the acute phase in those individuals who wish to continue being physically active, the results of such surgery are not given.

J.S. Torg, M.D.

The Piriformis Syndrome

Parziale JR, Hudgins TH, Fishman LM (Brown Univ, Providence, RI; Northwestern Univ, Chicago; Albert Einstein College of Medicine, New York)
Am J Orthop 25:819–823, 1996   4–3

Introduction.—Because the piriformis syndrome results in sciatic pain, a positive Lasègue sign, and tenderness at the sciatic notch, it can be misdiagnosed as sciatica or low back pain. The piriformis muscle passes through the sciatic notch along with the gluteal and sciatic nerves and the gluteal vessels. Four of the 6 possible anatomical variations of the sciatic nerve/piriformis muscle relationship have been confirmed.

Medical History and Symptoms.—Symptoms included buttock pain with or without radiation to the leg and pain exacerbated by activity or prolonged sitting particularly on hard surfaces, bowel movements, and intercourse for women.

The physical examination may reveal buttock tenderness, a spindle-shaped mass on pelvic or rectal examination, a positive Freiberg sign, and "Morton's foot."

Diagnostic Testing.—Computed tomography, MR imaging, and electromyography have been used for differential diagnosis. Compression of the sciatic nerve by an aneurysm, a fibrotic band, or hematoma must be ruled out, as must a herniated disk, spinal stenosis, posterior facet syndrome, pelvic tumor, or endometriosis.

Treatment.—Conservative treatment usually is satisfactory. Leg-length discrepancy can be corrected by using a heel lift; inflammation can be treated with nonsteroidal anti-inflammatory drugs, analgesics, and muscle relaxants. Physical therapy includes ultrasound treatments, stretching with internal rotation, hip adduction and flexion, pressure applied in the plane of the muscle, hip adductor strengthening exercises, coolant sprays, transrectal massage, and transcutaneous electric stimulation. More aggressive therapy requires local injections of anesthetic and corticosteroids. As a last resort, surgical release of the piriformis muscle can be performed.

Conclusion.—Piriformis syndrome is difficult to diagnose. Knowledge of the symptoms and techniques of differential diagnosis can improve the recognition and treatment of this cause of low back pain and sciatica.

▶ In the commentary to this article, H.S. Ahn, M.D., states, "The piriformis syndrome is somewhat controversial in that its diagnosis and treatment have not been well defined in the literature." The authors have presented a good review of the diagnosis and treatment of this syndrome. Runners who suffer from this syndrome should avoid running on "crowned" roads and be diligent with the prescribed flexibility exercises.

A simple diagnostic maneuver of having the patient lie on the unaffected side, hip flexed, knee resting on the table, and then contracting the piriformis by lifting and holding the knee several inches from the table was described by Beatty and commented on in the 1995 YEAR BOOK OF SPORTS MEDICINE.[1]

F.J. George, A.T.C., P.T.

Reference

1. 1995 YEAR BOOK OF SPORTS MEDICINE, pp 173–175.

Holmium:YAG Laser–Induced Aseptic Bone Necroses of the Femoral Condyle
Fink B, Schneider T, Braunstein S, et al (Heinrich Heine Univ of Düsseldorf, Germany; Clinic Lippe Detmold, Germany)
Arthroscopy 12:217–223, 1996   4–4

Introduction.—Cartilage necrosis caused by laser-controlled cartilage-ablation arthroplasties has been reported. Reported are 2 instances of holmium:YAG laser-induced aseptic femoral-condyle necrosis.

> *Case Report 1.*—A 57-year-old man had a 2-year history of stress-induced pains in the right medial knee joint that increased in intensity in December 1993. He underwent arthroscopy in January 1994, and a degenerative rupture of the medial meniscus and a third-degree chondromalacia of the medial femoral condyle was detected. A Ho:YAG laser-controlled partial resection of the meniscus and cartilage ablation were performed. Symptoms subsided, but stress-induced pain began in the medial knee joint in June 1994. In July, he had an extension deficit of the right knee joint of

10 degrees. Other than pain on extreme movements, physical examination of the right knee was unremarkable. Radiographs showed an oval osteolytic bone defect of the medial femoral condyle that was irregularly defined against the bone. Endoprosthetic replacement of the medial compartment was performed in August 1994. Aseptic bone necrosis of the femoral cartilage was seen on visual and histologic examination. The patient has fully recovered.

Case Report 2.—A 47-year-old man with psoriasis-associated arthritis experienced stress-induced pain in his right medial joint in August 1993. He was relieved of pain after undergoing arthroscopy with Ho:YAG laser-conducted cartilage ablation of the medial femoral condyle. In July 1994, the medial joint pain returned and was accompanied by joint effusion. Radiographs indicated gonarthrosis. An MRI in October 1994 showed avascular bone necroses and a lesion on the medial meniscus. Arthroscopy with subtotal resection of the torn posterior horn of the medial meniscus of the right knee was performed in November 1994. The medial condyle showed fourth-degree chondromalacia. The patient was able to walk without crutches in 1 week.

Conclusion.—Laser-controlled cartilage-ablation arthroplasties have their place in the treatment of chondromalacia. Distance between laser fiber and tissue, the angle of impact of the laser beam, time of influence of the laser on a certain region, and total count of laser pulses administered to a certain area are important factors in preventing the development of aseptic bone necrosis of the femoral head.

Osteonecrosis of the Knee Following Arthroscopic Laser Meniscectomy
Rozbruch SR, Wickiewicz TL, DiCarlo EF, et al (Cornell Univ, New York)
Arthroscopy 12:245–250, 1996   4–5

Introduction.—Causes of spontaneous osteonecrosis are thought to be idiopathic, vascular, or traumatic. Reported is a case history of 1 patient who experienced spontaneous osteonecrosis after undergoing an arthroscopic laser meniscectomy.

> *Case Report.*—Woman, 25, had a medial meniscal tear of the right knee from a fall on the ice in February 1992. In April 1992, she underwent an arthroscopic partial medial meniscectomy using a 60-W contact neodymium:yttrium aluminum garnet laser. She did well after surgery and physical therapy until she returned to sports activities. She experienced right medial pain that did not respond to a second course of physical therapy. An MRI revealed subchondral necrosis in the medial aspect of the medial tibial plateau with full-thickness chondral loss and osteonecrosis of the medial femoral condyle. She underwent arthroscopic débridement, but contin-

ued to have medial joint line pain, intermittent swelling, and a sensation of buckling of the knee. In March 1994, radiographs and MRI revealed frank osteonecrosis of the medial tibial plateau with marked subchondral collapse and considerable deformity of the adjacent articular cartilage. Two months later she underwent a joint-surface replacement of the medial tibial plateau with a fresh-frozen osteochondral meniscal allograft and an autograft dowel replacement of the necrotic lesion in the femoral condyle. Pathologic examination revealed centrally necrotic trabeculae with overlying viable bone with visible osteocytes. Postoperative anteroposterior radiograph revealed the medial plateau osteochondral allograft was fixed with AO 6.5-mm partially threaded cancellous screws and washers.

Conclusion.—As with any new technology introduced to surgery for its potential benefits, possible hazards must be reported and investigated. A lower power laser setting may have been more appropriate than the 60-W setting used for the patient described.

Delayed Articular Cartilage Slough: Two Cases Resulting From Holmium:YAG Laser Damage to Normal Articular Cartilage and a Review of the Literature
Thal R, Danziger MB, Kelly A (Town Ctr Orthopaedic Associates, Reston, Va; George Washington Univ, Washington, DC)
Arthroscopy 12:92–94, 1996   4–6

Introduction.—Reports have increased regarding unintended damage to adjacent soft tissue and cartilage after use of neodymium:YAG and holmium:YAG (Ho:YAG) lasers. Two case reports are presented, discussing patients with chondral damage and slough secondary to use of the Ho:YAG laser.

Case 1.—Woman, 50, had complaints of a locked knee after a twisting injury. A bucket handle tear of the lateral meniscus was found during arthroscopy and a partial lateral meniscectomy was performed with a 20-W Ho:YAG laser. The patient did not fully recover and had recurrent mechanical problems 6 months after surgery. She had a 3+ effusion and 10° mechanical block to full extension. The videotape of the first procedure revealed small burn marks on the lateral femoral condyle and intact articular cartilage. A second arthroscopic procedure showed multiple large cartilaginous loose fragments throughout the joint. Large areas of partial and full thickness cartilage defects were seen on the lateral condyle. The area was débrided and symptoms were resolved.

Case 2.—Woman, 35, had a 6-year history of intermittent right knee pain that did not respond to medical treatment. Arthroscopy revealed degenerative changes of the lateral tibial plateau and patella that were débrided with a motorized shaver. Five years later, she underwent a second arthroscopy for recurrent symptoms and grade III changes of the lateral tibial plateau and patella and partial lateral meniscus tear. The lateral femoral condyle was normal. A Hdmium:YAG laser was used to débride degenerative tissues and perform a partial lateral meniscectomy. Symptoms recurred 4 months later. She had a small effusion, significant patellofemoral pain, crepitus, and lateral joint line tenderness. Degenerative changes of the patella were seen on radiographs. Exercise was not helpful and symptoms worsened. Arthroscopy revealed degenerative changes of the lateral femoral condyle. The lateral tibial plateau and patella were debrided and a partial lateral meniscectomy was performed. Large loose fragments of cartilage from the patella and femoral condyle were removed. She had significant improvement at 3 months after the third arthroscopy.

Conclusion.—It is difficult to endorse the use of laser during arthroscopy of the knee with these findings and those of other case reports of osteonecrosis and cartilage sloughing.

▶ These 3 articles (abstracts 4–4, 4–5, and 4–6 bring our attention again to the potentially deleterious effects of laser energy used in the knee arthroscopically. These articles should not serve as a condemnation of this technology. Rather, it is important to understand the properties of laser energy. That is, each wavelength has specific tissue interaction. It is generally recognized that the Hdmium:YAG laser admits energy at a wavelength that is highly absorbed by meniscal tissue and cartilage, thus delivering less energy to the underlying bone. On the other hand, the neodymium:YAG laser admits light energy at a wavelength that is poorly absorbed by water and nonpigmented tissue such as meniscal and hyaline cartilage and presumably would have a more deleterious effect on the underlying bone. Garino[1] reported 5 cases with "osteonecrosis" of the knee after laser-assisted arthroscopic surgery. In these 2 cases a holmium-YAG laser was involved, thus raising the question of the role that surgical technique may contribute to these problems. The question raised by these various articles concerns the use of the term aseptic bone necrosis. Perhaps thermal necrosis would be more appropriate. It is important that these few anecdotal reports not serve as a condemnation of this technology. What should be emphasized is that the use of laser energy must be better understood by the surgeon.

J.S. Torg, M.D.

Reference

1. Garino JP, Lotke PA, Sapega AA, et al: Osteonecrosis of the knee following laser-assisted arthroscopic surgery: a report of six cases. *Arthroscopy* 11:467–474, 1995.

Patellar Tendon Ruptures

Matava MJ (Washington Univ, St Louis)
J Am Acad Orthop Surg 4:287–296, 1996   4–7

Background.—Rupture of the patellar tendon, a relatively uncommon injury, usually occurs in young, active persons during athletic events. The mechanism of injury is a violent contraction of the quadriceps muscle group resisted by the flexed knee. The rupture is usually the final stage of a degenerative tendinopathy resulting from repetitive microtrauma to the patellar tendon. The diagnosis and treatment of this injury were discussed.

Diagnosis and Treatment of Patellar Tendon Ruptures.—On physical examination, the hallmark of this injury is the patient's inability to actively extend the knee against gravity. The diagnosis of patellar tendon rupture is made on the basis of this finding along with the presence of a painful, palpable defect in the substance of the tendon and demonstration of patella alta on a lateral radiograph. To ensure optimal return of function, immediate surgical repair is recommended. A Bunnell-type repair is effective. Patients with a neglected rupture sometimes need preoperative patellar traction to overcome the contracted quadriceps muscle to enable tendon end reapproximation. Rarely, autogenous grafts or allograft tendons are needed to span the defect when local tissue is unavailable. Postoperatively, an aggressive rehabilitation program should emphasize early knee motion, quadriceps strengthening, and sport-specific functional rehabilitation. Outcomes are most closely related to the interval between injury and repair.

Conclusions.—Rupture of the patellar tendon is relatively uncommon, yet disabling. Immediate diagnosis and treatment are needed to ensure optimal outcomes and full return to an active lifestyle.

▶ This comprehensive review article emphasizes diagnosis and immediate surgery followed by an aggressive rehabilitation program to obtain maximum functional recovery for management of patella tendon ruptures. Importantly, delayed repair risks a compromised result with loss of full knee flexion and decreased quadriceps strength.

J.S. Torg, M.D.

Characteristics of the Leg Extensors in Male Volleyball Players With Jumper's Knee

Lian Ø, Engebretsen L, Øvrebø RV, et al (Norwegian Volleyball Federation, Rud, Norway; Univ of Minnesota, Minneapolis)
Am J Sports Med 24:380–385, 1996   4–8

Introduction.—Pain at the distal or proximal insertion of the patellar tendon or at the insertion of the quadriceps tendon is known as jumper's knee or patellar tendinitis. In volleyball players, the incidence of jumper's knee is related to the frequency of training sessions and playing on hard surfaces. It is not known why some athletes have problems with the high training volume and others remain uninjured. It may be that those athletes able to generate a high impulse during takeoff when jumping or running are at risk of injury from high repetitive loads on the leg extensor apparatus. The performance ability of leg extensors was tested in a group of well-conditioned male Norwegian volleyball players with jumper's knee, using a standardized program of jump and power tests. Results were compared with those of uninjured athletes.

Methods.—Twelve players who met criteria for jumper's knee and 12 matched controls underwent a testing program that included the following: a standing jump, a countermovement jump, a 15-second rebound jump test, a standing jump with a 20-kg load, and a standing jump with a load corresponding to one half of the athlete's body weight. A contact mat connected to an electronic timer was used to measure jump height and power.

Results.—Athletes from the patient and control groups came from the same teams, used the same types of shoes, and trained and played on similar gymnasium floors. Athletes in the patient group performed significantly better than controls in the countermovement jump, the standing jump with a 20-kg load, and the 15-second rebound jump test. Compared with controls, the patient group performed better in work done in countermovement and standing jumps and the difference between jump height and countermovement and standing jumps.

Discussion/Conclusion.—Athletes with jumper's knee performed better than well-matched controls without the injury in a standard series of jump and power tests. The risk of injury may be related to the load placed on the extensor apparatus during jumping, as indicated by the greater performance ability in the patient group, compared with controls. The injury may be an unhealed partial rupture, as it is possible that the risk of tendon tears is greater with load, not only with training frequency. The injured athletes must be able to generate a greater vertical impulse than controls to be able to jump higher. Because more than 50% of the work done in jumping is produced by knee extensors, it may be that the differences in jumping height reflect a true increase in the force transfer through the patellar tendon. Further investigation is needed to define the forces involved in jumping so that appropriate rehabilitation programs can be designed for injured high-performance athletes.

▶ This very revealing study indicates that athletes with jumper's knee jumped higher in jumps involving eccentric force generation, which results in greater stress to the patellar tendon and an increased chance of partial tears. Training and rehabilitation programs should include specific eccentric exercises, even in patients with recalcitrant tendinitis. The authors did state that they could not determine whether the problems occurred in the takeoff or the landing. Perhaps they may be a combination of both activities.

F.J. George, A.T.C., P.T.

Comparison of Intersegmental Tibiofemoral Joint Forces and Muscle Activity During Various Closed Kinetic Chain Exercises

Stuart MJ, Meglan DA, Lutz GE, et al (Mayo Clinic and Mayo Found, Rochester, Minn)

Am J Sports Med 24:792–799, 1996   4–9

Objective.—Closed kinetic strengthening exercises are considered safe for rehabilitation after knee ligament surgery. Results of a study analyzing the intersegmental forces at the tibiofemoral joint during the power squat, front squat, and lunge were presented.

Methods.—Six healthy male volunteers (average age, 26.6, years) with intact anterior cruciate ligaments performed 3 repetitions, each lasting 4 seconds, of the power squat, front squat, and lunge while holding a 223-N barbell with a 1- to 3-minute rest in between (Fig 1). Kinematics were measured using a 4-camera video system. Intersegmental resultant knee anterior-posterior shear force, compression-distraction force, and flexion-extension moment about the knee were calculated. Electromyographic activity of various muscle groups was measured.

Results.—During all 3 exercises, shear forces were directed posteriorly. Magnitude increased with flexion and decreased with extension, with maximal posterior shear of 495 N at 103 degrees of knee flexion for the lunge, a maximum of 295 N at 93 degrees for the power squat, and a maximum of 295 N at 97 degrees for the front squat. The lunge produced the maximum tibiofemoral compression forces. Flexion-extension moments were similar for all exercises. The lunge required increased quadriceps muscle involvement and decreased hamstring muscle involvement compared with the power and front squats. During the lunge, net extension moments at both 60 degrees and 90 degrees and quadriceps muscle

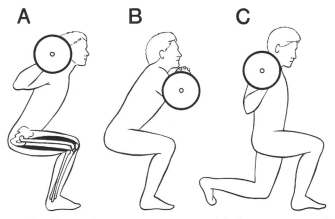

FIGURE 1.—Closed kinetic chain exercises: power squat (*left*), front squat (*center*), lunge (*right*). (Courtesy of Stuart MJ, Meglan DA, Lutz GE, et al: Comparison of intersegmental tibiofemoral joint forces and muscle activity during various closed kinetic chain exercises. *Am J Sports Med* 24:792–799, 1996).

electromyographic activity were significantly higher than those for the squat exercises.

Conclusion.—The intersegmental tibiofemoral forces and muscle activity generated in the power squat, front squat, and lunge are closed kinetic chain exercises that do not threaten the stability of the intact anterior cruciate ligament.

▶ Closed kinetic chain exercises for the lower extremity are performed when the foot is fixed and knee motion is accompanied by motion at the hip and ankle. Open kinetic chain exercises are performed when the foot is mobile and force application produces moments at the knee only, as these exercises may result in significant anterior cruciate ligament (ACL) strain. Closed kinetic chain exercises are thought to be safe for rehabilitation of the knee as the loads on the ACL are less.

The power squat, the front squat, and the lunge were examined to determine the stresses they produce on the ACL. It was reported that the shear forces in these exercises occur in a posterior direction and that the forces are not high enough to stress the normal posterior cruciate ligament and are not excessive in an ACL-intact knee. The use of these exercises in strengthening an ACL-injured or reconstructed knee will require further study, but provided the speed of movement is not excessive, this type of exercise may be relatively safe.

M.J.L. Alexander, Ph.D.

Timing and Intensity of Vastus Muscle Activity During Functional Activities in Subjects With and Without Patellofemoral Pain
Powers CM, Landel R, Perry J (Univ of Southern California, Los Angeles)
Phys Ther 76:946–955, 1996   4–10

Background.—Lateral patellar tracking and patellofemoral pain (PFP) may be caused partly by differences in intensity and timing of muscle activity between the vastus medialis and vastus lateralis muscles. Whether there are differences in the activity of the vastus muscles that would be suggestive of patellar instability in subjects with PFP was investigated.

Methods.—Twenty-six subjects with and 19 without PFP were included. The activity of the vastus medialis oblique, vastus medialis longus, vastus lateralis, and vastus intermedius muscles were recorded by fine-wire electromyography during walking, stair climbing, and walking on ramps. A 6-camera motion analysis system was used to assess knee motion.

Findings.—There were no differences in onset or cessation of muscle activity among the vastus muscles for either group, regardless of condition. Less activity of all vastus muscles for level and ramp walking was noted in subjects with PFP than in those without.

Conclusion.—Onset, cessation, and mean intensity of electromyographic activity of the vastus muscles did not differ during functional activities in either group. Thus, timing and intensity differences between the vastus medialis and vastus lateralis muscles are apparently unassociated with PFP.

▶ One of the interesting questions in sports medicine is whether the vastus medialis and vastus lateralis muscles can contract independently of one another, and whether each can be trained separately by altering the position of the lower leg relative to the knee. Some athletic therapists prescribe knee extension exercises with the lower leg laterally rotated to selectively train an atrophied vastus medialis, but there is little empirical evidence that this is effective. Other rehabilitation specialists suggest that because the vastus medialis and vastus lateralis muscles merge to form a common tendon, the quadriceps tendon, then quadriceps contraction engages all 4 heads of the muscle.

This study examined the intensity and onset of vastus lateralis and vastus medialis muscle activity in a group of subjects with and without PFP during several functional activities. They reported no differences in onset, cessation, or intensity of electromyographic activity in the 3 vastus muscles in the activities examined. This finding is not in agreement with those of other studies that have reported decreased vastus medialis activity associated with knee injury. The authors did note that their study did not include maximal force activities—such as might be seen in rehabilitation or strengthening situations—which may produce altered function between these muscles.

M.J.L. Alexander, Ph.D.

Surgical Correction of Medial Subluxation of the Patella
Hughston JC, Flandry F, Brinker MR, et al (Hughston Clinic, Columbus, Ga)
Am J Sports Med 24:486–491, 1996   4–11

Introduction.—Medial subluxation of the patella and its associated disability occurs most often as a result of a lateral retinacular release procedure. Results of a surgical technique used to correct medial patellar subluxation were presented (Fig 4).

Methods.—Sixty-five knees were repaired in 63 patients. Data regarding surgical reconstruction of the lateral patellotibial ligament were gathered from follow-up visits, telephone conversations, and medical records.

Results.—Average follow-up was 53.7 months. Of 63 patients, 44 (68%) reported improved functional status. Forty-nine (75%) patients reported subjective improvement after surgical correction. Fifty (80%) patients reported a good or excellent rating of the procedure. There were 16 (25%) complications. Six knees required a second repair after reinjury. Clinical outcome was not associated with patient age at the time of initial procedure, sex, or length of follow-up.

Conclusion.—Subjective satisfaction of 80% of patients who underwent surgical correction supports the use of this technique as an alternative treatment for painful iatrogenic medial subluxation of the patella.

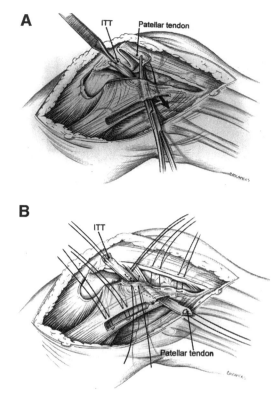

FIGURE 4.—Our current reconstruction method. **A,** A minor technical variation in which a strip of the iliotibial tract is rotated toward the patella and a strip of patellar tendon is rotated toward the lateral tibial tubercle. The strips of the iliotibial tract and patellar tendon (*arrow*) are routed deep to the iliopatellar band. **B,** Each strip retains a natural bony attachment, and the two strips are joined by side-to-side anastomosis. The defect from harvesting the strip of iliotibial tract is closed. This further allows for fine tuning of the tension in the reconstructed patellotibial ligament. (Courtesy of Hughston JC, Flandry F, Brinker MR, et al: Surgical correction of medial subluxation of the patella. *Am J Sports Med* 24:486–491, 1996.)

▶ In my view, medial subluxation of the patella caused by lateral retinacular release is a rare phenomenon, if it occurs at all. In view of the fact that both the diagnostic criteria for surgical intervention as well as the outcome analysis method were determined by the subjective evaluation of the examiner, both the validity of the results and conclusions must be questioned. As stated in the paper, "we have no equipment currently available that will validate our objective examination demonstrating the absence of medial patellar subluxation." Also of note is the fact that "this operation was not without complications," which occurred in 25% of the cases.

J.S. Torg, M.D.

Reflex Response Times of Vastus Medialis Oblique and Vastus Lateralis in Normal Subjects and in Subjects With Patellofemoral Pain Syndrome
Witvrouw E, Sneyers C, Lysens R, et al (Catholic Univ of Leuven, Belgium; Univ Hosp, Leuven, Belgium)
J Orthop Sports Phys Ther 24:160–165, 1996   4–12

Background.—The exact cause of patellofemoral pain is not known, but its occurrence secondary to patellar malalignment is generally accepted. Imbalance of the vastus medialis/vastus lateralis muscles has been implicated, but few published reports have substantiated the hypothesis. Whether patients with femoralpatellar pain syndrome (FPS) have an alteration in reflex response times of the vastus medialis oblique (VMO) and vastus lateralis (VL) muscles to a patellar tendon tap was examined.

Findings.—Participating were 80 healthy adults and 19 patients with FPS. In both groups, significant differences occurred between the VMO and VL reflex response times. The reflex response time of the VMO was significantly shorter than that of the VL in the controls; in patients with FPS, however, the VL fired significantly sooner than the VMO. These results indicate that a reversal has occurred in the firing pattern of the VMO and VL in patients with FPS. The reversal was observed in the injured and uninjured legs, with no significant difference in reflex response times between limbs.

Discussion.—The VMO is believed to have the singular functional role of medially tracking the patella; it is an antagonist to the effects of the VL in adjusting patellar alignment. The alterations in response time occurring in the patients with FPS are bound to affect the patellofemoral joint by disrupting the balance of the medial and lateral forces on the patella, thus creating patellar malalignment. These data suggest that the reversal of the firing sequence in patients with FPS is caused primarily by an increase in reflex response time of the VL. If so, retarding the VL, as opposed to accelerating the VMO reflex response time (which is already shorter in patients with FPS), would be more beneficial. Reflex response times in patients with FPS might be altered by the decrease in physical activity that typically accompanies this condition. Rehabilitation might alter reflex response times in patients with FPS, but further study on the topic is required.

▶ After reading the previous 2 abstracts (Abstracts 4–10 and 4–11), along with this study, there are many factors to consider when treating athletes with patellofemoral pain. The authors of this study suggest that patellofemoral pain syndrome is associated with disturbed neuromotor control of patellofemoral agonists. They recommend a rehabilitation program be designed to retard the firing of the VL rather than accelerating the VMO reflex response. Their reasoning is that both VL and VMO are already significantly shorter in the patient with patellofemoral pain.

F.J. George, A.T.C., P.T.

Biarticulating Two-dimensional Computer Model of the Human Patellofemoral Joint

Gill HS, O'Connor JJ (Univ of Oxford, England)
Clin Biomech 11:81–89, 1996   4–13

Introduction.—In the overall success of total knee replacement, the failure of prosthetic patellae is a significant factor, and about 50% of total knee replacement complications are caused by the patellofemoral joint. The kinematics and mechanics of the patella were related to the geometry and mechanics of the cruciate ligaments and the tibiofemoral joint. Two separate articulations on the model patella were included and represented the lateral facets and the median ridge, allowing modeling of the patellofemoral joint at high flexion angles.

Methods.—Geometric and force equilibrium constraints were used to calculate the orientation of the patella about its mediolateral axis in a biarticulating 2-dimensional model of the patellofemoral joint. An iterative numerical procedure was used to develop the equations from these constraints. The patellofemoral model was based on a rearrangement of

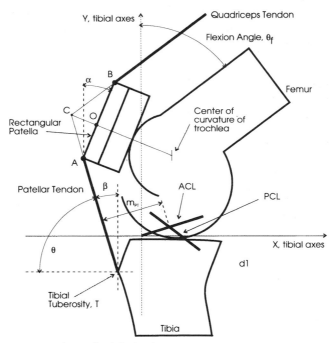

m_{pt} = moment arm of patellar tendon

FIGURE 2.—Schematic sagittal plane view of the knee. The x,y axes in the tibia lie parallel and perpendicular to the tibial plateau, with origin at the tibial insertion of the anterior cruciate ligament (*ACL*). *Abbreviation: PCL*, posterior cruciate ligament. (Courtesy of Gill HS, O'Connor JJ: Biarticulating two-dimensional computer model of the human patellofemoral joint. Reprinted from *Clin Biomech* 11:81–89, copyright 1996, with kind permission from Elsevier Science Ltd, The Boulevard, Langford Lane, Kidlington OX5 1GB UK.)

the terms in the geometric and the equilibrium equations to be functions of knee flexion angle and the patellar tendon angle. The iteration variable became the patellar tendon angle, and the equation variable was the flexion range from 2 degrees to 140 degrees in 1.5-degree steps (Fig 2).

Results.—The proximal rolling of the patella on the femur during flexion was explained and predicted by this model. Transfer of contact from the trochlea to the femoral condyles at high knee flexion angles was predicted by this model. The patellofemoral joint reaction force magnitude and the variation with flexion angle of the patellar mechanism angle are in agreement with previous results.

Conclusion.—Effects of surgical procedures can be investigated with the use of this model. During various activities, the internal joint forces can be calculated with this model. Replacement of the patellofemoral joint has been marred by problems of wear and deformation, and the necessity of incongruity in the functional geometry of the patellofemoral joint was explained by this model.

▶ The success of total knee replacement is often dependent on the geometry of the prosthetic patella. This study examined the mechanics of the patellofemoral joint by using a computer model of the rolling of the patella on the femur during flexion. This motion is not only simple sagittal plane motion but also rotation of the patella about a median axis, and it takes into consideration the contact points on the femur. This is a very complex mechanism because of the changing angles of pull of the patellar tendon and the quadriceps tendon on the patella, which continuously change the compressive forces on the femur. As might be expected, low contact stresses were predicted at low knee flexion angles, and at higher flexion angles larger contact stresses were predicted. Failure of patellar prostheses likely occurs as a result of activities with higher knee flexion angles, such as stair climbing.

M.J.L. Alexander, Ph.D.

Abduction-Adduction Moments at The Knee During Stair Ascent and Descent
Kowalk DL, Duncan JA, Vaughan CL (Univ of Virginia, Charlottesville)
J Biomech 29:383–388, 1996   4–14

Introduction.—When individuals walk on level ground, the plane that is perpendicular to their direction of progression can be considered to be the frontal plane, and the hip joint moment axes that are in this plane can be considered to be the flexion-extension and internal-external rotation axes (Fig 1). When individuals climb stairs, the moments applied about the axes should be considered to determine the flexion-extension and abduction-adduction axes. An anatomically consistent set of axes was recommended to determine joint moments and to examine the relative magnitude of the knee abduction-adduction moments in stair climbing.

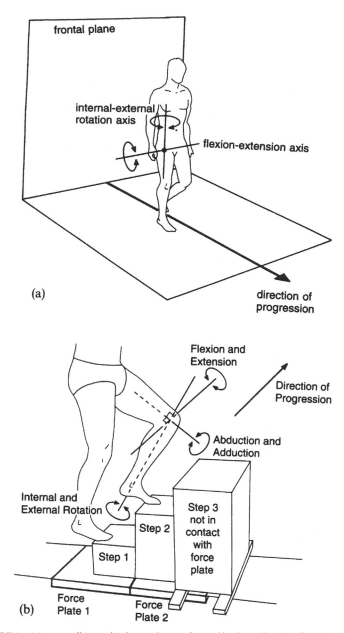

FIGURE 1.—(a), man walking on level ground moves forward by the application of joint moments about axes that are in the plane perpendicular to the intended direction of progression. In this example, it is the frontal plane, and the joint moment axes in this plane are the flexion-extension and internal-external rotation axes for the right hip. (b), location of the steps on the force platforms and definition of the knee joint references axes (Vaughan et al., 1992). Note that steps 1 and 2 were sensitive to reaction forces, whereas the ground and step 3 were not. The flexion-extension moment takes place about the mediolateral axis of the proximal segment (thigh). The internal-external rotation moment takes place about the longitudinal axis of the distal segment (calf). The abduction-adduction moment takes place about a floating axis that is perpendicular to the mediolateral and longitudinal axes (these axes are not normally perpendicular to each other). In this paper only the flexion-extension and abduction-adduction moments were evaluated. (Courtesy of Kowalk DL, Duncan JA, Vaughan CL: Abduction-adduction moments at the knee during stair ascent and descent. Reprinted from the *Journal of Biomechanics* 29:383–388, copyright 1996, with kind permission from Elsevier Science Ltd, The Boulevard, Langford Lane, Kidlington OX5 1GB UK.)

Methods.—Ten normal adults (6 men and 4 women) ranging in age from 22 to 40 years old with an average weight of 660 newtons, a right leg length of 0.962 m, and a height of 1.74 m participated in repeated trials of stair climbing to examine the relative magnitude of the knee abduction-adduction moments during stair climbing. A 4-camera video system and 2 forces plates incorporated within a flight of 3 stairs were used to collect data. To calculate the internal moments at the knee, the investigators used the inverse dynamics approach, and the moments were then normalized in magnitude and time.

Results.—For the first and second steps during stair ascent and descent, knee joint moments were similar in shape and magnitude. For stair ascent and descent, the extension moments (60–85 newton meters) were statistically larger than the abduction knee moments (25–45 newton meters), although they were comparable in magnitude. Throughout the stance, the moment patterns were exclusively abductor, which indicated that the ground reaction vector always passed medial to the knee joint center.

Conclusion.—When trying to understand the stability and function of the knee during stair climbing, investigators have found that the knee abduction-adduction moment is not in the primary plane of motion; however, its magnitude should not be ignored because it provides propulsion and mediolateral stability.

▶ Stair climbing is an important activity of daily living that has received increasing attention in recent years in terms of maintaining independent living for older individuals. The majority of the biomechanical studies of stair climbing have focussed on the knee moments in the flexion extension direction; however, the knee moments in the abduction-adduction direction are also important. The results indicated that the maximum knee abduction moment was statistically smaller than the extension moment for both ascent and descent. However, the abduction-adduction moments play an important role at the knee joint in that they provide both propulsion and mediolateral stability. The mediolateral stability at the knee joint is provided by the lateral collateral ligament and the iliotibial band; this moment is critical at 2 points in ascent and descent when the extension moment was close to 0. This paper emphasizes the importance of the integrity of ligaments and muscles in all aspects of a joint to maintain skill in activities of daily living and further supports activity programs for older adults.

M.J.L. Alexander, Ph.D.

Influences of Configuration Changes of the Patella on the Knee Extensor Mechanism
Cheng C-K, Yao N-K, Liu H-C, et al (Natl Yang Ming Univ, Taipei, Taiwan, Republic of China; Natl Taiwan Univ, Republic of China)
Clin Biomech 11:116–120, 1996   4–15

Introduction.—The patella performs a variety of important functions in the extensor mechanism of the knee, and a significant number of compli-

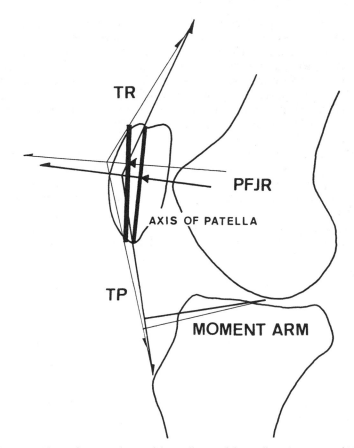

FIGURE 3.—The configuration change of the patella caused the patellar axis to move, which not only changed the moment arm of extensor mechanism but also influenced the forces involved in the extensor mechanism. *Abbreviations: TR,* quadriceps muscle force; *PFJR,* patellofemoral joint reaction force; *TP,* tension of the patella tendon. (Courtesy of Cheng C-K, Yao N-K, Liu H-C, et al: Influences of configuration changes of the patella on the knee extensor mechanism. *Clin Biomech* 11:116–120, copyright 1996, with kind permission from Elsevier Science Ltd, The Boulevard, Langford Lane, Kidlington OX5 1GB UK.)

cations of total knee arthroplasty are related to patellofemoral problems. The influence of patella thickness and forward/backward tilting of the patella on function was analyzed biomechanically.

Methods.—Study participants were 6 healthy adult volunteers, 3 men and 3 women with an average age of 20 years. Normal patellar tracking in the sagittal plane was obtained by recording and digitizing knee extension with fluoroscopy. Based on the averaged normal patellar tracking data, the position of patellar axis was adjusted by translation and rotation to simulate different patellar configuration changes. The extensor moment was assumed to remain constant before and after the patellar configuration was changed. According to a balance beam model, the quadriceps muscle force, the tension of the patellar tendon, and the patellofemoral joint reaction force (PFJR) should be in equilibrium; thus, the ratio between any 2 forces can be estimated (Fig 3).

Results.—When patellar thickness decreased, quadriceps force increased but PFJR decreased; the reverse was observed with thickening of the patella. With backward tilting of the patella, the quadriceps force and PFJR decreased and the patellar tendon/quadriceps force ratio increased. Thus, backward tilting produced a better mechanical advantage of force transmission of patella. Forward tilting led to the opposite effect.

Conclusions.—Because the configuration changes of the patella affect the force distribution on the patellofemoral joint, these changes are important in designing prostheses and in performing total knee arthroplasty. For older patients with weak quadriceps muscles, the patella can be tilted backward to increase the mechanical advantage of force transmission. In younger patients with relatively strong quadriceps, the chance of implant failure can be reduced by decreasing patellar thickness and PFJR. Patellar thickness should be at least 15 mm, however, to avoid the risk of fracture.

▶ The role of the patella in the biomechanical functioning of the knee joint is unquestioned. As noted in this paper, its major functions include maintaining a mechanical advantage for the quadriceps by increasing its moment arm; decreasing friction; protecting the joint from trauma; and preventing additional wear of the quadriceps tendon. Total knee replacement surgery is now common, and requires greater knowledge of patellar mechanics for successful replacement. One common complication of knee replacement is patellar subluxation and dislocation. This study examined the influences of patellar thickness and patellar tilting on function. One interesting finding was that PFJR (I disagree Au) will decrease when patellar thickness decreases in younger patients, because it is often assumed that a thicker patella will increase the distance to the axis and decrease the muscle force required for any given torque. The authors further suggest that the patella be tilted backward for older patients, to increase the length of the moment arm and increase the mechanical advantage of the mechanism.

M.J.L. Alexander, Ph.D.

Long-term Evaluation of the Elmslie-Trillat-Maquet Procedure for Patellofemoral Dysfunction
Naranja RJ Jr, Reilly PJ, Kuhlman JR, et al (Univ of Pennsylvania, Philadelphia; Gate Orthopaedics, Warwick, RI; Statesville Med Group, NC; et al)
Am J Sports Med 24:779–784, 1996   4–16

Introduction.—There is no consensus on optimal treatment of patellofemoral dysfunction. Described are results of a new surgical technique for treating patellofemoral pain or instability or both.

Surgical Technique.—The technique combines the Elmslie-Trillat procedure to medialize the tibial tubercle and the Maquet procedure, which raises the tibial tubercle anteriorly (Fig 1). The technique is detailed in the original article.

Methods.—Fifty-five knees of 51 patients who underwent Elmslie-Trillat-Maquet procedures were reviewed retrospectively. Mean patient age at follow-up was 27.5 years. Preoperatively, patients reported patellofemoral pain, instability, or both in 17, 24, and 14 knees, respectively. Outcome was evaluated at a mean follow-up of 74.2 months with the Fulkerson's functional knee score and patient questionnaires.

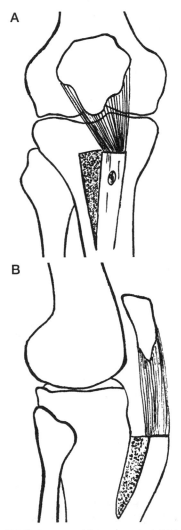

FIGURE 1.—**A**, Lateral-medial displacement of the osteotomized tibial tubercle pedicle (Elmslie-Trillat portion of the procedure). **B**, One-centimeter elevation affected by placement of cortiocancellous graft obtained from original osteotomy site (Maquet portion of the procedure). (Courtesy of Naranja RJ Jr, Reilly PJ, Kulman JR, et al: Long-term evaluation of the Elmslie-Trillat-Maquet procedure for patello-femoral dysfunction. *Am J Sports Med* 24:779–784, 1996.)

Result.—Patients reported results to be excellent in 9 (16%) knees, good in 24 (44%) knees, and fair in 13 (24%) knees for an overall total of improvement in 46 (84%) knees. Improvement with Fulkerson's functional knee score was: excellent in 19 (35%) knees, good in 10 (18%) knees, and fair in 11 (20%) knees for an overall improvement of 73% (40 knees). Average pain score improved from 7.2 preoperatively to 4.2 postoperatively. Outcome was significantly better in younger than older patients. Better results were seen in patients who had instability rather than pain and in those with more than 2 preoperative dislocations, compared with those with 1 or no dislocations. Patients with better surgical outcome had significantly fewer medial and lateral tibiofemoral compartment changes than those with a greater degree of degenerative changes.

Conclusion.—Overall subjective and objective improvement was 84% and 73%, respectively, for patients undergoing the Elmslie-Trillat-Maquet procedure for patellofemoral dysfunction. Risk factors for poorer outcome were age greater than 31.5 years, fewer than 2 dislocations, medial or lateral tibiofemoral compartment chondromalacia more than grade I, and presence of 2 or more conditions.

Functional Treatment of Patellar Dislocation in an Athletic Population
Garth WP Jr, Pomphrey M Jr, Merrill K (Univ of Alabama, Birmingham; St Louis, Mo; Univ of South Carolina, Charleston)
Am J Sports Med 24:785–791, 1996   4–17

Objective.—Outcome after rehabilitation without previous immobilization in the nonoperative treatment of patellar dislocation is inconsistent, particularly in athletes. Because of recent reports that early mobilization increases ligament strength whereas periods of immobilization slow recovery, a protocol of immediate functional rehabilitation with bracing after patellar dislocation was initiated. Results of a follow-up study evaluating outcomes after 2 years and identifying risk factors that adversely affect prognosis are presented.

Methods.—Radiographic examinations were conducted at the initial and follow-up visits for an average of 46.2 months after onset of rehabilitation without prior immobilization in 68 patients (19 women), aged 7 to 35, with a history of patellar dislocations in 79 knees. Most injuries occurred during contact sports, running, cheerleading, and dancing, with the knee flexed and the foot in a weight-bearing position. Patients were divided into those who were seen within 1 month of an acute episode (group I, *n* = 39 knees) and those who had never been treated or rehabilitated (group II, *n* = 30 knees).

Results.—Good or excellent stability results were achieved in 39 acute knee injuries and 15 chronic knee injuries. Both subjective and objective assessments of stability were better in group I than in group II. Sixteen patients were dissatisfied with results, including 10 patients who had surgery on 11 knees. Six group I and 12 group II patients (26%) had recurrent instability after rehabilitation. Earlier onset of instability, female sex, anatomic predisposition to instability, and bilateral instability were significantly associated with fair or poor results. Association between age and bilaterality, sex and bilaterality, and anatomic predisposition and bilaterality were significantly related to fair or poor outcome.

Conclusion.—A majority of patients' patellar dislocations respond satisfactorily to functional rehabilitation without prior immobilization. Predisposing risk factors for poorer outcome included earlier onset of instability, female sex, anatomic predisposition to instability, and bilateral instability.

Clinical Significance.—Patients with patellar dislocation and predisposing risk factors for patellar instability generally have poorer outcomes after functional rehabilitation without prior immobilization.

▶ This is an excellent paper that makes a very strong case for the success of conservative management of patellar dislocation in a specific population. That is, 72% of the patients were male with "slightly less anatomic predisposition to patellar instability." Also, the authors regard significant patellar femoral incongruity after patella dislocation as an indication for early surgical management. They define such incongruity as that which may result from osteochondral fractures with persistent marked lateral patellar subluxation. They also conclude that "the athlete with mild or no predisposition to patellar instability who sustains patellar dislocation and yet persists with symptoms or has recurrence of instability despite adequate rehabilitation probably stands to gain the most from surgical stabilization."

J.S. Torg, M.D.

Osteochondritis Dissecans

Schenck RC Jr, Goodnight JM (Univ of Texas, San Antonio)
J Bone Joint Surg Am 78A:439–456, 1996   4–18

Introduction.—Osteochondritis dissecans, an injury or condition usually affecting children between the ages of 5 and 15 who have open physes and older adolescents who have closed physes, results in separation of cartilage and subchondral bone. The entity includes osteochondral fractures, osteonecrosis, accessory centers of ossification, osteochondrosis, and hereditary epiphyseal dysplasia. Operative treatments including drilling, fixation of the lesion, and grafting have been described in the literature.

Osteochondritis Dissecans of the Knee.—Early symptoms are variable and intermittent but can include activity-related pain and swelling. Adult osteochondritis dissecans is usually the result of an unhealed lesion that formed during childhood. The lesion typically appears as a well-defined area of sclerotic subchondral bone affecting the lateral aspect of the medial femoral condyle and commonly included the weight-bearing surfaces. Using the anteroposterior radiograph, Cahill and Berg have developed a classification system based on the extent of the lesion. Technetium uptake studies, which demonstrate a relationship between degree of osseus uptake and healing potential, are used to describe lesion stages. MRI and CT are used in preoperative planning to visualize any loose bone fragments that may be present. Osteochondritis dissecans may result from indirect trauma, osteochondral fractures of the lateral femoral condyle after reduction of the patella, stress fracture, or possibly indirect microtrauma. Although some families demonstrate a predisposition for osteochondritis dissecans, no genetic link has been found. Lesions result when, after trauma, normal cartilage is not regenerated but instead is replaced by mesenchymal tissue that is converted into fibrocartilage that eventually undergoes endochondral ossification. Operative indications include loose fragments, symptoms that persist after conservative management, bone scans, and MRI studies. Excision and use of allogenic and autogenous grafts usually yields poor results.

Osteochondritis Dissecans of the Ankle.—The lesions are usually asymptomatic transchondral fractures that failed to heal, although patients may have no history of trauma. Medial lesions and lateral lesions were shaped differently but both had a necrotic osseous area.

Osteochondritis Dissecans of the Elbow.—Characterized by joint pain, swelling, and limited mobility, this condition usually results from overuse that is possibly caused by ischemia. A diagnosis can generally be made from plain radiographs. Treatment consists of débridement, removal of loose fragments, and revascularization stimulated by drilling the crater with a Kirschner wire.

Conclusion.—Osteochondritis dissecans appears to arise from many factors related to trauma. Knee lesions usually respond well to conservative treatment. Symptomatic lesions require arthroscopic surgery and protected weight bearing. Osteochondritis dissecans of the ankle can appear either posteromedially or anterolaterally. Osteochondritis dissecans of the elbow is commonly an overuse injury. Both ankle and elbow lesions respond to débridement and curettage or drilling.

▶ This is an excellent comprehensive review of the current concepts dealing with osteochondritis dissecans. The original article is recommended reading for the interested practitioner.

J.S. Torg, M.D.

Chondral Delamination of the Knee in Soccer Players
Levy AS, Lohnes J, Sculley S, et al (Duke Univ, Durham, NC)
Am J Sports Med 24:634–639, 1996   4–19

Introduction.—Knee injuries account for approximately 20% of all injuries to soccer players. Many studies have discussed cruciate and meniscal injuries, but there is little information on injuries to the articular cartilage. Isolated chondral injuries appear to be increasing in frequency

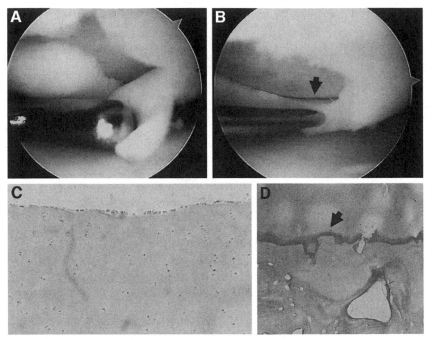

FIGURE 1.—A, arthroscopic view of the medial femoral condyle in a 22-year-old female soccer player. The chondral delamination flap is identified at tip of probe. B, the same arthroscopic view after removal of the delamination flap. Further delamination (*arrow*) extends past the border. C, a histologic section (original magnification, X400) of the delamination flap in the same patient. The surface and superficial layers appear normal. D, a histologic section (original magnification, X400) of the delamination border from the same patient, demonstrating failure at the tidemark (*arrow*). (Courtesy of Levy AS, Lohnes J, Sculley S, et al: Chondral delamination of the knee in soccer players. Am J Sports Med 24:634–639, 1996.)

and may result from disruption of the deep cartilage ultrastructure by large shear forces. Records of a group of soccer players were reviewed for the diagnosis, treatment, and outcome of isolated chondral lesions.

Methods.—Fifteen soccer players with 23 isolated chondral lesions were studied. All competed at Division I collegiate, national select, or professional levels. The athletes were evaluated by physical examination, MRI, and diagnostic arthroscopy. All chondral lesions were débrided to a stable margin, and the calcified cartilage base was removed. After surgery patients were treated with cryotherapy and aggressive physical therapy, followed by a 4-phase rehabilitation program. Outcome was graded with a scoring system based on the presence of pain, swelling, and locking with strenuous activity.

Results.—Before diagnosis and treatment, all players reported pain that limited activity. Effusions occurred in 48% of cases, joint line tenderness in 33%, and crepitus in 19%. Preoperative MRI had a sensitivity of 21%, correctly identifying the chondral lesions seen at arthroscopic examination in 5 knees. The average interval between symptom onset and arthroscopic examination was 3 months. Lesions were seen on the medial femoral condyle in 8 patients, the patella in 6, the lateral femoral condyle in 6, and the trochlea in 3. There was a relationship between lesion site and the type of motions than resulted in pain. Biopsies of cartilage flaps showed the surface and superficial layers to be normal (Fig 1), whereas calcified cartilage remained with the subchondral bone at the delamination border. The athletes were able to return to play at an average of 10.8 weeks. Outcome at 1-year follow-up was excellent in 6 cases and good in 9; no outcomes were judged fair or poor. A new lesion developed in 4 patients after return to play. All underwent repeat arthroscopic procedures, and 1 year after their last débridement, 2 have a good outcome and 2 a fair outcome.

Discussion.—The high velocities and repetitive pivoting decelerations that occur in soccer place extreme stress on the articular cartilage of the knee. Arthroscopic probing of the articular surface is needed for a definitive diagnosis of chondral delamination. Early functional results of débridement appear to compare favorably with those of autologous transplantation.

▶ It is important to note that the authors defined an excellent result to be one in which there was no pain, swelling, or locking with strenuous activity, whereas a good result had mild aching with strenuous activity but no swelling or locking. Apparently, follow-up was short; all knees were graded 1 year after surgery. Thus, it is appropriately concluded that "caution...is recommended when treating articular cartilage injuries because no long-term data exists as to whether any treatment modality can prevent the development of degenerative joint disease."

J.S. Torg, M.D.

Local Anesthesia in Outpatient Knee Arthroscopy: A Comparison of Efficacy and Cost
Lintner S, Shawen S, Lohnes J, et al (Duke Univ, Durham, NC)
Arthroscopy 12:482–488, 1996   4–20

Objective.—Knee arthroscopy, 1 of the most common orthopedic procedures, is increasingly being performed as an outpatient procedure. Use of local anesthesia is becoming more common. Results of prospective and retrospective reviews comparing the efficacy, safety, patient satisfaction, and cost benefits of local anesthesia, general, and regional anesthesia are presented.

> *Technique.*—With the patient under sufficient local anesthesia (0.5% lidocaine and 0.125% bupivacaine with epinephrine) to produce a large skin wheal when injected subcutaneously, injected into deeper tissues, and injected intraarticularly through the anterolateral site, a capsular incision is made and enlarged to accommodate instrumentation. Arthroscopy is performed, and the patient is removed to ambulatory surgery.

Retrospective Study.—Operative records of 256 orthoscopic knee surgeries were reviewed for patient age, sex, type of anesthesia, surgical procedure, operative time, total anesthesia time, drugs administered and their cost, need for supplemental anesthesia, postanesthesia care unit (PACU) duration and cost, ambulatory surgery unit (ASU) duration and cost, and complications. These data were analyzed using the Kruskal-Wallis nonparametric analysis of variance test.

Prospective Study.—The operative technique described was used for 100 consecutive outpatients, data identical to those listed above were collected, and a patient satisfaction questionnaire was obtained at 1 week after surgery. This information was compared with results from the retrospective review.

Results.—In the retrospective study, surgery was performed with use of general anesthetic in 69 patients, regional anesthetic in 62, and local in 125. Nonoperative procedure times averaged 57, 69, and 34 minutes, respectively. Average drug, PACU, ASU, and recovery room costs were $1,181, $1,164, and $230, respectively. Complication rates were 27.5%, 25.8%, and 1.6%, respectively. The times and dollar values calculated for the local anesthesia group were significantly different from the those calculated for the other 2 groups. None of the patients in the prospective group required conversion to general anesthesia. Only 1 patient in the prospective group was dissatisfied with the local anesthesia and would not select it again.

Conclusion.—Performing knee arthroscopy with the patient under local anesthesia is a cost-effective, safe, and effective procedure. Patient satisfaction with the use of local anesthesia was high.

Knee Arthroscopy: A Cost Analysis of General and Local Anesthesia
Trieshmann HW Jr (Orthopaedic Surgery & Sports Medicine Ctr, Newport News, Va)
Arthroscopy 12:60–63, 1996   4–21

Objective.—A retrospective review of patients undergoing outpatient knee arthroscopy was conducted to determine whether local anesthesia yields cost savings compared with general anesthesia. Local anesthesia is known to be effective, safe, and well accepted by patients, but its cost savings have not been documented.

Methods.—During a 6-month period, 73 patients had outpatient knee arthroscopy performed by a single surgeon at the study institution. Demographic data, type of procedure, and operating room time were recorded for each patient. Itemized charges were provided by the hospital.

Results.—Forty-eight patients elected local anesthesia, 5 elected general anesthesia, and 20 received general anesthesia because of the nature of their surgical procedure. The elective general and local anesthesia groups were similar in type of surgery, age, and gender. None of the patients who elected local anesthesia required conversion to general anesthesia, and no patient in either group had to be hospitalized overnight because of post-operative complications. Total hospital charges averaged $2,995 for general anesthesia and $2,377 for local anesthesia, a statistically significant difference. Significant reductions in anesthesia equipment charges and recovery room charges accounted for the savings with local anesthesia. Local anesthesia was also associated with statistically significant reductions in operating room time and surgery time.

Discussion.—In this series of patients undergoing outpatient knee arthroscopy, local anesthesia was associated with an average reduction in overall charges of $600 compared with general anesthesia. The absence of a recovery room charge and reduced anesthesia equipment charges were the most important factors in cost reduction. Costs might be lowered further if similar patients (without medical diagnoses and not requiring complex procedures) underwent knee arthroscopy with local anesthesia and in a less expensive physical environment than a hospital.

▶ We previously published an article demonstrating the efficacy of local anesthesia for surgical arthroscopy of the knee.[1] Our observations coincided with those reported in these two studies. Specifically, surgical arthroscopy with the patient under local anesthesia with IV sedation is both safe and well accepted by patients. It appears that with the factor of increased cost-effectiveness demonstrated, in the hands of the experienced arthroscopic surgeon, this should be the anesthesia of choice.

J.S. Torg, M.D.

Reference

1. Yacobucci GN, Bruce R, Conahan TJ, et al: Arthroscopic surgery of the knee under general anesthesia. *Arthroscopy* 6:311–314, 1990.

Unstable Knees in Unstable Times
Keller RB (Maine Med Assessment Found, Manchester)
Am J Sports Med 24:570–574, 1996   4–22

Background.—All physicians should be concerned about the future of health care. In a special lecture, the author addresses 4 related issues affecting the medical profession: changes in medical practice, physician profiling, outcomes research, and the physician workforce.

Changes in Medical Practice.—Recent years have seen tremendous advances in orthopedic diagnosis and treatment, with accompanying increases in cost to the health care system. Failed attempts at national health care reform left the way open to a business-driven, competitive market with a focus on cutting costs. The changes taking place in this environment are beyond the control of the physician and surgeon.

Physician Profiling.—Physician profiling is the use of information about a physician's practice by health care organizations to make decisions about credentialing, reimbursement, and other matters. Although this information can be valuable and useful, it is often not applied properly. Geographic variations in the frequency with which a procedure is performed may be used to label that procedure "discretionary." With poor-quality data, apparent divergences may actually be nonsignificant. In an area of controversy, such as anterior cruciate ligament surgery, plan directors are likely to opt for the least expensive protocol and come up with guidelines to enforce them.

Outcomes Research.—In the face of these threats to autonomy and credibility, the author sees outcomes research as the physician's best weapon. The way to find out what patients think of a procedure is to ask them. Reliable instruments and methods are needed to collect accurate and statistically significant data. Four regionally based outcomes assessment instruments are now available from the American Academy of Orthopaedic Surgeons Committee on Outcome Studies: pediatrics, spine, and upper and lower extremity. The information obtained from patients can be combined with other utilization data to reliably measure the results and outcomes of care.

Physician Workforce.—The final issue is the over supply of specialist and subspecialist physicians in the United States. In particular, the number of orthopedic medicine sports medicine graduates has jumped in recent years. If a buyer's market for surgical services develops, health plans will be in an even stronger position to dictate the terms. In the absence of a federal mandate, any effort to reduce the physician workforce must come from individual programs and physicians. The necessary downsizing is likely to be very difficult.

Discussion.—Four key issues that promise to have a major, potentially negative impact on medical and orthopedic practice were reviewed. Physicians must take the opportunities offered by the current situation and study how they practice, address variations in practice and treatment patterns, conduct high-quality, coordinated outcomes research, and deal with the problems posed by the physician workforce.

▶ This paper represents the Kennedy Lecture presented by Dr. Keller at the meeting of the American Orthopaedic Society for Sports Medicine in Atlanta, Georgia in February 1996. It clearly outlines 4 problematic areas that the orthopaedic surgeon specializing in sports medicine faces and is recommended reading.

J.S. Torg, M.D.

The Future of Anterior Cruciate Ligament Restoration
Dye SF (Univ of California, San Francisco)
Clin Orthop 325:130–139, 1996   4–23

Introduction.—An injured knee has its own unique anatomic, kinematic, physiologic, and treatment factors that contribute to its function. The current status of anatomy, kinematics, and physiology must be considered for the anterior cruciate ligament (ACL)–deficient knee before offering possible future therapeutic directions.

Anatomy/Kinematics.—The complexity of the knee makes it difficult to recreate the anatomic structure of the ACL. Currently, the following are not being recreated in ACL restorations: the broad asymmetrical femoral and tibial foot prints of the ACL origin and insertion; the normal pattern of mixed large and small fibrils; complex transition zones of fibrocartilage and calcified cartilage; neurologic systems that are important in sensory/proprioceptive function; and full biomechanical integrity. Normal recruitment patterns of ACL fibers under load have not been observed in ACL-reconstructed knees. Knee proprioception and functional outcome are closely correlated in knees that have undergone ACL reconstruction.

Physiology.—Homeostasis of the components of a living knee is necessary for normal long-term function. There are few known treatment options to control or enhance an individual's molecular and cellular maintenance and reparative mechanisms.

Goals of Treatment.—In the distant future, the ultimate goal of treatment is full restoration. This may be achieved through genetic manipulation. The midterm future goals include the use of resorbable stents with incorporated bioactive growth factors with the potential to induce normal ACL anatomy without traditional autograft or allograft. Goals for the near future focus on developing more benign autografts and allografts and absorbable fixation of the graft to bone. Graft placement can be enhanced through development of 3-dimensional arthroscopic visualization and robotic surgical techniques. Nonsurgical factors for improving treatment and management of the ACL include control of muscle atrophy, enhancement of cerebellar-proprioceptive rehabilitation, and better bracing techniques.

Conclusion.—The basic principle of any treatment approach must be to achieve the greatest functional range of load acceptance and transference with the least degree of risk to the patient.

▶ Although many in the field believe that the "problem" presented by the anterior cruciate ligament has been solved by current technology and surgical techniques, I agree with the author that the future holds yet greater potential. I would take issue, however, with his belief that a use for artificial grafts is not foreseen. Certainly, the experience with Gore-Tex was unfortunate. However, it appears to this observer that the design of the implant alone doomed it to failure. We have had an experience using a high density polyethylene woven graft with encouraging results. Unfortunately, this device is also no longer available.

J.S. Torg, M.D.

Failure of Anterior Cruciate Ligament Reconstruction

Corsetti JR, Jackson DW (Southern California Ctr for Sports Medicine, Long Beach; Long Beach Mem Med Ctr, Calif)
Clin Orthop 323:42–49, 1996   4–24

Introduction.—Successful reconstruction of the anterior cruciate ligament (ACL) depends on several factors, including choice and cross-sectional area of graft tissue, graft position, fixation, tensioning, and postoperative rehabilitation. The complex interactions that affect the biologic behavior of ACL replacement tissue in its new environment are discussed.

Biologic Remodeling and Biomechanical Incorporation.—Autograft and allograft ACL replacement tissues both undergo a similar remodeling process of avascular necrosis, cellular repopulation, collagen remodeling, and maturation. There is a loss of graft strength at completion of the remodeling process that is related to diminished graft function. The role of the various biologic factors that affect ultimate graft incorporation and function are less understood than biomechanical factors. Biologic incorporation depends on optimal positioning, tensioning, and postoperative protection from deleterious stress as the graft incorporates.

Graft Tensioning.—It is likely that the loss of strength in ACL grafts during remodeling is partly from the inability to reproduce physiologic tension and position precisely. Initial ACL graft tension has significant and lasting effects on the biomechanical properties of the knee. Undertensioning can lead to laxity and overtensioning can lead to restricted knee motion. The precise tension at which an ACL substitute is implanted is currently unknown.

Conclusion.—The ultimate function of the reconstructed ACL ligament depends on a combination of biologic and mechanical factors. Optimal functioning of the graft is contingent on its ability to perform in a new biomechanical and biologic environment.

▶ This is a less than comprehensive review in that the authors have failed to deal with the problem of inaccurate tunnel positioning. On the basis of my experience with ACL revision surgery, this is the most common cause of graft failure. Specifically, if the femoral tunnel is placed too far anterior, the graft lengthens in flexion, whereas if the tibial tunnel is placed too far posterior, it lengthens in extension. Anterior placement of the tibial tunnel results in graft impingement.

J.S. Torg, M.D.

Compartment Syndrome After Arthroscopic Surgery of Knee: A Report of Two Cases Managed Nonoperatively

Kaper BP, Carr CF, Shirreffs TG (Dartmouth Hitchcock Med Ctr, Lebanon, NH)
Am J Sports Med 25:123–125, 1997   4–25

Background.—Acute compartment syndrome is one of the most devastating potential complications of knee arthroscopic surgery. In the 2 patients described below, apparent compartment syndrome of the leg after arthroscopic procedures of the knee was managed conservatively.

Case Reports.—Man, 24, had injured his knee in a mountain bike accident 1 year earlier. Findings were consistent with an anterior cruciate ligament (ACL)-deficient knee, and an arthroscopic repair was planned. During the procedure, an old midsubstance tear and meniscal tears in the posterior horn of the medial and lateral menisci were found. Reconstruction of the ACL was accomplished with a bone-patellar tendon-bone autograft secured with 2 cannulated interference screws. The tourniquet was applied for 2 hours and 11 minutes. Postoperatively, the left side of the calf was tense to palpation. Compartment pressures in all 4 compartments of the leg, recorded intraoperatively, exceeded 120 mm Hg. The diastolic pressure was 60 mm Hg. Palpable dorsalis pedis and posterior tibialis pulses were noted clinically. The patient was awakened but reported no pain with passive stretch of the ankle or great toe. In the recovery room, the leg was elevated and ice applied to the knee and calf. Compartment pressures measured 1 and 4 hours postoperatively declined significantly. By the fourth hour, the calf was completely soft. No further signs or symptoms suggesting compartment syndrome occurred overnight, and the next day the patient was discharged home. His recovery was uneventful.

Case 2.—Man, 19, was a varsity football player who sustained a hyperextension injury to his left knee. Five days later, arthroscopic surgery was performed and the suspected diagnosis of posterior instability confirmed. He also had an avulsion fracture of the tibial insertion of the posterior cruciate ligament (PCL) and a radial tear of the anterior horn of the lateral meniscus. At this point, the patient's calf was palpated and found to be quite tense. The tourniquet was deflated. Palpable pulses were felt distally. Pressures in all 4 compartments were found to exceed 100 mm Hg. The procedure was stopped, and the patient was awakened and taken to the recovery room. No additional objective or subjective findings suggesting compartment syndrome were noted. During the next 6 hours, the extremity was elevated and monitored serially. At the end of the observation period, the calf was soft. The neurologic findings were still within normal limits. The patient subsequently recovered, and the surgical repairs were completed.

Conclusions.—Emergency fasciotomies are apparently not absolutely indicated when compartment pressures are increased after arthroscopic procedures on the knee. Observing the patient in the recovery room with serial assessments and repeat measures of compartment pressures may be adequate.

An Experimental Assessment of the Risk of Compartment Syndrome During Knee Arthroscopy

Ekman EF, Poehling GG (Wake Forest Univ, Winston-Salem, NC)
Arthroscopy 12:193–199, 1996   4–26

Background.—The development of compartment syndrome after arthroscopy has been reported. The risk of this complication associated with arthroscopy, especially when mechanical infusion systems are used, was investigated.

Methods.—Twelve hind limbs in 6 live pigs were subjected to 2 standardized capsulotomies to allow free extravasation of fluid. An additional 3 limbs were studied as shams.

Findings.—The mean maximum compartment pressure during fluid infusion was 78.8 mm Hg. When the interrelationships of infusion time, maximum compartment pressures, time of resolution of increased pressures, and intraarticular pressures were compared, significant variability was noted. Increased compartment pressures quickly resolved when fluid infusion was stopped. Postoperatively, all nerve conduction findings were normal. Electromyographic analysis yielded normal findings in the biceps, gracilis, abductor digiti quinti, and adductor digiti segundi. Though electromyographic assessment of the tibialis anterior and extensor digitorum brevis showed 1+ fibrillation, this finding was noted in the sham studies with the tourniquet alone. There was no evidence of myonecrosis on muscle biopsies. In addition, 5 of the 6 swine ambulated with no problem the first day after surgery, and the sixth limped for 2 days.

Findings.—These experimental data show that, in this swine model, the risk of sequelae from compartment syndrome during arthroscopy is minimal. This risk appears to be minimal even when significant fluid extravasation and increased compartment pressures have occurred.

▶ Having had several experiences with both "rock hard" thighs and calves during routine arthroscopic procedures, I am fully appreciative of the relevance of these 2 articles (abstracts 4–25 and 4–26). Although such occurrences are clearly a cause for concern, my own experience has been to turn off the pump and complete the procedure with irrigation solutions running at gravity flow. All cases usually resolve within an hour or 2 without residual morbidity. However, 1 of my patients did have a deep vein thrombosis develop postoperatively.

J.S. Torg, M.D.

Neuromuscular Performance Characteristics in Elite Female Athletes

Huston LJ, Wojtys EM (Univ of Michigan, Ann Arbor)
Am J Sports Med 24:427–436, 1996   4–27

Background.—There is great concern over the recent epidemic of severe knee injuries in female athletes. Rates of anterior cruciate ligament injury

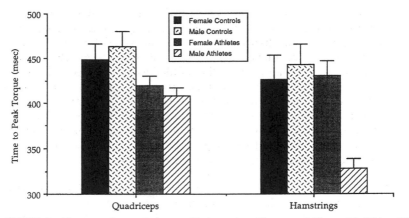

FIGURE 3.—Time-to-peak torque data at 60 degrees/sec. (Courtesy of Huston LJ, Wojtys EM: Neuromuscular performance characteristics in elite female athletes. *Am J Sports Med* 24:427–436, 1996.)

up to eight-fold higher than in male athletes have been reported. This study sought to identify neuromuscular factors predisposing to knee injuries in female athletes.

Methods.—The study included 40 active, healthy volunteers (26 men and 14 women); 40 Division I female athletes in various sports; and 60 male college football players. All participants were free of knee abnormalities. Testing included evaluation of knee function and activity level, arthrometer measurement of anterior tibial translation, strength and endurance testing using an isokinetic dynamometer, and an anterior tibial translation stress test. The anterior tibial translation test included a relaxed test, in which the subjects were asked not to contract their muscles in response to an anteriorly directed force, and a response test, in which subjects were to resist the force as soon as they felt tibial movement. Athletic and nonathletic women and men were compared for anterior tibial laxity; isokinetic measurements of strength, endurance, time-to-peak torque, muscle reaction time, and muscle recruitment order preferences.

Results.—Knee laxity testing showed that the knees of the athletes were tighter than those of the nonathletes, and that women's knees were looser than men's knees. Both groups of women had weaker quadriceps and hamstring muscles at 60 degrees/sec, even after normalization for body weight. The athletic groups had better muscle endurance in knee extension and flexion. After normalization for body weight, the women in both groups still had lesser endurance than their male counterparts. There were no differences between groups in time-to-peak torque in knee extension (Fig 3). However, average knee flexion time-to-peak torque was slower in female athletes than in male athletes. When tested at 240 degrees/sec, the female athletes had significantly slower peak torque times than the male athletes. The main muscle recruitment order in the female athletes was quadriceps-hamstring-gastrocnemius, whereas all other groups followed a hamstring-quadriceps-gastrocnemius pattern.

Conclusion.—Female athletes tended to use the quadriceps and gastrocnemius muscles to resist anterior tibial translation, whereas men more often recruited the hamstring muscle for initial knee stabilization. On isokinetic testing, time to hamstring peak torque was slower for female athletes than for male athletes. Female athletes had weaker knee extension and flexion strength and lower endurance rates than male athletes and male nonathletes. Greater strength of the lower-extremity muscles did not correlate with shorter muscle reaction times. The knees of women were generally laxer than the knees of men; the knees of athletes were tighter than the knees of controls. The findings may aid in understanding the difference in knee injury rates between men and women.

▶ The higher incidence of anterior cruciate ligament injuries among female athletes compared with males is a concern to all of us in the sports medicine field. These authors suggest that an imbalance in strength between the hamstrings and quadriceps may be 1 factor explaining the higher injury rate among women. Among other data, the authors report that the 5 strongest female athletes had a recruitment pattern favoring the use of the hamstrings first, as men do, whereas the 5 weakest women depended on the quadriceps. The obvious question is whether a muscle conditioning program designed to strengthen the hamstrings can alter the pattern of recruitment and decrease the incidence of anterior cruciate ligament injuries.

B.L. Drinkwater, Ph.D.

Age, Fat-Free Weight, and Isokinetic Peak Torque in High School Female Gymnasts

Housh TJ, Johnson GO, Housh DJ, et al (Univ of Nebraska-Lincoln)
Med Sci Sports Exerc 28:610–613, 1996   4–28

Introduction.—Increases in fat-free weight (FFW) and strength are observed during childhood and adolescence. Recent reports indicate an age effect for increases in peak torque in young female and male runners and high school wrestlers not accounted for by changes in FFW. The covariate influence of FFW on age-related increases in isokinetic peak torque were evaluated for leg flexion and extension in 72 high school female gymnasts.

Methods.—Preseason measurements of isokinetic leg flexion and extension strength were taken using a calibrated Cybex II dynamometer at 30, 180, and 300 degrees/sec. Body composition was measured via underwater weighing. Relative fat and FFW were calculated mathematically.

Results.—There was a significant correlation between age and leg flexion and extension peak torque. Leg flexion and extension were also significantly correlated with FFW. Significant first-order partial correlations were observed for leg extension at 30, 180, and 300 degrees/sec but not for leg flexion.

Conclusion.—The age-related increases in leg extension peak torque at 30, 180, and 300 degrees/sec could not be accounted for by changes in

FFW in this cohort of female high school gymnasts. It may be that factors other than FFW—such as increases in muscle mass per unit of FFW or neural maturation—may augment strength increases in female athletes during adolescence.

▶ One of the most surprising results of this study was finding that peak torque in leg flexion and extension strength was not as high for these gymnasts as that reported for female track and field athletes, basketball and soccer players, and alpine skiers. Whether athletes in those sports spend more time in the weight room or whether the difference is related to the specific demands of the sport was not discussed. It is interesting to note that whereas the increase in leg flexion peak torque could be accounted for by the increase in FFW, there were additional factors associated with the increase in leg extension strength. The authors suggest the possibility that these factors are neural in origin or can be accounted for by an increase in muscle mass per unit of FFW. The conclusion in the Huston and Wojty article (abstract 9–28) that women rely more on their quadriceps than their hamstring muscles to stabilize their knees during anterior tibial translation would suggest a closer look at this discrepancy in strength and recruitment of the hamstrings and quadriceps in relation to the anterior cruciate ligament injury question.

B.L. Drinkwater, Ph.D.

Prospective Validation of a Decision Rule for the Use of Radiography in Acute Knee Injuries
Stiell IG, Greenberg GH, Wells GA, et al (Univ of Ottawa, Ont, Canada)
JAMA 275:611–615, 1996   4–29

Background.—Most patients seen in United States' emergency departments with acute knee trauma undergo plain radiography. However, only 6% actually have a fracture. A previously derived decision rule for the use of radiography in such patients was validated.

Methods.—A convenience sample of 1,096 adults with acute knee injuries was included in the prospective study. Patients were assessed for 14 clinical variables that were components of the decision rule or felt to be of possible value for refining it. The decision rule states that a radiograph is only necessary for patients aged 55 years or older, patients with tenderness at the head of the fibula, patients with isolated tenderness of the patella, patients unable to flex to 90 degrees, and patients unable to bear weight both immediately and in the emergency department. The presence of 1 or more of these findings indicated radiography.

Findings.—The sensitivity of this decision rule for identifying 63 clinically important fractures was 1.0. Physicians correctly interpreted the rule in 96% of their examinations. The potential relative decrease in the use of radiography was an estimated 28%. The probability of fracture when the decision rule did not indicate radiography was 0. Attempts to refine the rule increased specificity but resulted in an unacceptable loss of sensitivity. *Conclusions.*—The decision rule described has a 100% sensitivity for identifying knee fractures. This reliable, acceptable tool may help decrease the use of radiography in patients with acute knee injury.

▶ Most noteworthy is the statement that "the current medicolegal climate of North American medical practice does not foster the most efficient use of diagnostic tests." It should be pointed out that the "decision rule" has not been tested in patients younger than 18 years and should not be applied to the pediatric population. Perhaps the term "guidelines" rather than "rule" would be more appropriate for this particular approach to patient evaluation.

J.S. Torg, M.D.

Reactions of Meniscal Tissue After Arthroscopic Laser Application: An In Vivo Study Using Five Different Laser Systems
Bernard M, Grouthues-Spork M, Hertel P, et al (Martin-Luther-Krankenhaus, Berlin; Universitätsklinikum Rudolf-Virchow der Humboldt Universität, Berlin)
Arthroscopy 12:441–451, 1996   4–30

Background.—The effect of laser radiation on meniscal tissue has been explored in many clinical and in vitro studies. However, the real extent of tissue damage caused by laser irradiation can only be determined in long-term in vivo studies.

Methods.—Arthroscopic meniscal cuts were made in the anterior horn of the medial meniscus of 72 pig knees. Five groups of pigs were operated on with 5 different laser systems, including the Neodym:YAG 1440 nm wavelength, Nd:YAG 1064 nm wavelength, Excimer, Holmium:YAG, and CO_2. In a sixth group, mechanical punches were used.

Findings.—All laser systems produced more damage to the meniscal tissue than the mechanical instruments. This damage consisted of a biological tissue reaction characterized by a necrotic zone that surrounded the meniscus cut. This necrotic zone was not visible intraoperatively. It was observed at 2, 6, and 12 weeks after sugery. These necrotic zones ranged in diameter from 1.5 to 9 mm. No necrotic zones in surrounding tissue were visible after meniscus cuts with mechanical instruments. Laser cuts in the meniscus resulted in more extensive healing reaction than did mechanical instrument cuts. The Nd:YAG 1064 nm, Ho:YAG, and CO_2 lasers caused incomplete healing, as the tissue repair showed by tissue growing from the synovial edge into the defect only. The Nd:YAG 1440 nm wavelength and Excimer resulted in tissue growing from the synovial edge and remodeling of original meniscal tissue manifested by reduction in the necrotic zone.

Conclusions.—Laser-related damage to meniscus tissue is much greater than can be seen during surgery. It is much greater than that caused by mechanical punches. The tissue's healing reaction is more extensive after laser application than after mechanical instruments. In vitro studies on laser-related tissue damage do not fully describe the effects of lasers on living tissue.

▶ To be emphasized is the conclusion that "Many findings of this study cannot be explained completely and further long-term in vivo investigations on laser effects are necessary."

J.S. Torg, M.D.

MRI of Anterior Cruciate Ligament Healing
Ihara H, Miwa M, Dya K, et al (Kyushu Rosai Hosp, Japan)
J Comput Assist Tomogr 20:317–321, 1996   4–31

Objective.—MRI has not been previously used to evaluate anterior cruciate ligament (ACL) healing. Results of a study evaluated the use of MRI in order to track healing of the ACL when it is treated conservatively by early protective motion.

Methods.—MRI was used to evaluate consecutive acute complete intra-ligamentous ruptures of the ACL in 50 patients (21 women), aged 15 to 63, before and 3 months after nonoperative conservative treatment. Tears occurred during sports activities in 45 patients. MRI reevaluations were performed in 29 patients at 11 months and in 7 at 24 months. The MRI image of the treated ACL was classified into 4 grades based on band size, type, and intensity. The treated ACL was evaluated arthroscopically using a probe and categorized into 4 grades based on continuity, tautness, and thickness. Agreement between arthroscopic and MRI findings were evaluated using Spearman correlation coefficients.

Treatment.—The knee was fitted with a brace with a traction system and treated using early continuous passive motion followed by dynamic joint control training progressing to full weight-bearing after 3 weeks, and brace removal at 3 or 4 months.

Results.—After 3 months 21 patients had a grade 1 MR assessment, 16 a grade 2, 4 a grade 3, and 9 a grade 4. After 11 months, 14 had a grade 1 MR assessment, 8 a grade 2, 3 a grade 3, and 4 a grade 4. The relationship between 3- and 11-month MR assessments was significant. At 24 months, the MR assessments showed 5 patients with a grade 1 result, 1 with a grade 2, and 1 with a grade 3 (Fig 3). Arthroscopic assessments showed 29 patients with a grade 1 rating, 10 with a grade 2, 6 with a grade 3, and 5 with a grade 4. Radiographic results showed 31 patients with a grade 1 assessment, 14 with a grade 2, 1 with a grade 3, and 4 with a grade 4. MR assessments were significantly related to both arthroscopic evaluations and stress radiographic images.

Conclusion.—MRI assessments of conservatively treated ACL healing agree well with radiographic and arthroscopic evaluations.

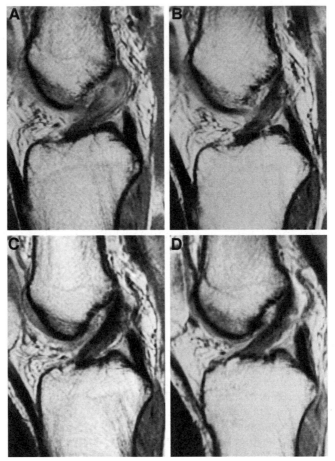

FIGURE 3.—MR image (sagittal proton density SE 2,000/20) taken the third day after the injury, shows a tear from the femoral attachment of the ACL (A). After 3 month treatment, normal-sized straight band spotted with high signal intensity (B) is seen. MR images post 11 (C) and post 24 (D) months show a well defined normal-sized straight band having homogeneous low signal intensity, stable with time. (Courtesy of Ihara H, Miwa M, Dya K, et al: MRI of anterior cruciate ligament healing. *J Comput Assist Tomogr* 20:317–321, 1996).

▶ Clinically, the sine qua non of anterior cruciate ligament integrity is the knee's ability to withstand the stress of vigorous physical activity including cutting maneuvers without locking, giving way, effusion or experiencing reinjury. These parameters, of course, were not evaluated. Thus, although the authors have demonstrated evidence of healing as manifested by magnetic resonant imaging, they fail to demonstrate clinical healing.

J.S. Torg, M.D.

A Comparison of Accuracy Between Clinical Examination and Magnetic Resonance Imaging in the Diagnosis of Meniscal and Anterior Cruciate Ligament Tears

Rose NE, Gold SM (Harbor-UCLA Med Ctr, Torrance, Calif)
Arthroscopy 12:398–405, 1996   4–32

Introduction.—Most patients with acute knee pain undergo arthroscopic surgery within 6 months, regardless of magnetic resonance imaging (MRI) findings. The value and cost-effectiveness of MRI in clinical decision-making for meniscal and anterior cruciate ligament (ACL) injuries are under question. The accuracy of clinical examination and MRI in the diagnosis of meniscal and ACL tears was compared with that of arthroscopy.

Methods.—Of 154 patients evaluated, 100 underwent preoperative clinical examination and MRI, and 54 patients underwent clinical examination alone. Accuracy of clinical and MRI findings was determined by arthroscopic findings. Sensitivity, specificity, positive predictive values (PPV), and negative predictive values (NPV) were calculated.

Results.—The accuracy, sensitivity, specificity, PPV, and NPV, respectively, for patients undergoing both clinical evaluation and MRI for medial and lateral meniscal tears, were 72%, 57%, 92%, 90%, and 62% for MRI and 79%, 79%, 79%, 83%, and 74% for clinical examination. There were no significant differences between clinical examination and MRI for any of these values. MRI contributed to treatment in 16 of 100 patients. In 54 patients who were evaluated by clinical examination alone, the accuracy, sensitivity, specificity, PPV, and NPV did not differ significantly from those calculated for the first 100 patients. The accuracy of MRI and clinical examination for ACL tears was 98% and 99%, respectively. Clinical examination and MRI were in complete agreement and correct for 97% of ACL tears.

Conclusion.—The MRI evaluation rarely added information to a careful history and physical examination in patients with acute knee injuries. Only certain circumstances justify the expense of an MRI for meniscal and ACL tears.

A Prospective Study Comparing the Accuracy of the Clinical Diagnosis of Meniscus Tear With Magnetic Resonance Imaging and Its Effect on Clinical Outcome

Miller GK (Northwestern Univ, Evanston, Ill; Windy City Orthopedics and Sports Medicine, Evanston, Ill)
Arthroscopy 12:406–413, 1996   4–33

Introduction.—It is not known if preoperative MRI improves diagnostic accuracy once a diagnosis of torn meniscus has been made, based on clinical findings. Fifty-seven consecutive knees were evaluated by MRI to determine if it could improve accuracy in patients with initial clinical diagnosis of torn meniscus.

Methods.—A clinical diagnosis of torn meniscus was made by the operating surgeon in this single-blind, prospective investigation. All patients underwent preoperative MRI. Clinical and MRI findings were confirmed by arthroscopy.

Results.—The diagnostic accuracy of clinical examination and MRI was 80.7% and 73.7%, respectively. Clinical diagnosis and MRI correctly identified hemarthrosis in 60.0% and 44.5% of patients, respectively. Blind reliance on MRI alone would have resulted in inappropriate treatment in 35.1% of knees. Arthroscopy frequently found additional pathology not identified by MRI.

Conclusion.—The MRI is unlikely to prevent unnecessary surgery. If used as a diagnostic gold standard, MRI will misdirect surgery in 1 of 3 patients. Elimination of MRI in the diagnosis of torn meniscus will save large amounts of money without compromising patients' care. An MRI may be a useful adjunct to clinical examination in select patients, but surgeons must be aware of its limitations and potential sources of error.

▶ These two studies (Abstracts 4–32 and 4–33) support the findings of Gelb, et al.[1] that MRI is not a cost-effective method of evaluating knee injuries compared with a skilled examiner, is overused, adds little to the overall treatment plan for most patients, and should not replace a careful history and physical examination.

J.S. Torg, M.D.

Reference

1. Gelb HJ, Glasgow SG, Sapega AA, et al: Magnetic resonance imaging of knee disorders. Clinical value and cost-effectiveness in a sports medicine practice. *Am J Sports Med* 24:99–103, 1996.

Gender Differences in Anterior Cruciate Ligament Injury Rates in Wisconsin Intercollegiate Basketball

Oliphant JG, Drawbert JP (Univ of Wisconsin, Eau Claire)
J Athletic Train 31:245–247, 1996   4–34

Background.—The incidence of anterior cruciate ligament (ACL) injuries in female basketball players has in recent years exceeded that of male basketball players. The ACL injury rate for male and female intercollegiate basketball players in Wisconsin was determined and various possible contributing factors were examined.

Methods.—Surveys (22) were sent to certified athletic trainers at 22 Wisconsin colleges and universities having both a men's and a women's intercollegiate basketball team. Number of injuries and data regarding these injuries were sought for the previous 5 years. Seventeen of the 22 surveys were returned.

Results.—The rate of ACL injury among basketball players was 2.3 times higher for women than for men. The factors of contact/noncontact mechanism, game or practice, time of season, and right or left hand dominance did not prove significant.

Conclusions.—The difference in ACL injury rate between basketball players of different sexes is significant. Further studies are necessary to determine the cause of this difference. Female basketball players may be more susceptible to injury because of initiating the sport at a later age or with less strength, or because of practicing a style of play that is less "up-tempo" than that normally practiced by men. Screening to detect athletes at higher risk of ACL, with the option of subsequent increased strength or movement training, would be desirable.

▶ Women athletes participating in basketball and soccer are at a greater risk for ACL injuries than their male counterparts. Many different etiologic factors have been presented, which may or may not be the reason for a gender difference in these injuries. Women participating in these sports should do specific quadriceps, gastrocnemius, and hamstring strength training, also agility and specific movement drills, which may help prevent some of these injuries.

F.J. George, A.T.C., P.T.

Knee Injury Patterns Among Men and Women in Collegiate Basketball and Soccer: NCAA Data and Review of Literature
Arendt E, Dick R (Univ of Minnesota, Minneapolis; Natl Collegiate Athletic Assoc, Overland Park, Ks)
Am J Sports Med 23:694–701, 1995   4–35

Purpose.—Previous studies have reported higher rates of anterior cruciate ligament (ACL) injuries in female basketball and handball players than in men playing the same sports. These studies have had sample and methodologic shortcomings, however. The incidence of ACL injuries in a broad sample of female and male athletes was assessed to test the hypothesis that women are at higher risk for ACL injury.

Methods.—The study used data from the voluntary National Collegiate Athletic Association (NCAA) Injury Surveillance System from 1989 to 1993 for the sports of soccer and basketball. A random sample of injuries was selected, with at least 10% representation of each NCAA division and region. Reportable injuries were those related to an organized practice or game, requiring medical attention, and restricting the athlete's activity for 1 or more days. The unit of risk was an athlete-exposure, defined as 1 athlete participating in 1 practice or game in which there is the possibility of injury. The injury rate was expressed as number of injuries per 1,000 athlete-exposures.

Results.—Female soccer players had more knee injuries than male soccer players, whether assessed by injury rate or as a percentage of all injuries.

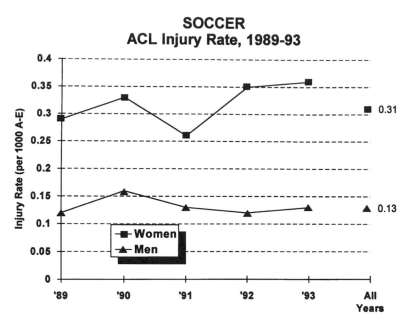

FIGURE 1.—Anterior cruciate ligament injury rate among male and female soccer players during the 5-year study. (Courtesy of Arendt E, Dick R: Knee injury patterns among men and women in collegiate basketball and soccer: NCAA data and review of literature. *Am J Sports Med* 23:694–701, 1995.)

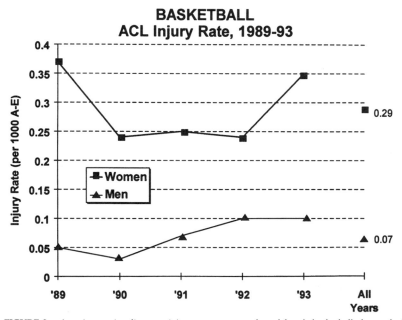

FIGURE 2.—Anterior cruciate ligament injury rate among male and female basketball players during the 5-year study. (Courtesy of Arendt E, Dick R: Knee injury patterns among men and women in collegiate basketball and soccer: NCAA data and review of literature. *Am J Sports Med* 23:694–701, 1995.)

The rate of ACL injuries was 0.31 in women's soccer compared with 0.13 in men's soccer (Fig 1). The rate of cartilage tears was also higher for women, 0.34 vs. 0.19. For female soccer players, ACL injuries were most likely to involve "no apparent contact" followed by "player contact," whereas the order was reversed for male soccer players. The knee injury rate was higher for female than for male basketball players. The rate of ACL injury was 0.29 for women vs. 0.07 for men; the rate of torn cartilage was 0.29 for women vs. 0.13 for men (Fig 2).

Conclusion.—Female soccer and basketball players are at higher risk of ACL injuries than men in the same sports. The cause is probably multifactorial. It may include extrinsic factors such as muscle strength, experience, and conditioning, and intrinsic factors such as ligament size, limb alignment, and joint laxity. Explanations for the sex-specific factors related to ACL injury may help in developing preventive interventions.

▶ Any doubt that there are more knee injuries among female athletes than male athletes should be put to rest by this study. Hopefully, this will lead to increased attention to determining what factors are responsible for the higher incidence of knee injuries—and ACL injuries in particular—among women. The authors believe the cause of these injuries is multifactorial. Fortunately, many of the contributing factors they list—such as muscle strength, skill, and conditioning—are amenable to change. Whether attention to these factors will reduce the incidence of these injuries remains to be seen.

B.L. Drinkwater, Ph.D.

Combined Injuries of the Anterior Cruciate and Medial Collateral Ligaments of the Knee: Effect of Treatment on Stability and Function of the Joint

Hillard-Sembell D, Daniel DM, Stone ML, et al (San Diego Kaiser Med Ctr, Calif)
J Bone Joint Surg Am 78A:169–176, 1996   4–36

Introduction.—Combined injuries of the medial collateral and anterior cruciate ligaments have been treated by various methods, and there is little consensus on the best management. To determine whether an injury of the medial collateral ligament alters the result of reconstruction of the anterior cruciate ligament, 66 patients were retrospectively studied.

Methods.—The study group included 41 men and 25 women (mean age, 35 years). Most were injured during sports activities. All patients were examined within 14 days after the injury and all had valgus instability. Eleven underwent reconstruction of the anterior cruciate ligament and repair of the medial collateral ligament (all within 2 weeks after the injury), 33 had reconstruction of the anterior cruciate ligament only (21 within 2 weeks after the injury), and 22 were treated nonoperatively. Operative treatment was recommended for patients younger than 30 years who regularly participated in sports. Conservative treatment consisted of immobilization, followed by a brace, home exercise, and a 3-month delay in return to sports. Follow-up evaluations included a questionnaire to assess symptoms and level of impairment, functional tests, and clinical examination of range of motion and stability of the joint.

Results.—The mean follow-up interval was 45 months. Clinical examinations showed no signs of valgus instability. Stress roentgenograms, available for 60 patients, showed injured vs. uninjured knees to have a mean difference of 1.3 mm in medial joint space. Eight patients had evidence of instability; the opening of the medial joint space was more than 2.5 mm greater in the injured knee of these patients. Four had not had surgery, 2 had reconstruction of the anterior cruciate ligament only, and 2 had both ligaments repaired. Patients who had a combined ligamentous injury and reconstruction of the anterior cruciate ligament only were compared with other patients who had reconstruction of an isolated tear of the anterior cruciate ligament. With a mean follow-up of 35 months, these 2 groups did not differ in anterior displacement, impairment of function, level of sports participation, strength, or results of the 1-leg hop for distance test.

Conclusion.—In patients with combined injuries of the anterior cruciate and medial collateral ligaments of the knee and mild or moderate valgus instability, the medial collateral ligament does not need to be repaired when the anterior cruciate ligament is reconstructed.

▶ The observations and conclusions of the authors are in keeping with my own clinical experience.

J.S. Torg, M.D.

The Relationship Between Static Posture and ACL Injury in Female Athletes
Loudon JK, Jenkins W, Loudon KL (Univ of Kansas, Kansas City; East Carolina Univ, Greenville, NC)
J Orthop Sports Phys Ther 24:91–97, 1996   4–37

Objective.—Injuries to the knee and the anterior cruciate ligament (ACL) are common in women athletes. Biomechanical deviations of the legs may contribute to the greater risk of injury of women. A static posture consisting of anterior pelvic tilt and knee joint hyperextension may contribute to the risk of injury. The effect of postural faults on noncontact ACL injury in women athletes was studied.

Methods.—Pelvic position, femoral anteversion, hamstring length, standing sagittal knee extension, standing knee angle in the frontal plane, the navicular drop test, and subtalar joint neutral position were determined for 20 women aged 16–41 years, with 1 ACL injury treated surgically in 8 patients and nonsurgically in 12, and 20 age-matched controls. Data between groups were compared statistically.

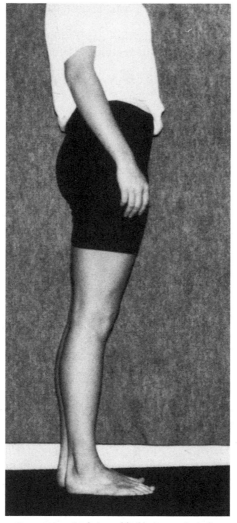

FIGURE 2.—Faulty static posture; sagittal view of faulty posture, including anteriorly tilted pelvis and knee joint hyperextension. (Courtesy of Loudon JK, Jenkins W, Louden KL: The relationship between static posture and ACL injury in female athletes. *J Orthop Sports Phys Ther* 24[2]:91–97, 1996).

Results.—A postural model that may predispose female athletes to ACL injuries includes an anterior pelvic tilt, internal rotation of the hip, increased valgus at the knee, recurvatum of the knee, and excessive subtalar joint pronation (Fig 2). Female athletes with ACL injuries had significantly shorter hamstrings than did female athletes without injury. Female athletes with ACL injuries had greater navicular drop test scores than did uninjured female athletes. Female athletes with subtalar joint pronation and knee recurvatum were at higher risk of ACL injury than female athletes with pronation only. Treatment should include correcting posture, wearing appropriate shoes and orthotics, and training to move in patterns that minimize injury.

Conclusion.—Knee hyperextension with subtalar joint pronation increases the risk of ACL injury in female athletes.

▶ The authors have identified components of static posture in female athletes that may predispose them to ACL injuries. They describe these components as knee recurvatum, excessive navicular drop, and excessive subtalar joint pronation. If female athletes with these problems are identified, they may benefit from correction of these postural faults through training, exercises, and the use of orthotics and proper footwear. The importance of training and coaching athletes to prevent injuries cannot be stressed enough. Please refer to a study done by Ettlinger et al. and abstracted in the 1996 YEAR BOOK OF SPORTS MEDICINE, with my comments.[1]

F.J. George, A.T.C., P.T.

Reference

1. 1996 YEAR BOOK OF SPORTS MEDICINE, pp 44–46.

Arthroscopically Assisted Reconstruction of the Anterior Cruciate Ligament: A Prospective Randomized Analysis of the Techniques
O'Neill DB (St John Sports Medicine Ctr, Nassau Bay, Tex)
J Bone Joint Surg Am 78A:803–813, 1996   4–38

Background.—Rupture of the anterior cruciate ligament (ACL) has been successfully treated with both open and arthroscopically assisted reconstruction techniques. The outcome of arthroscopically assisted reconstruction of the ACL with a semitendinosus-gracilis graft, arthroscopically assisted reconstruction of the ACL with a patellar ligament graft, and endoscopic reconstruction with a patellar ligament graft were compared in a prospective, randomized study of 127 patients with ACL rupture.

Methods.—The study group consisted of 125 patients with ACL rupture who underwent reconstruction from 1989 and 1992. Group I included 40 patients who underwent arthroscopically assisted reconstruction of the ACL with a semitendinosus-gracilis graft; group II included 40 patients who underwent arthroscopically assisted reconstruction with a patellar ligament graft; and group III included 45 patients who underwent endoscopic reconstruction with a patellar graft. There were no significant differences in age, sex, athletic activity, interval between injury and reconstruction, previous procedures, and associated injuries among the 3 groups. All patients followed the same postoperative rehabilitation regimen. The knee was evaluated at follow-up by radiographs, dynamometer, KT-2000 arthrometer, and functional tests.

Results.—The difference in laxity between the involved and the contralateral knee was 3 mm or less in 83% of group I, 93% of group II, and

87% of group III. It was 2 mm or less in 75% of group I, 78% of group II, and 78% of group III. Normal athletic activity was resumed by 88% of group I, 95% of group II, and 89% of group III. Four grafts failed due to trauma. One graft in group I and 1 in group III had at least 7 mm difference in laxity between the 2 knees. There were fewer additional operative procedures performed on group III patients. Patients in Group II returned to the highest level of athletic activity of the 3 groups. There were no significant differences in the overall outcomes among these 3 treatment groups. There were no significant differences in outcome between acute and late reconstructions, including those performed with a semitendinosus-gracilis graft. Patient age had no significant effect on outcome.

Conclusions.—A series of 125 patients with ruptures of the ACL underwent reconstruction by either arthroscopically assisted reconstruction with an autogenous semitendinosus-gracilis graft, arthroscopically assisted reconstruction with a patellar ligament graft, or endoscopic reconstruction with a patellar ligament graft. In this patient series, there were no significant differences in outcome among these 3 groups, nor between acute and delayed reconstructions. This study is continuing with additional patients and longer follow-up to determine whether this will reveal any differences in outcome among these 3 procedures for treating rupture of the ACL.

▶ This paper brings to our attention several interesting points. First, contrary to prevailing thought, the semitendinosus-gracilis graft was successful whether it was performed on an acutely or chronically unstable knee. Postoperative rehabilitation was similar, with immediate full range of knee motion and full weight- bearing regardless of technique employed. Although not statistically significant, 96% of the knees with the tendon grafts were rated as having normal or near-normal function, as opposed to 88% of those with infrapatellar-bone-tendon-bone.

J.S. Torg, M.D.

Classification and Management of Arthrofibrosis of the Knee After Anterior Cruciate Ligament Reconstruction
Shelbourne KD, Patel DV, Martini DJ (Methodist Sports Medicine Ctr, Indianapolis, Ind)
Am J Sports Med 24:857–862, 1996   4–39

Introduction.—Arthrofibrosis of the knee develops in some patients after anterior cruciate ligament (ACL) reconstruction. The evaluation and treatment of such patients could be enhanced by a grading system based on clinical findings. A group of 72 patients with disabling knee arthrofibrosis provided data for a simple and practical grading system for managing arthrofibrosis of the knee after ACL reconstruction.

Methods.—The patients were treated between 1983 and 1993 by a single surgeon. All had symptoms of persistent anterior knee pain and stiffness and were unable to return to their previous levels of activity. None experienced improvement after a rehabilitation protocol or with use of an extension board or extension casts. Four levels of arthrofibrosis were identified: 25 patients had <10 degrees of extension loss and normal flexion (type 1); 16 had >10 degrees of extension loss and normal flexion (type 2); 15 had >10 degrees of extension loss and >25 degrees of flexion loss with decreased medial and lateral movement of the patella and no patellar infera (type 3); and 16 had >10 degrees of extension loss, ≥30 degrees of flexion loss, and objective patella infera with marked patellar tightness (type 4). All patients underwent outpatient arthroscopic surgery.

Results.—The mean interval between the initial ACL surgery and arthroscopic scar resection was 12.5 months. Patients were followed up for an average of 35 months after scar resection. The mean range of motion was improved in all types of arthrofibrosis. Seven patients with type III and 13 with type 4 arthrofibrosis lacked full symmetrical flexion. Full extension was achieved by 88% of patients with type 1, 81% of patients with type 2, 80% of patients with type 3, and 69% of patients with type 4 arthrofibrosis. All reported subjective improvement in knee stiffness, self-assessment, and functional activity scores. All patients with types 2, 3, and 4 arthrofibrosis required anterior scar resection down to the proximal tibia; those with types 3 or 4 required medial and lateral capsular releases and knee manipulation. Serial extension casting was used postoperatively in all cases of types 2, 3, and 4 arthrofibrosis. No complications resulted from the scar resection procedure.

Conclusion.—Arthrofibrosis can be a disabling complication after ACL surgery. Patients have pain, impaired knee function, and restriction in their activities. A classification system based on loss of motion and patellar tightness and contracture compared with the opposite, normal knee provides guidelines for individualized treatment.

▶ The authors have successfully categorized and outlined the treatment regimen for pathologic periarticular and intraarticular scar formation associated with arthrofibrosis after ACL reconstruction. It is pointed out that in a group of uninjured athletes, men averaged 5 degrees and women averaged 6 degrees of hyperextension. The authors believe that for patients undergoing ACL reconstruction, the goal is to restore full extension, including hyperextension, compared with the opposite knee. Thus, they have defined arthrofibrosis as any symptomatic limitation in knee motion compared with the normal contralateral knee. The point is well taken that arthrofibrosis after ACL surgery can result from a variety of pathologic abnormalities and that a thorough understanding of the problem and a systematic approach to its management can lead to a satisfactory result.

J.S. Torg, M.D.

Reconstruction of the Anterior Cruciate Ligament With Human Allograft: Comparison of Early and Late Results

Noyes FR, Barber-Westin SD (Cincinnati Sportsmedicine and Orthopedic Ctr, Ohio; Deaconess Hosp, Cincinnati, Ohio)
J Bone Joint Surg Am 78A:524–537, 1996   4–40

Background.—Data on any changes in the long term are needed to determine the ability of allografts to provide long-term stability and function of the knee. The long-term outcomes of surgical treatment with 1 of 2 types of allograft for acute ruptures of the anterior cruciate ligament in 1 series were reported.

Methods and Findings.—Sixty-eight patients who had undergone reconstruction of an acute rupture of the anterior cruciate ligament with a fascia lata or bone-patellar ligament-bone allograft were assessed at 2–4 years and again at 5–9 years after surgery. At the first follow-up assessment, 78% of the patients tested using an arthrometer at 89 newtons had less than 3 mm of increased anterior-posterior displacement compared with that of the contralateral limb. At the second assessment, this finding was present in 79%. Arthrometric and pivot-shift-test findings indicated that 48% of the 64 grafts were considered functional at the first assessment; 22%, partially functional; and 3%, failures. At the second assessment, 50% of the 68 grafts were functional; 19%, partially functional; and 7%, failures. Ninety-three percent of the patients had no palpable patellofemoral crepitus and 7% had moderate crepitus at the first evaluation, compared with 75% and 24%, respectively, at the second evaluation. Severe crepitus was noted at this time in 1%. At the first assessment, outcomes were judged to be excellent or good in 60% of patients, fair in 33%, and poor in 6%. At the second assessment, these proportions were 66%, 26%, and 7%, respectively.

Conclusion.—These data show that favorable long-term outcomes can be achieved with allografts in this patient population. However, arthroscopically assisted reconstruction with a bone–patellar ligament–bone autogenous graft is recommended as the treatment of choice for acute rupture of the anterior cruciate ligament.

▶ This report gives a comparison of short- and long-term follow-up of the results in 68 patients who had received either a fascia lata or a bone–patellar ligament–bone allograft to replace an anterior cruciate ligament. It presents the follow-up evaluation after 5–9 years (mean, 7 years) postoperatively. As there were no decreases in the function of the knee in the long-term follow up, it was concluded that allografts provide good long-term replacements for the anterior cruciate ligament. However, allografts are no longer used as anterior cruciate ligament replacements because of the cost and the risk of disease transmission; the authors note that they currently recommend reconstruction with autogenous bone–patellar ligament–bone grafts. No mention was made of the current practice of many surgeons of using 1 of the hamstring tendons as an anterior cruciate ligament replacement, to avoid the weakening effect on the patellar tendon.

M.J.L. Alexander, Ph.D.

Long-term Survival of Chondrocytes in an Osteochondral Articular Cartilage Allograft: A Case Report
Convery FR, Akeson WH, Amiel D, et al (Univ of California, San Diego)
J Bone Joint Surg Am 78A:1082–1088, 1996   4–41

Introduction.—Although osteochondral allografts have not gained widespread acceptance, many younger patients are referred for the procedure after nonoperative treatment has failed and when prosthetic arthroplasty or arthrodesis of the affected joint is not appropriate. The case presented here is accompanied by a description of the histologic characteristics, viability of the chondrocytes, and biochemical changes in an osteochondral allograft specimen that had been in situ for 10 years.

> *Case Report.*—Man, 28, worked as a mail carrier and had injured his left knee while playing baseball. Arthroscopic débridement relieved the symptoms, and the patient was told he had a large defect of cartilage and bone in the left medial femoral condyle. Eighteen months later, symptoms persisted with activity and a second arthroscopic procedure failed to relieve his pain. The patient was then referred for osteochondral allografting to fill a defect (Fig 1). At this time, a loose body was removed from the weight-bearing surface of the left medial femoral condyle and was replaced anatomically with a fresh osteochondral shell allograft.
>
> Approximately 8 years after this procedure, persistent pain caused the man to retire with a disability pension from his job as a mail carrier. Two years later, a second allograft was inserted after roentgenograms showed a transverse fracture and collapse of the allograft. Autogenous bone was placed in the crater and the defect filled with a fresh allograft of cartilage and subchondral bone. Histologic and biochemical analyses were performed on the initial allograft.

Discussion.—This patient's graft failed as a result of resorption of the transplanted subchondral allograft bone rather than of metabolic activity of the articular cartilage. In contrast to the technique used in this case, additional autogenous bone graft is now placed beneath the allograft to fill the gap between the host bed and the allograft. It appears that the allograft's collapse was relatively recent and that it had remained functional until the collapse. Although viable chondrocytes were present 10 years after transplantation, it is uncertain whether living chondrocytes are required for a successful clinical result. Findings suggest that a fresh osteo-

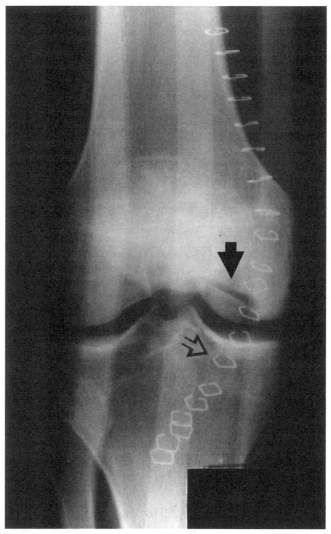

FIGURE 1.—Anteroposterior roentgenogram of the knee, made in 1982, after the initial allograft procedure. The transplanted allograft is identified by the *open arrow*. There is a gap between the allograft and the host bone *(solid arrow)*. (Courtesy of Convery FR, Akeson WH, Amiel D, et al: Long-term survival of chondrocytes in an osteochondral articular cartilage allograft: A case report. *J Bone Joint Surg Am* 78A:1082–1088, 1996.)

chondral allograft is a viable alternative to arthrodesis or prosthetic arthroplasty to reconstruct defects of articular cartilage.

▶ This study examined the controversial question of the use of allografts in repair of articular cartilage defects. This type of treatment is not commonly used in recent years, because of the lack of appropriate donors, fear of transmitted disease, and uncertainty regarding possible immune responses to the allograft. This study was a case report of a young man who received an osteochondral allograft for a baseball injury to the knee joint. After 8 years, he had a transverse fracture and collapse of the allograft; so a second allograft was inserted. The authors reported that the allograft failed as a result of resorption of the transplanted subchondral allograft bone; there was no evidence of revascularization of the subchondral bone of the allograft. They noted that they were unable to determine whether it was a successful clinical result, because the bone implant failed but the articular cartilage had viable chondrocytes 10 years later. They concluded that the use of a fresh osteochondral allograft to reconstruct articular cartilage defects is a viable alternative treatment to arthrodesis or prosthetic arthroplasty.

M.J.L. Alexander, Ph.D.

Anterior Cruciate Ligament Functional Brace Use in Sports
Wojtys EM, Kothari SU, Huston LJ (Univ of Michigan, Ann Arbor)
Am J Sports Med 24:539–546, 1996   4–42

Introduction.—Objective results of independent brace testing and subjective testimonials of brace users and manufacturers are not in agreement regarding the clinical role of functional braces. Clinical trials indicate that functional knee braces are not capable of eliminating most pathologic anteroposterior translation or internal-external rotation in the anterior cruciate ligament (ACL)-deficient knee. It may be hazardous to allow patients with unstable ACL deficient knees to participate in sports because they are at risk for further injury. The effect of bracing on neuromuscular function, anterior tibial translation, and isometric performance was evaluated in 5 consecutive patients with chronic, complete tears of the ACL.

Methods.—Six popular braces were evaluated in a special anterior tibial translation stress test. Research subjects' knees were placed in a device that allowed anterior tibial translation. With and without braces, isokinetic performance and neuromuscular function were monitored in the medial and lateral quadriceps, medial and lateral hamstring, and gastrocnemius muscles.

Results.—Medial and lateral quadriceps spinal cord reflex response time was significantly improved using all 6 braces. In the hamstrings, the spinal reflex in the lateral hamstring muscle was improved using all 6 braces. The medial hamstring muscle response time was improved with 3 braces and slowed with the other 3 braces. Gastrocnemius muscle response time was relatively unchanged. The intermediate response time was slowed in most muscle groups with the use of a brace. Voluntary muscle reaction times were generally slowed by knee braces in the quadriceps and hamstring muscles. Anterior tibial translation was decreased by an average of 33.1% from baseline during muscles-relaxed tests. The braces reduced anterior tibial translation by an average of 80.1% from baseline during the muscles-contracted tests. This reduction in anterior tibial translation was significant for both sets of muscles tests. Isokinetic testing showed that brace application decreases hamstring muscle performance in each of 4 hamstring mucle variables.

Conclusion.—Brace use was associated with improvement in spinal level muscle reaction times, particularly in the quadriceps muscle. Use of some braces seemed to consistently decrease muscle reaction times at the voluntary level. Anterior tibial translation was significantly reduced with bracing.

Clinical Significance.—Tibial control was improved at low levels of force. It is not known what degree of control is present at higher, functional levels. With the delays in voluntary muscle reaction times, there is a question regarding which is most important—tibial control or muscle inhibition. It would be helpful to have data on the ACL strain-reducing capabilities of braces in the reconstructed knee. More research is needed to answer the important questions regarding the role of functional bracing after ACL injury or surgery.

▶ The authors raise some serious questions regarding the use of functional knee braces in ACL-deficient or postoperative knees. Further studies must be done to determine whether anterior translation can be reduced with these braces and whether the braces do inhibit muscle function. If this hypothesis is true, then it must be determined which of these factors is more important in the ACL-deficient knee. Is it safe to inhibit muscle function if anterior translation is reduced? Are we helping or hurting our patients by recommending these braces?

F.J. George, A.T.C., P.T.

Long-term Followup of the Untreated Isolated Posterior Cruciate Ligament-Deficient Knee
Boynton MD, Tietjens BR (Eastwood Orthopaedic Clinic, Auckland, New Zealand; Med College of Wisconsin, Milwaukee)
Am J Sports Med 24:306–310, 1996   4–43

Background.—The natural history of knees with posterior cruciate ligament (PCL) disruption with no other ligamentous injury has not been well documented. Such information is needed before surgical reconstruction of the isolated PCL-deficient knee can be recommended.

Methods.—Thirty-eight patients with isolated PCL-deficient knees were evaluated at a mean of 13.4 years after injury. Each patient filled out a standardized questionnaire and underwent physical assessment as well as radiography of both knees.

Findings.—Twenty-one percent of the patients underwent surgery for meniscal injuries after PCL injury. On a 50-point scale, the mean score for function was 34.4 for patients with meniscal operations and 40 for those without. Eighty-one percent of the 30 patients with isolated PCL-deficient knees with normal menisci had at least occasional pain, and 56% had at least occasional swelling. Articular degeneration on radiographs increased as length of time from injury increased.

Conclusions.—The prognosis for isolated PCL-deficient knees appears to vary. Some patients have significant symptoms and articular deterioration, whereas others essentially have no symptoms, retaining their usual knee function.

▶ This is a well-documented study with adequate long-term follow-up. The authors have certainly accomplished the purpose of the study, which was "... to increase our understanding of the symptoms and functional and articular surface changes experienced by patients with isolated PCL-deficient knees." They also imply that we must first understand the natural history of the problem before recommending surgical reconstruction of the isolated PCL-deficient knee. Unfortunately, the observations and conclusions do not contribute further insight into the important issue of who, if anyone, should have a ligamentous reconstruction.

J.S. Torg, M.D.

The Effect of Femoral Tunnel Position and Graft Tensioning Technique on Posterior Laxity of the Posterior Cruciate Ligament-Reconstructed Knee

Burns WC II, Draganich LF, Pyevich M, et al (Univ of Chicago)
Am J Sports Med 23:424–430, 1995   4–44

Introduction.—The posterior cruciate ligament (PCL) is known to play an important role in preventing abnormal posterior laxity of the knee. However, the natural history of PCL deficiency is unclear; most studies of PCL reconstruction have found that posterior laxity is not completely eliminated. The role of knee flexion angle during tensioning of PCL grafts has not been well studied. Cadaver knees were studied to determine the effects of femoral tunnel position and graft tensioning technique on posterior laxity.

Methods.—Seven cadaver knees were mounted in an anterior-posterior laxity testing machine. Each PCL was transected at the level of the tibial attachment, then reconstructed. A specially designed alignment jig was used to locate the isometric femoral tunnel site. Two more femoral tunnels were placed 5 mm proximal and distal to this site. Two different techniques of graft tensioning were compared as well: tensioning at 90 degrees of knee flexion while applying a 156 N anterior drawer force to the tibia, and tensioning with the knee in full extension without an anterior drawer force.

Results.—Graft tension decreased with knee flexion with the graft in the proximal femoral tunnel. With the graft in the distal femoral tunnel, the opposite was true: graft tension increased with knee flexion. Graft placement in the isometric femoral tunnel led to nearly isometric graft tension from 0 to 90 degrees of knee flexion. Graft tensioning in flexion with an anterior drawer force restored normal posterior stability at 0 to 90 degrees for the distal femoral tunnel position, at 0 to 75 degrees for the isometric tunnel position, and at 0 to 45 degrees for the proximal tunnel position. When the graft was tensioned with the knee in extension and without an anterior drawer force, posterior translation was significantly abnormal between 15 and 90 degrees for all femoral tunnel positions.

Conclusions.—In the PCL-reconstructed knee, the graft positioning technique is a major contributor to the posterior stability produced by the patellar tendon reconstruction technique used in this study. Posterior stability is improved when the graft is tensioned at 90 degrees with an anterior drawer force of 156 N than when the graft is tensioned at full extension. Placing the femoral tunnel in a more distal position appears to improve posterior stability at increased angles of flexion.

▶ This paper was the winner of the American Orthopedic Society For Sports Medicine 1994 Cabaud Award. An in vitro bench study, it raises the question, "Why should tensioning the graft at 90 degrees of knee flexion with an anterior drawer force result in better posterior stability?" It is stated that "the answer appears to lay in the practical details of graft tensioning." To this observer, the specifics of their explanation are conjectural and not necessarily convincing.

J.S. Torg, M.D.

Primary Repair for Posterior Cruciate Ligament Injuries
Richter M, Kiefer H, Hehl G, et al (Univ of Ulm, Germany)
Am J Sports Med 24:298–305, 1996   4–45

Background.—Posterior cruciate ligament (PCL) injuries with associated ligamentous injuries are treated operatively. The treatment of isolated PCL rupture remains controversial. A clinical retrospective study was performed to examine long-term results of primary repair of PCL injuries.

Methods.—Between 1981 and 1988, 58 patients underwent primary repair of acute PCL injuries. Of these 58 patients, 53 were available for follow-up and were included in this review. There were 40 men and 13 women aged 18 to 61 years. Among these patients, 16 had isolated PCL ruptures, 16 had complex injuries with either capsular or collateral ligament involvement, and 21 had both posterior and anterior cruciate ligament ruptures. In this series of patients, 46 were treated with transosseus multiple-loop sutures and 7 with bony avulsions were treated with screw osteosynthesis. The average follow-up period was 7.5 years. All patients were evaluated by questionnaire, clinical examination, KT-1000 arthrometer, functional testing, radiographs and Cybex II isokinetic strength analysis. The results of this evaluation were assessed according to the International Knee Documentation Committee (IKDC) evaluation form and Lysholm score.

Results.—The mean Lysholm score in this patient group was 82.4. Of the 53 patients, 38 returned to preinjury levels of activity, 35 had normal subjective assessments, 41 were normal on the IKDC knee evaluation form, and 46 had normal posterior drawer tests. There was a 10% decrease in quadriceps muscle strength in the affected limb by Cybex isokinetic strength analysis. Distal ligamentous ruptures, lack of athletic activity and temporary olecranization were associated with poor results, whereas bony avulsions, mid or proximal ruptures, and athletic activity were associated with good results.

Conclusions.—In a group of 53 patients with PCL injuries, primary repair was associated with good long-term results in the majority of patients, although not all could return to preinjury levels of activity. In this group, primary repair appeared to provide better results than have been reported for patients treated nonoperatively, even in those patients with isolated PCL injuries. Primary repair of distal ligamentous PCL ruptures was associated with poor results. These injuries should be treated by another method, such as free patellar tendon grafting.

▶ It is generally accepted that isolated tears of the PCL do well without reconstruction, whereas those injuries with associated ligamentous disruption and multiplane instability become problematic. It is interesting to note that the results of this study indicate that the results after primary repair did not depend on the existence of associated ligamentous injuries but rather on the location of the PCL failure. This, I believe, is an original observation. In view of the fact that this was a retrospective study lacking a control group with conservative treatment, the conclusion that primary repair provides better subjective and objective results compared with nonoperative treatment is not valid.

J.S. Torg, M.D.

Analysis of Skiing Accidents Involving Combined Injuries to the Medial Collateral and Anterior Cruciate Ligaments
Hull ML (Univ of California, Davis)
Am J Sports Med 25:35–40, 1997   4–46

Background.—The knee is the structure at greatest risk for injury during alpine skiing. Most of these knee injuries involve the ligaments, particularly the anterior cruciate (ACL) and the medial collateral (MCL) ligaments. A review of the literature was conducted to critically assess the ability of 2-mode release bindings to prevent MCL and ACL injuries.

Study Design.—A literature review was conducted.

Findings.—The studies reviewed suggest that the MCL is the primary restraint and the ACL a weaker, secondary restraint to both valgus and external axial moments. External axial moment is reported to be more damaging because injury could occur at a lower level of loading than for valgus moment. The axial moment transmitted by the knee was reported to be strongly related to the lateral force at the toe. The varus-valgus moment at the knee was weakly related to lateral toe force but strongly related to new medial-lateral boot sole force. This implies that 2-mode bindings offer sufficient release sensitivity to protect skiers against knee injuries caused by transmission of external axial moment loads.

Conclusions.—Alpine skiers frequently injure medial knee structures. These injuries can be accompanied by ACL injuries. The MCL is the primary constraint for both external axial and valgus moments, with the ACL a weaker, secondary constraint. An external axial moment is more damaging than a valgus moment. Two-mode bindings, if used and maintained properly, offer good release sensitivity to external axial moments transmitted by the knee.

▶ The stated purpose of this article was "to critically assess the ability of 2-mode release bindings to protect skiers against combined MCL/ACL injuries." Because this is a review article with no original data, it appears that this is a difficult goal to accomplish. I am not sure that in the injury mechanism involving external axial and valgus moments the MCL is the primary restraint and the ACL is a weak, secondary restraint, becoming a primary restraint only after the MCL is ruptured. This is in variance with the clinical observation that the most frequent injury resulting from this mechanism in skiers is isolated rupture of the ACL.

J.S. Torg, M.D.

The Biceps Femoris Muscle Complex at the Knee: Its Anatomy and Injury Patterns Associated With Acute Anterolateral-Anteromedial Rotatory Instability

Terry GC, LaPrade RF (Hughston Clinic, Columbus, Ga)
Am J Sports Med 24:2–8, 1996   4–47

Objective.—Biceps femoris muscle injury has been linked to acute knee instability. However, the patterns of injury to the biceps femoris have never been explored. An anatomical and clinical study was performed to analyze the anatomy of the biceps femoris muscle complex at the knee, to determine the incidence of biceps femoris muscle injury in patients with acute knee injuries, and to describe a surgical approach to the biceps femoris muscle.

Anatomical Findings.—On dissection of 30 cadaveric knees, 5 main components of the long arm of the biceps femoris were identified: a reflected arm, a direct arm, an anterior arm, and a lateral and anterior aponeurosis. The 6 main components of the short head of the biceps femoris are a capsular arm, a confluens of the biceps and the capsulo-osseous layer of the iliotibial tract, a direct arm, an anterior arm, and a lateral aponeurosis (Fig 4).

Clinical Findings.—Eighty-two consecutive patients undergoing surgical treatment for acute knee injuries with evidence of anterolateral-anterome-

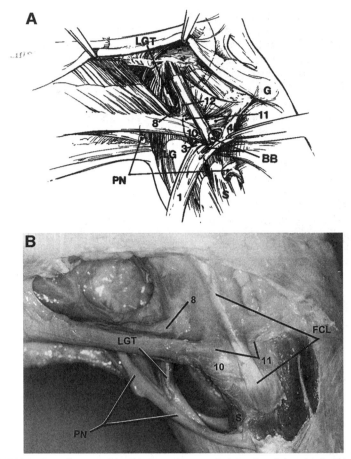

FIGURE 4.—Lateral aspect of the right knee. **A,** anatomical drawing of short head of biceps femoris muscle. Long head components—proximal tendon (*1*), direct arm (*3*), and anterior arm (*4*)—are retracted. Components of the short head of the biceps femoris muscle visible here were the capsular arm (*8*), direct arm (*10*), anterior arm (*11*), and lateral aponeurosis (*12*). *Abbreviations: LGT,* lateral gastrocnemius tendon; *G,* Gerdy's tubercle; *BB,* bicipital bursa; *S,* soleus muscle; *LG,* lateral gastrocnemius muscle; *PN,* peroneal nerve. **B,** deep and capsulo-osseous layers of the iliotibial tract with long head of the biceps femoris muscle removed. Short head of the biceps femoris muscle's capsular arm (*8*), direct arm (*10*), and anterior arm (*11*). *Abbreviations: FCL,* fibular collateral ligament; *S,* soleus muscle; *LGT,* lateral gastrocnemius tendon; *PN,* peroneal nerve. (Courtesy of Terry GC, LaPrade RF: The biceps femoris muscle complex at the knee: Its anatomy and injury patterns associated with acute anterolateral-anteromedial rotatory instability. *Am J Sports Med* 24:2–8, 1996.)

dial rotatory instability were studied as well. Seventy-two percent of knees had injuries to part of the biceps femoris muscle complex, and 35% had injuries to multiple components of this complex. Of the 92 total injuries, 89 were in the short head of the biceps femoris and 3 in the long head. Patients with increased anterior translation with the knee in 25 degrees of flexion on the Lachman test were likely to have injury of the biceps-capsulo-osseous iliotibial tract confluens. Those with adduction laxity in 30 degrees of flexion often had a Segond fracture. Three fascial incisions were used to identify the deep structures of the biceps femoris complex: a primary incision between the posterior edge of the lateral intermuscular septum and the short head of the biceps femoris muscle, a second incision posterior to the biceps tendon and parallel to the peroneal nerve, and an iliotibial tract–splitting incision.

Conclusion.—Acute knee injuries with anterolateral-anteromedial rotatory instability are commonly associated with injury to the biceps femoris muscle complex. The findings underscore the important contributions of the dynamic knee stabilizers to the normal limits on knee function. Although it is difficult to assess the effect of the biceps femoris muscles on knee instability in vivo, it is a major contributor to static and dynamic stability and proprioception.

▶ The biceps femoris muscle complex is known primarily as one of the hamstring group with major roles in producing knee flexion and hip extension. The biceps femoris also assists in lateral rotation of the flexed knee. The biceps femoris muscle has important roles in knee stability, as it prevents anterior translation of the lower leg complex, as well as stabilizing the lateral side of the knee with the lateral collateral ligaments.

Examination of patients with acute anterior translation instability revealed that 72% of 82 injured knees had injury to a component of the biceps femoris muscle. The most commonly injured component was found to be the capsular arm of the short head, followed by the biceps attachment to the iliotibial tract. These injuries produced marked increases in anterior translation and adduction laxity. The biceps femoris muscle is an important static and dynamic stabilizer of the lateral side of the knee.

M.J.L. Alexander, Ph.D.

The Effect of Open and Closed Chain Exercise and Knee Joint Position on Patellar Tracking in Lateral Patellar Compression Syndrome
Doucette SA, Child DD (Mountain West Physical Therapy, Logan, Utah; Western Med Ctr, Logan, Utah)
J Orthop Sports Phys Ther 23:104–110, 1996   4–48

Background.—Few objective data address the optimal form of exercise for rehabilitation of patellar dysfunction. Closed chain quadriceps strengthening exercises—such as the squat, leg press, and step exercises—are considered more functional than open chain exercises because physiologic load is normal through the skeletal system, muscle contractions are synergistic, and normal proprioceptive feedback mechanisms are used. In an open chain condition, the quadriceps acts as a knee extensor; in a closed chain condition, it is a decelerator of knee flexion and an anterior stabilizer. The effect of open and closed chain exercise and knee joint position on patellar tracking in lateral patellar compression syndrome (LPCS) was evaluated.

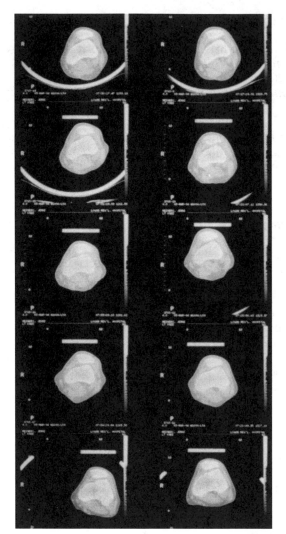

FIGURE 5.—Axial view radiographic comparison of the patellofemoral joint in 1 patient with open chain muscle condition (**left**) and closed chain muscle condition (**right**). From *top to bottom*: 0, 10, 20, 30, and 40 degrees of knee flexion. (Courtesy of Doucette SA, Child DD: The effect of open and closed chain exercise and knee joint position on patellar tracking in lateral patellar compression syndrome. *J Orthop Sports Phys Ther* 23:104–110, 1996.)

Methods.—The patellofemoral joints of 16 patients with LPCS were evaluated by CT scanning with the leg in 3 muscle conditions and at 5 knee angles. Congruence angles were determined to evaluate patellar tracking.

Results.—At 0, 10, and 20 degrees of knee flexion, congruence was improved more with the relaxed and closed chain conditions than with the open chain condition (Fig 5). After 30 degrees of knee flexion, open chain strengthening techniques appeared to be most appropriate. Patellar congruence progressively improved from 1 to 40 degrees of knee flexion with all 3 muscle conditions.

Discussion.—At knee flexions greater than 30 degrees, patellar tracking appears unaffected by exercise type, although open chain activities may cause less patellofemoral stress and more vastus medialis oblique muscle (VMO) electromyographic activity at larger angles. Leg press may be tolerated better than leg extension in functional ranges of motion by patients with patellofemoral joint arthritis, because of the lower patellofemoral joint stresses produced. For strengthening of the VMO in patients with LPCS, closed chain exercise allows better patellar positioning and less joint irritation in functional ranges of motion. Open chain strengthening techniques should be avoided during the first 30 degrees of knee range of motion unless a proper one-to-one relationship of VMO to vastus lateralis can be ensured with electromyographic feedback techniques. Radiography with open chain contractions could produce false positive subluxators because of lack of synergistic muscle contraction and lower-extremity biomechanical adaptations.

▶ Developing an effective rehabilitation program for patients with LPCS has been very difficult. Many factors must be considered including anatomical, biomechanical, and functional issues. A general approach would include strengthening of the VMO and stretching of the lateral structures, external appliances, nonsteroidal anti-inflammatory drugs, modalities, and bio feedback. This study indicates that closed chain exercises should be used from 0–20 degrees of knee flexion and open chain exercises should be used after 30 degrees of knee flexion. The authors have used CT scanning to evaluate patella maltracking and to support their claims. This study should be read together with the following study.

F.J. George, A.T.C., P.T.

The Role of Quadriceps Exercise in the Treatment of Patellofemoral Pain Syndrome
Callaghan MJ, Oldham JA (Royal Liverpool Univ, England; Manchester Univ, England)
Sports Med 2:384–391, 1996   4–49

Background.—Patellofemoral pain syndrome (PFPS) is common, and the most frequently chosen method of conservative treatment is exercise. However, no consensus exists among clinicians and researchers regarding the most beneficial type of exercise. Published recommendations for PFPS treatment usually center on the strengthening of the quadriceps through various methods. The value of some of these exercise regimens was questioned.

Quadriceps Exercise.—Patients with PFPS generally have few clinical abnormalities, and the origin of PFPS is uncertain. Isometric quadriceps exercise with the knee in full extension is standard in lower limb rehabilitation, but isometric exercise neither selectively fatigues nor exercises the vastus medialis oblique muscle (VMO). Inner range exercise (short arc exercise; terminal extension exercise) has been suggested for PFPS because of low contact forces at the patellofemoral joint. This method can be detrimental to patients with patellar instability, however, because the patella is at its most unstable during this arc of movement. Although some studies have shown improvement in PFPS with straight leg raise exercises, it was proposed that this method may not be the most effective for PFPS. Closed kinetic chain exercises have been proposed for rehabilitation in PFPS, primarily because of purported eccentric training of the quadriceps, but minimal research documents the amount of muscle activity occurring with these techniques. Eccentric exercises for the quadriceps have also been suggested.

Vastus Medialis Oblique Activation.—Selective dysfunction or insufficiency of certain components of the quadriceps has been suggested as a cause of PFPS, and selective enhancement of VMO contraction by altering knee and hip position has been suggested as a means of rehabilitation. The work of Bose et al. indicated that hip adduction in conjunction with quadriceps contraction should enhance VMO contraction and strength, but subsequent clinical studies yielded conflicting results. The work of Hodges and Richardson provided support for selective enhancement of the VMO using hip adduction in addition to quadriceps contraction in the weight-bearing situation.

Conclusion.—Methodologic flaws hamper comparisons of these studies; further research is needed to achieve consensus. Current anatomical and physiologic knowledge does, however, indicate that generalized quadriceps exercises should be adapted and modified to be more specific for rehabilitation of patients with PFPS.

▶ This study should be read with the previous study. As mentioned in the previous comments, a major component of rehabilitation in these patients is VMO strengthening. Exercises that were previously thought to isolate or improve VMO function selectively have been proven to be ineffective. The combination of hip adduction in a closed chain position with quadriceps contraction has a higher VMO:vastus lateralis ratio than in a non–weight-bearing position.[1]

F.J. George A.T.C., P.T.

Reference

1. Hodges PW, Richardson CA: The influence of isometric hip adduction on quadriceps femoris activity. *Scand J Rehabil Med* 25:57–62, 1993.

Arthroscopic Anterior Cruciate Ligament Transection Induces Canine Osteoarthritis
Marshall KW, Chan ADM (Univ of Toronto)
J Rheumatol 23:338–343, 1996   4–50

Background.—The canine model of osteoarthritis (OA) has contributed most to our understanding of the pathogenesis of OA. To induce OA, the anterior cruciate ligament (ACL) is transected by either a percutaneous

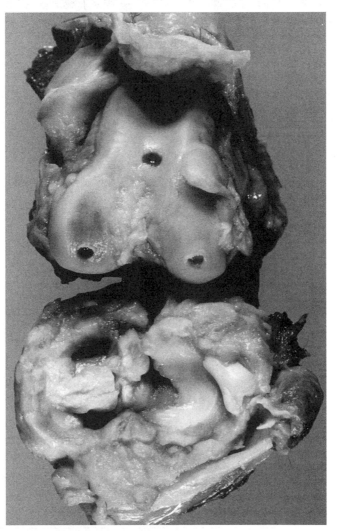

FIGURE 2.—Gross pathology specimen. Left knee 4 months after transection of the anterior cruciate ligament, showing grade 3 changes to the weight-bearing area of the medial femoral condyle, osteophytes along the outer margins of the condyles, and a medial meniscal tear. Holes in the center of articular surfaces are harvest sites for histologic analysis. (Courtesy of Marshall KW, Chan ADM: Arthroscopic anterior cruciate ligament transection induces canine osteoarthritis. *J Rheumatol* 23:338–343, 1996.)

stab incision or an open arthrotomy procedure. Both of these techniques have their limitations. The percutaneous stab does not allow direct visualization, whereas the arthrotomy technique requires extensive tissue dissection. To get around these difficulties, OA can be induced using fiberoptic arthroscopic technology, which permits direct visualization while minimizing surgical dissection. The effectiveness of this technique in the induction of canine OA was assessed.

Methods.—Six adult mongrel dogs were anesthetized and the left hind limb ACL was completely transected with arthroscopic scissors under direct visual control. Injury to other intra-articular structures was avoided.

Results.—All animals could bear full weight on the operated limb within 24 hours and had a normal gait by the second postoperative week. By sacrifice at 2, 4, or 6 months postoperatively, no limp was detected. Both ACL transected and intact knees were examined from each animal. Gross (Fig 2) and histologic examination revealed that OA was induced by this technique in every ACL transected knee. No degenerative OA changes were observed in any contralateral knee.

Conclusions.—Arthroscopic transection of the ACL is an effective method to induce osteoarthritis in dogs. The direct visualization and minimal invasiveness of this technique make it the preferred method of inducing ACL transection to create a canine model of OA.

▶ It has been previously suggested that injury to the ACL will produce early degenerative changes to the knee joint surfaces. In this study, the ACL of the left knee of a group of 6 dogs was transected arthroscopically, with care taken not to damage the joint surfaces during the procedure. All the injured knees sustained osteoarthritis, whereas the intact knees exhibited no degenerative changes. The timing of the degenerative changes included: initial roughening of the medial tibial surface, pitting of the cartilage over the femoral condyles, followed by fibrillation and meniscal tears, and fragmentation of the medial femoral condyle. These severe changes indicated the importance of the stabilization of the ACL in maintaining the integrity of the knee joint surfaces. Patients with a complete ACL tear are at risk for these degenerative changes and should be considered for prompt ACL repair if age and activity levels are appropriate.

M.J.L. Alexander, Ph.D.

Primary Repair Plus Intra-articular Iliotibial Band Augmentation in the Treatment of an Acute Anterior Cruciate Ligament Rupture: A Follow-up Study of 70 Patients
Natri A, Järvinen M, Kannus P (UKK Inst, Tampere, Finland; Univ Hosp, Tampere, Finland)
Arch Orthop Trauma Surg 115:22–27, 1996   4–51

Introduction.—Abnormal kinematic and major degenerative changes are often the causes of anterior cruciate ligament (ACL)-deficient knees. A previous study showed that patients who were treated conservatively did poorly at follow-up and had a high frequency of chronic symptomatic instability, meniscal tears, muscle atrophy, and posttraumatic osteoarthrosis. Optimistic results have been reported for surgical treatment of acute ACL deformities. Results of acute ACL ruptures treated with a modified Marshall method using the iliotibial band as the source of intra-articular augmentation were evaluated.

Methods.—There were 90 patients with an acute ACL rupture who were treated with the multiple suture technique and iliotibial band augmentation. Seventy were examined at a mean of 3.5 years after the operation with clinical examinations, laxity tests, radiologic examinations, questionnaires, and isokinetic muscle strength testing. Most of the frequently involved injuries were caused by downhill skiing (18 patients), followed by soccer and volleyball.

Results.—There were 55 patients at follow-up (79%) who were satisfied with the results; 53 were found to be excellent or good (75%). Full knee extension was found in 58 patients (83%), and full knee flexion was found in 40 patients (57%). There was an average 14% strength deficit in isokinetic knee extension in the operated knee compared with the uninjured knee and a 6% deficit in flexion at the speed of 60 degrees per second. Forty of the 44 patients (91%) who were active in sports before their injuries were able to return to sports. Thigh muscle atrophy and quadriceps weakness were associated with a flexion deficit of 5 degrees or more and slow and high speed of the isokinetic movement.

Conclusion.—Primary repair of the ligament with intra-articular iliotibial band augmentation seems to be a good method to restore the functional capacity of the injured knee in an acute rupture of the ACL.

▶ There remains much debate in the sports medicine literature regarding the most effective treatment of the acute ACL rupture. Although the bone–patellar tendon–bone repair has been the treatment of choice in the past, other popular tissue replacements have included the semimembranosus, semitendinosus, gracilis, and iliotibial bands. This study reported the use of the iliotibial band to augment the suturing of the ACL to repair ruptures in 90 patients, although it has been criticized as having inadequate initial strength. The authors reported that 79% of their patients were satisfied with the repair and had excellent or good functional results. Some patients had knee laxity, some restrictions in knee joint movements, and an average strength deficit of 6% to 14%. A major problem reported was a flexion deficit of the operated knee, which may be alleviated by more aggressive rehabilitation. The iliotibial band repair does avoid postoperative weakness of the patellar tendon complex and should be considered a satisfactory augmentation tissue.

M.J.L. Alexander, Ph.D.

Electromyographic and Kinematic Analysis of Graded Treadmill Walking and the Implications for Knee Rehabilitation

Lange GW, Hintermeister RA, Schlegel T, et al (Steadman Hawkins Sports Medicine Found, Vail, Colo; Steadman Hawkins Clinic, Englewood, Colo)
J Orthop Sports Phys Ther 23:294–301, 1996   4–52

Introduction.—Knee rehabilitation must consider not only quadriceps and hamstring training but also the proper range of motion and cardiovascular conditioning. Exercises performed between 30 and 60 degrees of knee flexion are believed to avoid excessive strain on the anterior cruciate ligament while reducing patellofemoral pain. To see whether certain exercises would be appropriate for knee rehabilitation, the muscle activity, joint angles, and heart rate involved in uphill walking were studied.

Methods.—The study included 6 healthy men with an average age of 28.5 years. The men walked at self-selected speeds at 3 grades—0%, 12%, and 24%—for measurement of ankle, knee, and hip angles; heart rate; and electromyographic (EMG) activity of the quadriceps and hamstrings. The goal of the study was to measure muscle activation at the different treadmill grades and to identify the grade or grades at which knee range of motion would not cause further joint compromise.

Results.—Significant increases in average and peak EMG activity were noted for the vastus medialis oblique muscles (125% and 154%, respectively), vastus lateralis (109% and 139%), and biceps femoris (53% and 46%). No significant change was noted for the medial hamstrings. As grade increased, so did maximum knee flexion at heel strike. Heart rate increased with grade, even though the participants selected slower walking speeds at higher grades.

Conclusions.—Quadriceps and hamstring muscle activity increase with steepness of grade during treadmill walking. This type of exercise provides a progressively increasing intensity for the knee muscles. The EMG findings are consistent with, but do not prove, a strengthening effect. For minimizing patellofemoral joint reaction forces and relieving anterior cruciate ligament strain, a grade of just greater than 12% may be the most appropriate for knee rehabilitation.

▶ The authors address the clinician's dilemma of rehabilitating an anterior cruciate ligament reconstructed knee and avoiding patellofemoral joint problems. They believe a solution to the problem is to exercise in the range of 30 to 60 degrees of knee flexion. To achieve this with a treadmill, they suggest exercising at a slightly greater than 12% (6.8 degrees) grade at a self-selected speed.

The authors comment that although there is significant increase in EMG activity, this may not necessarily suggest a strengthening effect. They do believe that graded walking meets the parameters of specificity of training because it provides a functional exercise of affected joints, within appropriate ranges of motion, in a controlled environment, thereby affording the reconstructed knee a degree of protection.

Please read this study with the following study (Abstract 4–53).

F.J. George, A.T.C., P.T.

Recovery of Muscle Strength Following Arthroscopic Meniscectomy
Matthews P, St-Pierre DMM (North Country Hosp, Newport, Vt; McGill Univ, Montréal)
J Orthop Sports Phys Ther 23:18–26, 1996   4–53

Objective.—Although it is believed that exercise can facilitate recovery of muscle strength and size after a period of disuse, the extent of this recovery in individuals without supervised exercise training is not known. Results of an investigation of the time course of spontaneous recovery of muscle torque in the first 3 months after arthroscopic partial meniscectomy were presented.

Methods.—Knee stability, flexor and extensor strength (at 60, 120, 180, and 240 degrees/sec), range of motion, and pain were measured (using either a Cybex II+ or a Cybex II isokinetic device) before and at 2-week intervals for 12 weeks after partial meniscectomy in 22 patients (5 women) aged 20–49 years. Patients were given a home program of rehabilitation exercises. Torque measurements of the involved side were statistically compared with measurements of the noninvolved side.

Results.—Fourteen patients had injured the dominant leg, and 18 required postoperative medication for several days. Patients took an average of 20.5 days to return to work. Initially involved quadriceps were significantly weaker than noninvolved quadriceps at 60 degrees/sec. Peak torques for involved quadriceps were significantly smaller 2 weeks after surgery at all speeds; they had returned to preoperative levels by 4–6 weeks after surgery but were still significantly weaker than those on the noninvolved side at both 60 and 120 degrees/sec. Although hamstring strength was comparable on the involved and noninvolved sides before surgery, at 2 weeks after surgery torque was significantly smaller for the involved side at both 60 and 120 degrees/sec. By 4 weeks, the hamstrings had recovered. Activity decreased significantly after surgery and did not increase significantly until 12 weeks after surgery. There was no relationship between pain and torque or pain and activity level.

Conclusion.—After meniscectomy, hamstrings were fully recovered by week 4, but quadriceps had not fully recovered after 12 weeks for patients on home exercise programs. Supervised rehabilitation appears to be necessary for these patients to regain balanced quadriceps strength.

▶ The ability of a muscle group to recover to full strength after arthroscopic surgery would seem to depend on a supervised training program with strict adherence by the subjects. The subjects in this study were not given supervised rehabilitation but simply returned to their normal activity levels as pain and mobility allowed. This group of patients was able to recover their quadriceps strength to presurgery levels by 4–6 weeks after surgery, whereas the hamstrings were fully recovered by 4 weeks post surgery. However, there were significant quadriceps deficits in strength preoperatively, likely resulting from the fact that symptoms caused by the meniscus tear had been present an average of 2 years before surgery. Even after 12 weeks post surgery, there was significant quadriceps muscle weakness, which suggests that supervised rehabilitation may be required for patients to attain balanced strength between injured and noninjured limbs.

M.J.L. Alexander, Ph.D.

Rehabilitation Following Allograft Meniscal Transplantation: A Review of the Literature and Case Study
Fritz JM, Irrgang JJ, Harner CD (Univ of Pittsburgh, Pa)
J Orthop Sports Phys Ther 24:98–106, 1996   4–54

Introduction.—Meniscal transplantation has recently been developed and used to treat meniscal injuries. The research regarding meniscal function and the effects of meniscectomy and the development of meniscal transplantation were reviewed. A case study emphasizing postoperative rehabilitation guidelines was presented.

Meniscectomy.—Early surgical treatment of the menisci was total meniscectomy because the menisci were considered functionless. Thinking changed after reports of the harmful long-term effects of meniscectomy were published. These findings and the introduction of arthroscopic techniques led to the development of partial meniscectomy. Subsequent reports indicated that the severity of post–partial meniscectomy changes were correlated with the amount of meniscal tissue removed. Recent emphasis on meniscal repair has resulted in success rates of 90% at 3–5 years of follow-up.

Allograft Meniscal Transplantation.—Healing of meniscal tissue is enhanced when it is attached to a well-vascularized periphery. Animal trials indicate that meniscal allografts can heal to the recipient's vascular periphery and can slow the degenerative process, compared with meniscectomized knees. Grafts must be chosen from the same side and compartment as the recipient's and can be implanted fresh from the donor. The preferred method of graft preservation is cryopreservation. Because there is a risk of disease transmission (i.e., a 1 in a million risk of HIV transmission from screened donors), many tissue banks use irradiation as a secondary sterilization. For implantation, bone plugs must be left intact on the meniscal horns of the graft. With an open or arthroscopic procedure, tibial tunnels are drilled for the bone blocks, and the periphery of the meniscus is sutured to the capsule This procedure was first performed in humans in 1984. Reports indicate that 85% to 95% of transplanted menisci heal to the capsule and have a grossly normal appearance. Three of a series of 25 patients with clinical failures required reoperation for removal of the transplanted meniscus because of loosening from the capsule and decreased vascularity.

Rehabilitation.—Postoperative rehabilitation has not been fully developed in the literature. Most reports call for use of a brace on the involved knee, 5–6 weeks of non–weight-bearing, and immediate range-of-motion exercises or use of a continuous passive motion machine. Gait training without the extension brace begins at 6 weeks after operation. Closed kinetic chain activities are limited to a 0- 60-degree range of flexion and proprioceptive training is emphasized. Quadriceps strength and endurance is emphasized before initiating functional progression. Because the quadriceps function eccentrically as shock absorbers during functional activities, compromised quadriceps may affect the menisci. The involved knee should be monitored for evidence of overtraining.

> *Case Report.*—Man, 28, injured his right knee while playing basketball at age 20 years. An arthroscopic total medial meniscectomy was performed 2 years later. He experienced increased episodes of instability and subsequently was given a diagnosis of a chronic grade III anterior cruciate ligament (ACL) tear. Minimal degenerative changes were detected in the medial compartment, using 45-degree flexion weight-bearing radiographs. He underwent ACL reconstruction using an allograft patellar tendon at age 23. At age 27, he experienced medial pain and swelling after playing football. There was no knee instability, but radiographs showed degenerative changes in the medial compartment. He underwent arthroscopic fresh frozen, nonirradiated medial meniscus transplantation using a posteromedial incision. The patient underwent 4 phases of rehabilitation: maximum protection (0–8 weeks), moderate protection (8–12 weeks), minimum protection (3–9 months), and return to activity (9 months+).

Conclusion.—Patients are more likely to benefit from a transplantation procedure early in the degenerative process. The ACL deficiency and meniscal pathology are often addressed concurrently. The approach to rehabilitation described here after combined meniscal and ACL reconstruction is more aggressive than isolated meniscal transplant, but similar to ACL rehabilitation. Exceptions include the following: maintaining the knee in extension in the first 4 weeks after surgery with flexion limited to 90 degrees, delay of closed kinetic chain activities until 4 weeks postoperatively, isolated hamstring exercises for 8 weeks, and delay of return to functional activities until 9 months after surgery. The long-term success of meniscal transplantation will be tested by its ability to cease or slow the degenerative process observed in meniscectomized knees.

▶ This excellent article reviews the importance of knee menisci and their function in assisting load transmission, shock absorption, joint lubrication, and joint stability. The authors outline a protocol for allograft meniscal transplantation and a postoperative rehabilitation program. They explain that progression through this program is based on the individual patient's clinical presentation and readiness to move to the next phase of the program. Progression is based on the achievement of certain criteria, such as the ability to do a straight leg raise without extension lag or normal gait without an assistive device or patellofemoral complaints.

F.J. George, A.T.C., P.T.

Oxygen Consumption, Heart Rate, and Rating of Perceived Exertion in Young Adult Women During Backward Walking at Different Speeds
Clarkson E, Cameron S, Osmon P, et al (DeWitt Army Community Hosp, Fort Belvoir, Va; Keesler Med Ctr, Keesler Air Force Base, Miss; Brooke Army Med Ctr, Fort Sam Houston, Tex; et al)
J Orthop Sports Phys Ther 25:113–118, 1997   4–55

Background.—For patients with knee problems, backward walking is a useful way to maintain cardiovascular conditioning while reducing forces on the knee during rehabilitation. In addition to reducing compressive forces at the patellofemoral joint, backward walking also may prevent overstretching of the anterior cruciate ligament. The relation of backward walking speed with oxygen consumption and heart rate has previously been established in men. This study attempted to do the same in women.

Methods.—The study included 25 healthy women 21–35 years of age, with no musculoskeletal pathologic findings. All performed a backward walking test and a graded exercise test. The backward walking tests were done at speeds of 0.96, 1.20, 1.43, 1.67, and 1.91 m/sec in random order. Relations among treadmill speed, heart rate, and oxygen consumption were analyzed.

Results.—The analysis found a curvilinear relation between speed and oxygen consumption and between speed and heart rate. In contrast, the relation between heart rate and oxygen consumption was linear. Equations were developed for use in prescribing backward walking speed according to oxygen consumption or heart rate. For a specific training VO_2, the equation was: $V = 0.06 \dot{V}O_2 - 0.00056 \dot{V}O_2{}^2 + 0.26$ where V is backward walking speed in m/sec. For a prescribed heart rate, the equation was: $V = 0.0096\ HR + 0.04$.

Conclusions.—Relations between backward walking speed and oxygen consumption and heart rate were determined in women. This information will permit appropriate prescription of backward walking speed for women undergoing knee rehabilitation. The clinician should bear in mind that backward walking can place high physical and metabolic demands on the body.

▶ As the authors state, there has been very little research on the benefits of backward walking as a treatment technique. Suggestions have been made that it is beneficial in treating patellofemoral pain syndrome and anterior cruciate ligament–injured knees. The authors do caution clinicians to be aware of the potentially high physical and metabolic demands of backward walking.

Please read this abstract with the previous study (Abstract 4–54).

F.J. George, A.T.C., P.T.

Exertional Compartment Syndrome of the Leg: Steps for Expedient Return to Activity
Edwards P, Myerson MS (Union Mem Hosp, Baltimore, Md)
Physician Sportsmed 24:31–38, 44–46, 1996   4–56

Background.—Exertional compartment syndrome (ECS) is characterized by exercise-induced pain and swelling relieved by rest, with weakness and paresthesia in some patients. The most common site of involvement is the leg. Exertional compartment syndrome of the leg was discussed.

Anatomy and Pathophysiology.—Four osseofascial compartments, each surrounded by a relatively inelastic fascial covering and containing a major nerve, are found in the leg. The chronic form of the syndrome is much more common than the acute form. The syndrome is associated with increased pressure while the muscles are relaxed. Skeletal muscle is perfused during muscle relaxation only. Relaxation pressures of greater than 35–45 mm Hg result in reduced blood flow and acute myoneural ischemia typical of an acute compartment syndrome.

Two theories have been proposed to explain the cause of increased relaxation pressure in ECS. The first theory stipulates that normal compartmental volume can increase 20% with exercise because of fiber swelling and increased intracompartmental blood volume; thus, muscles may hyperatrophy in conditioned athletes. The second theory is the mechanical damage theory, which stipulates that eccentric exercise causes myofiber damage. Repetitive eccentric contraction results in increased osmotic pressure in the compartment, subsequently leading to increased capillary relaxation pressure and decreased blood flow. Typically, chronic ECS develops in well-conditioned athletes younger than 40 years of age. When athletes with chronic ECS markedly increase their training, acute ECS may develop. The anterior compartment is involved in 45% of chronic ECS cases and the deep posterior compartment in 40%.

Clinical Presentation and Diagnosis.—Patients with chronic ECS report a gradual onset of aching leg pain and a feeling of fullness. Pain related to activity begins at a predictable time after exercise initiation or after a certain intensity level is reached. The pain is completely relieved by rest, usually within 20 minutes of finishing exercise, and recurs when exercise is begun. Intracompartmental pressure needs to be measured to confirm the diagnosis of ECS. Postexercise pressures alone can be used but only if the exercise reproduces the patient's symptoms.

Treatment.—Immediate fasciotomy is indicated after the diagnosis of acute ECS associated with high compartment pressure. Initially, nonoperative treatment is almost always appropriate for patients with chronic

ECS. Fasciotomy is recommended for such patients if symptoms persist for more than 3 months. Generally, athletes are able to return to sports participation by 8–12 weeks with no pain or with greatly improved symptoms.

▶ Here is a comprehensive, practical article on a vexing problem for some athletes. The leg is the most common site of ECS, which is marked by exercise-induced pain and swelling (sometimes with weakness and paresthesia) that resolves quickly with rest. The leg has 4 osseofascial compartments, each surrounded by relatively inelastic fascial covering and containing a major nerve. Chronic ECS is far more common than the acute form and usually occurs in fit athletes under age 40 years. The 2 theories of causation are covered in this discussion, as is the typical clinical presentation.

To confirm the diagnosis, postexercise intracompartmental pressure must be shown to be elevated and is valid only if exercise reproduces the patient's symptoms. Conservative therapy is outlined in the paper; however, it often fails and then fasciotomy is recommended. Long-term results of fasciotomy for ECS of the leg were covered in the 1994 YEAR BOOK OF SPORTS MEDICINE.[1]

E.R. Eichner, M.D.

Reference

1. 1994 YEAR BOOK OF SPORTS MEDICINE, pp. 169–170.

Analysis of Failed Surgical Management of Fractures of the Base of the Fifth Metatarsal Distal to the Tuberosity: The Jones Fracture
Glasgow MT, Naranja RJ Jr, Glasgow SG, et al (Dekalb County Orthopaedics, III; Univ of Pennsylvania, Philadelphia)
Foot Ankle Int 17:449–457, 1996   4–57

Background.—To date, only one failure of surgical management of fractures of the base of the fifth metatarsal distal to the tuberosity has been reported. Eleven cases of surgically managed Jones fractures complicated by refracture, delayed union, or nonunion were reported.

Methods and Findings.—The 11 patients included 9 men and 2 women, aged 14 to 26 years. All had acute fractures characterized by a narrow fracture line and absence of intramedullary sclerosis on radiographs. Surgery was complicated by delayed union in 3 patients, refracture in 7, and nonunion in 1. Intramedullary screw fixation was performed in 6 patients and inlaid corticocancellous bone graft in 5. In the former group, not using a 4.5 mm ASIF malleolar screw for internal fixation was associated with failure. In the latter group, failure was associated with undersized corticocancellous grafts and incomplete reaming of the medullary canal. Early return to vigorous physical activity appeared to have played a role in delayed union and refracture in both groups.

Conclusions.—Delayed union, nonunion, or refracture can complicate surgical treatment for Jones fractures. Meticulous operative technique is needed. The best outcomes can be ensured by following established guidelines.

▶ This article makes two important points. First, surgical treatment of Jones fractures may result in delayed union, nonunion, or refracture. Second, to ensure best results, the surgical technique should be meticulous and follow established, previously published guidelines.

J.S. Torg, M.D.

The Bicycle Spoke Injury: An Avoidable Accident?
D'Souza LG, Hynes DE, McManus F, et al (Children's Hosp, Dublin)
Foot Ankle Int 17:170–173, 1996   4–58

Objective.—Although the bicycle is a common mode of transportation and improvements in construction have been made, the design of the wheel has remained unchanged. Results of a prospective study of bicycle spoke injuries to children over a 12-month period are reported.

Methods.—Between November 1992 and October 1993, 71 children (27 girls), aged 20 months to 13 years, were treated in the emergency department of The Children's Hospital for foot and ankle injuries caused by bicycle spokes. A biomechanical study conducted in a wind resistance tunnel examined the differences in wind resistance and turbulence between a flat cover without holes and a mesh cover over the wheel to prevent the child's foot from getting caught in the wheel spokes.

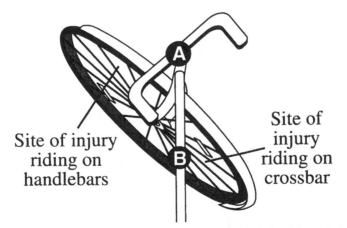

Site of injury riding on handlebars

Site of injury riding on crossbar

FIGURE 1.—**A** , Site of injury when the passenger is sitting astride the handlebars. The front wheel turns to the left and the left foot is injured by the spokes. **B**, Site of injury when the passenger is sitting astride the crossbar. The front wheel turns to the left and the right foot is caught by the spokes. (Courtesy of D'Souza LG, Hynes DE, McManus F, et al: The bicycle spoke injury: an avoidable accident? *Foot Ankle Int* 17:170–173, 1996. Reprinted with permission from D'Souza LG, Hynes DE, McManus F, et al: The bicycle spoke injury: an avoidable accident? *Foot and Ankle International* 17:170–176, 1996.)

Results.—Bicycle spoke injuries accounted for 8.52% of all ankle and foot injuries to children. Four of the injured children were riding a child's bike. The remaining 67 were passengers on an adult bike when they were hurt; 48 were riding on the crossbar, 4 on the handlebars, and 19 in a carrier, and all were injured on the front wheel. All injuries were classified as contusions or superficial abrasions ($n = 45$), skin loss ($n = 10$), skin laceration ($n = 4$), or undisplaced fractures ($n = 12$). Whether the right or left foot was injured depended on where the child was riding (Fig 1). The 3 types of injuries incurred included laceration from the spokes, crush injuries from impingement between the wheel and the fork of the bicycle, and shearing injuries resulting from a combination of these 2 injuries. The mesh wheel cover had less wind resistance than the solid cover.

Conclusion.—Bicycle spoke injuries to ankles and feet occur by 3 mechanisms and can be prevented by using a mesh wheel cover.

▶ It is interesting to note that there were 3 mechanisms responsible for the injuries. Lacerations occurred from the knifelike action of the bicycle spokes. Crushing injuries were from impingement between the wheel and the fork of the bike. Shearing injuries occurred from a combination of these two forces. Certainly the suggestion that these injuries can be prevented if the bicycles were fitted with guards is appropriate. Of course a more direct approach would be an educational program to discourage youngsters from traveling on the crossbar or handlebar.

J.S. Torg, M.D.

Risk Factors for Stress Fractures in Track and Field Athletes
Bennell KL, Malcolm SA, Thomas SA, et al (Univ of Melbourne, Australia; La Trobe Univ, Melbourne, Australia; St Vincent's Hosp, Melbourne, Australia; et al)
Am J Sports Med 24:810–818, 1996   4–59

Introduction.—Considerable interference with training and competition accompanies athletes with stress fractures, which occur with repetitive mechanical loading, bone remodeling, and microdamage accumulation playing roles. Risk factors for stress fracture include soft tissue composition, low bone density, dietary insufficiency, menstrual disturbances, and excessive training. The differences in these risk factors between male and female athletes were assessed in this 12-month prospective study. The ability of risk factors to predict the likelihood of a stress fracture was also evaluated.

Methods.—There were 53 female and 58 male track and field athletes, ages 17 to 26 years, who participated in this study. Dual-energy radiographic absorptiometry and anthropometric techniques were used to measure total bone mineral content, regional bone density, and soft tissue composition. Training of the athletes included running, interval, hill, plyometric, skill, stretching, and cross-training. Questionnaires were used to assess menstrual characteristics, current dietary intake, and training. A physical therapist performed a clinical biomechanical assessment.

Results.—With most injuries located in the tibia, the incidence of stress fractures during the study was 21.1%. The occurrence of stress fractures in men could not be predicted by any of the risk factors. However, in women, risk factors were able to predict stress fractures, including lower bone density, a history of menstrual disturbance, less lean mass in the lower limb, a lower-fat diet, and a discrepancy in leg length. A significantly later age of menarche, fewer menses in the year preceding the study, and a lower menstrual index indicating fewer menses per year since menarche were associated with female athletes who sustained a stress fracture. The best independent predictors of stress fractures in women were age of menarche and calf girth, according to multiple logistic regression. Eighty percent of the female athletes were correctly assigned into their respective stress fracture or nonstress fracture groups with this bivariate model.

Conclusion.—Female athletes most at risk for this overuse bone injury may possibly be identified with these risk factors.

▶ Certainly, this attempt to identify risk factors for stress fractures is, for the most part, a credible effort. However, the 21% incidence of stress fractures reported in this study is extremely high. This is perhaps explained on what, to this observer, was a liberal interpretation of both the triple-phase isotope bone scan and computed tomographic scans. As the authors emphasize, "these results suggest that it may be possible to identify female athletes most at risk for overuse bone injury."

J.S. Torg, M.D.

The Popliteofibular Ligament: Rediscovery of a Key Element in Posterolateral Stability
Maynard MJ, Deng X, Wickiewicz TL, et al (Hosp for Special Surgery, New York)
Am J Sports Med 24:311–316, 1996   4–60

Background.—In the face of ongoing debate over the anatomy and function of the posterolateral corner of the knee, there is no accepted treatment of choice for posterolateral instability, either acute or chronic. The authors' cadaver studies have suggested that the popliteofibular ligament serves as a strong, direct attachment between the popliteal tendon and fibula. The presence of the popliteofibular ligament and its role in posterolateral stability were studied.

Findings.—Dissection identified the popliteofibular ligament in 20 of 20 knees. The popliteofibular ligament averaged 47 mm in length and 6.9 mm^2 in cross-sectional area, compared to 53.4 mm and 7.2 mm^2, respectively, for the lateral collateral ligament. On biomechanical testing to failure in response to varus stress, the lateral collateral ligament was the first structure to fail, followed by the popliteofibular ligament, and finally the popliteus muscle belly. Average maximal force to failure was 425 N for the popliteofibular ligament vs. 747 N for the lateral collateral ligament.

Conclusions.—The popliteofibular ligament exists in the human knee and plays a role in posterolateral stability. The authors are considering reconstruction of the popliteofibular ligament for patients with injury to the posterolateral corner of the knee. This may prove more appropriate than femur-to-tibia reconstruction.

▶ This paper was the winner of the American Orthopedic Society for Sports Medicine 1994 O'Donahue Award. The potential clinical relevance of the authors' observation is the potential role of the popliteofibular ligament in the surgical approach to posterolateral corner instability. Specifically, the authors state that they are considering restoration of the popliteofibular ligament. They propose that reconstructing the tendon from the femur to the fibula might be more appropriate than the femur to tibia reconstruction that they have used in the past.

J.S. Torg, M.D.

Intramedullary Nailing for Chronic Tibial Stress Fractures
Chang PS, Harris RM (Womack Army Med Ctr, Ft Bragg, NC)
Am J Sports Med 24:688–692, 1996   4–61

Background.—Chronic tibial stress fracture usually occurs in athletes or military personnel and can interfere with these professions. This report describes a review of 5 patients who underwent intramedullary tibial nailing for chronic stress fracture at Womack Army Medical Center from 1991 to 1994.

Methods.—The indication for surgery was chronic midanterior tibial stress fracture that was recalcitrant to nonoperative therapy for at least 1 year. The patients underwent closed, reamed intramedullary nailing of the tibia with the Russell-Taylor system. The outcome was evaluated by patient interview. The average follow-up period was 21 months.

Results.—All 5 patients in this series had unusually narrow medullary canals, thickened anterior cortex, and a linear unicortical fracture on the anterior or tension side. All patients reported improvement. Of the 5 cases, 2 could return to unlimited pain-free running and 3 had limited pain-free running and minor pain with vigorous activity.

Conclusions.—Five patients with chronic tibial stress fractures were treated by intramedullary nailing and the results were reviewed. The results of this treatment in this limited series of patients were good to excellent. This suggests that intramedullary nailing should be considered for patients with chronic tibial stress fracture who do not improve with long-term nonoperative treatment.

▶ This particular lesion, delayed union of a stress fracture of the anterior tibial cortex, has been appropriately named the "dreaded black line" by

Bergfeld. In view of the fact that the results of this study are somewhat equivocal in that "all patients reported improvement in their symptoms and could return to limited running," the effectiveness of intramedullary nailing can be appropriately questioned. My own approach to this problem has been to saucerize the area of the cortical defect through a small anterior incision. Actually, the lesion itself involves only half of the thickened tibial cortex and rarely is more than a centimeter in width. With regard to results, sometimes it works, sometimes it doesn't.

J.S. Torg, M.D.

A Study of Intrinsic Factors in Patients With Stress Fractures of the Tibia

Ekenman I, Tsai-Felländer L, Westblad P, et al (Huddinge Univ, Sweden)

Foot Ankle Int 17:477–482, 1996   4–62

Background.—Stress reactions to the bone, or stress fractures, are common overuse injuries in athletes. The bone that is most frequently involved in stress fracture is the tibia. The cause of stress fracture of the tibia is not well understood. To understand the cause of this injury, intrinsic factors were examined in 29 consecutive patients with unilateral stress fracture of the tibia.

Methods.—The study group consisted of 29 consecutive patients with unilateral, documented stress fracture of the tibia. Of these, 15 were elite athletes and 14 were recreational athletes. There were 5 men and 5 women with anterior stress fractures and 6 men and 13 women with posteromedial stress fractures. Anthropometry, range of motion, isokinetic plantar flexor muscle performance, and gait pattern were analyzed in this study with the uninjured leg as the control. The study group was also compared with an uninjured reference group, which consisted of 18 elite athletes and 12 sedentary volunteers.

Results.—The 10 anterior stress fractures of the tibia were localized to the push-off/landing leg in 9 of 10 of the athletes in this study group, whereas the 19 posteromedial injuries were distributed between both legs. There were no significant systematic differences in anthropomorphy, range of motion, gait pattern, or isokinetic plantar flexor muscle peak torque and endurance between injured and uninjured legs or between the study group and the reference group.

Conclusions.—Other than the predominance of injury to the push-off/landing leg in those with anterior stress fracture of the tibia, no intrinsic factor was found to be associated with the occurrence of stress fracture of the tibia in this study.

▶ The conclusion that no one intrinsic factor was found to be associated with the occurrence of a stress fracture of the tibia is in keeping with my own clinical experience.

J.S. Torg, M.D.

Clinical and Sonographic Evaluation of the Risk of Rupture in the Achilles Tendon

Nehrer S, Breitenseher M, Brodner W, et al (Univ of Vienna)
Arch Orthop Trauma Surg 116:14–18, 1997   4–63

Introduction.—Chronic pain in the region of the Achilles tendon may indicate progressive degeneration of the tendon. Previous studies have reported that 97% of spontaneously ruptured tendons exhibit histopathologic signs of degeneration. To identify characteristics predictive of rupture, researchers studied the clinical course and sonograms of 36 patients with achillodynia.

Methods.—The patient group included 26 men and 10 women with a mean age of 43 years. All had painful symptoms in the region of the Achilles tendon, but none had a definite clinical diagnosis of acute tendon rupture. Sonographic examinations of 72 tendons were obtained in the sagittal plane of the entire length of the tendons as well as transverse sections. Tendons were analyzed and graded for swelling, abnormal structure, and thickness. An average of 48 months after the first evaluation, clinical and sonographic follow-up investigations were performed.

Results.—Clinically symptomatic tendons were present bilaterally in 12 patients, on the right side in 13, and on the left side in 11. All patients had pain on loading. Sonography revealed normal findings in 39 of 48 symptomatic tendons. All 39 of these tendons showed a homogenous fibrillar structure on sagittal scans; a honeycomb pattern was seen on transverse scans. Tendon thickness ranged from 4 to 6 mm. Abnormalities of tendon structure and thickness were observed in 33 tendons. Sonography had a sensitivity of 0.58 and a specificity of 0.72. At follow-up, 7 tendons had spontaneously ruptured. Initial sonograms in these 7 cases exhibited a high-grade thickening in 4, moderate thickening in 2, and a diameter between 6 and 8 mm in 1. No tendon initially classified as normal ruptured during follow-up. Patients without sonographic changes responded to conservative treatment. Sonographic follow-up showed progression to a higher grade of tendon degeneration in 30 patients. Clinical outcome was rated as excellent or good in 23 tendons and fair or poor in 25. Only 11 patients returned to full sporting activity.

Conclusion.—Sonography was able to determine the thickness and echotexture of these symptomatic Achilles tendons, allowing risk for rupture and response to conservative treatment to be estimated. Outcome was significantly better for patients without sonographic changes.

▶ The observation that all tendons in this study were symptomatic before rupture is not in keeping with the literature or my own clinical experience. However, this is certainly an interesting observation. Of note, the authors point out that a long-term clinical and sonographic follow-up of patients with and without achillodynia is necessary to evaluate the predicted value of these findings.

J.S. Torg, M.D.

Stable Lateral Malleolar Fractures Treated With Aircast Ankle Brace and DonJoy R.O.M.-Walker Brace: A Prospective Randomized Study

Brink O, Staunstrup H, Sommer J (Aarhus Univ, Denmark)

Foot Ankle Int 17:679–684, 1996   4–64

Objective.—Lauge-Hansen supination-eversion stage II ankle fractures are the most common fractures of the fibula. The preferred method of treatment is closed without reduction. Traditional immobilization in a below-the-knee walking cast usually leaves some joint stiffness after the cast is removed. To determine if a different type of immobilization might reduce the stiffness, the Aircast Air-Stirrup ankle brace and the DonJoy's R.O.M.-Walker were compared for comfort, range of motion, pain, swelling, and level of activity.

Methods.—Either the Aircast ($40) or the DonJoy ($110) ankle brace was used to immobilize isolated SE-II ankle fractures in 66 patients (28 men) aged 18 to 84 years. Patients were full weight-bearing, wearing the brace day and night for 4 weeks and omitting the brace at night thereafter. Patients were reviewed at 1, 4, and 12 weeks. Braces were statistically compared with the *t*-test and Mann-Whitney rank test.

Results.—Average bracing times for the Aircast and DonJoy were 39 and 35 days, respectively. Patients scored the Aircast significantly higher for comfort and ease of use, although both braces had high scores. Pain intensity for both groups significantly decreased between 1 and 4 weeks. At 4 weeks, 70% of Aircast users and 78% of DonJoy users had no pain walking. Inflammation significantly decreased for both groups between weeks 1 and 4 but was significantly less in the DonJoy users. The average time to return to work was 6 weeks. At 12 weeks, 1 Aircast and 1 DonJoy user had a displaced fracture. All fractures were united at 12 weeks. At 12 weeks there was no difference in range of motion, pain, swelling, ambulation, or inflammation scores.

Conclusion.—Both braces significantly reduced pain by 4 weeks. Patients returned to work by 6 weeks on average. All ankles had united by 12 weeks. the Aircast brace was rated more comfortable and easier to use than the DonJoy brace, but the DonJoy brace provided more pain relief, increased range of motion, a slightly earlier return to walking.

▶ I fully concur with the observations and conclusions of the authors regarding the recommended use of either the Aircast ankle brace or DonJoy R.O.M.-Walker brace for stable lateral malleolar fractures.

J.S. Torg, M.D.

Reflex Sympathetic Dystrophy and Pain Dysfunction in the Lower Extremity

Lindenfeld TN, Bach BR Jr, Wojtys EM (Deaconess Hosp, Cincinnati, Ohio; Rush Presbyterian St Luke's Med Ctr, Chicago; Univ of Michigan, Ann Arbor)
J Bone Joint Surg Am 78A:1936–1944, 1996   4–65

Introduction.—Early treatment of stiff and painful knees is key to creating the best chance of success in patients with reflex sympathetic dystrophy (RSD) and pain dysfunction in the lower extremity. Diagnosis and treatment of sympathetically maintained pain is described.

Diagnosis.—The diagnosis of RSD should be considered in patients with a stiff, swollen extremity out of proportion to the underlying mechanical problem. Sympathetically maintained pain usually begins within 6 weeks of what may be a seemingly simple injury. The pain follows a non-anatomical distribution (ie, does not follow the distribution of a single peripheral nerve and is often described as burning in nature). Patients may experience: color changes in the extremity, increased sweating, intolerance to cold, allodynia, and hyperpathia. Later changes include: dystrophic, smooth, shiny skin; osteoporosis; fast growing and brittle nails; hypertrichosis; muscular and subcutaneous atrophy; extra-articular swelling; and joint contractures. The best method for determining sympathetically maintained pain is sympathetic blockade.

Treatment.—The 3 treatment approaches for systematically maintained pain are: lumbar sympathetic blockade (through use of blocks or surgery), pharmacological therapy, and physical therapy. Blocks can provide sympathetic pain relief for longer periods of time than pharmacologic agents. The more complete and long-lasting pain relief obtained from a lumbar sympathetic block, the better the chances for recovery. Orally administered corticosteroids, non-steroidal anti-inflammatory agents, and narcotics are the drugs of choice. Benzodiazepines are not recommended. Physical therapy is important to management, but patients with sympathetically maintained pain must be progressed slowly with strengthening and range-of-motion exercises. Ice packs should be avoided. Moist heat may be helpful in reducing pain and stiffness.

Conclusion.—Reflex sympathetic dystrophy should be suspected in patients with pain and stiffness out of proportion to causative insult. Early treatment is crucial. Lumbar sympathetic blockade can be used to confirm diagnosis and treat symptoms. Successful outcome is enhanced by a multidisciplinary approach.

▶ An excellent review article. The original is recommended reading for the interested practitioner. Importantly, the authors point out that RSD of the lower extremity frequently does not manifest all of the possible symptoms and occurs more commonly than is currently recognized. Also, the key to successful management is early diagnosis and treatment. Successful management may require the skill of the anesthesiologist, physical therapist, and physicians experienced in the use of multiple drug therapy.

J.S. Torg, M.D.

Ankle Arthroscopy: Outcome in 79 Consecutive Patients

Amendola A, Petrik J, Webster-Bogaert S (London Health Sciences Centre, Ont, Canada)
Arthroscopy 12:565–573, 1996   4–66

Objective.—There are few studies assessing the results of ankle arthroscopy. Results of a review of 79 ankle arthroscopies (28 female subjects), for patients aged 16 to 56, performed with noninvasive distraction and current surgical technique with visual analog scales to assess the benefits and risks of the procedure were presented.

Methods.—Preoperative, postoperative, and at least 2 years of follow-up data from 79 consecutive ankle arthroscopies performed between August 1991 and April 1993 were prospectively reviewed. Demographic data and visual analog scores were compiled and diagnostic and therapeutic outcomes assessed. Variables were compared with a 2-tailed paired *t* test for means.

Results.—Patients had symptoms for an average of 43 months before surgery. Ankle arthroscopies were performed because conservative nonoperative treatment had failed. A therapeutic procedure performed in 44 patients failed in 8 as a result of osteomyelitis in 3, diffuse pigmented villonodular synovitis in 1, osteochondral lesion of the lateral dome of the talus in 1, anterior soft tissue impingement or synovitis in 2, and posttraumatic chondromalacia in 1. Procedures performed for therapeutic and diagnostic reasons in 35 patients failed in 8 because of posttalar neck fracture in 1, talar dome chondromalacia in 2, post–ankle fracture arthrofibrosis in 3, and post–ankle fracture osteoarthritis in 2. Visual analog scores were lower for patients with diffuse osteoarthritis for chondromalacia, Worker's compensation or litigation cases, and postfracture scar and higher for patients with localized osteochondral lesions of the talar dome, soft tissue or bony impingement, and lateral plica. Postoperative complications included 2 patients with a deep peroneal nerve injury and 1 with a superficial lateral peroneal nerve injury.

Conclusion.—Arthroscopic ankle surgery is diagnostically and therapeutically beneficial for patients with localized ankle joint problems. Worker's compensation patients, patients with litigation, and those with osteoarthritis, chondromalacia, or synovitis benefitted less from the procedure.

▶ This is one of the few studies evaluating outcome after arthroscopic surgery of the ankle joint: A prospective study with average follow-up of 2.5 years (range 2.0 to 3.0 years). Results were determined by using a visual analog scale that attempts to determine the patient's subjective response to the procedure. As would be expected, those patients with diffuse disease processes such as osteoarthritis, chondromalacia, or synovitis and worker's compensation or litigation cases did not see significant improvement.

J.S. Torg, M.D.

Ankle Flexibility and Injury Patterns in Dancers

Weisler ER, Hunter DM, Martin DF, et al (Wake Forest Univ, Winston-Salem, NC)
Am J Sports Med 24:754–757, 1996   4–67

Background.—Dancers experience the same type of overuse injuries seen in other athletes, although they also have some unique injury patterns. One factor in dance injuries is the dancer's focus on artistic perfection over physical conditioning. Lower limb injuries in dancers were correlated with ankle range of motion measurements and injury history.

Methods.—The prospective study included 148 students at an arts school; 101 were studying ballet and 47 were studying modern dance. At the beginning of the year, ankle flexibility measurements were obtained. An injury history was taken as well; 28% of the dancers reported previous ankle sprains. The students were then followed for lower limb injuries requiring attention from health care personnel.

Results.—During the follow-up period, 63.5% of the dancers had at least 1 injury. Thirty-nine percent of the injuries were to the ankle, 23% to the foot, 18% to the knee, and 20% to the hip or thigh. Tendinitis, knee strains, and ankle sprains were the most common types of injuries. Two thirds of the injured dancers were studying ballet. Students with a history of lower extremity injuries had lower dorsiflexion measurements and were more likely to experience new injuries. Injury risk was unrelated to age, years of training, body mass index, sex, or ankle range of motion. Flexibility at the ankle and the metatarsophalangeal joint was greater for female students.

Conclusion.—The risk of injury in dancers is apparently unaffected by ankle range of motion. Neither is injury risk related to sex, body mass index, or years of training. Ankle range of motion is greater for female dancers and for modern vs. ballet dancers.

▶ There are some inconsistencies in this paper. First, it is stated that "Previously injured dancers had significantly lower ankle dorsiflexion measurements on the corresponding lower limbs." Elsewhere, the results indicate that "The only statistically significant result was that a reported previous injury was predictive of a new injury." Then the authors conclude that the "data did not support the hypothesis that ankle range of motion abnormalities serve as predictors for future injuries." Also, the authors did not attempt the statistical correlation of the recurrence of a specific injury to the occurrence of a new injury. To be noted, the definition of an injury, whether a recurrence or acute, did not involve a determination of severity.

J.S. Torg, M.D.

The Foot and Ankle: An Overview of Arthrokinematics and Selected Joint Techniques

Loudon JK, Bell SL (Univ of Kansas, Kansas City)
J Athletic Train 31:173–178, 1996   4–68

Background.—Ankle injuries are common athletic injuries. Immobilization of an ankle sprain can cause adhesion formation and joint capsule shortening in several joints. These tissue changes may alter joint arthrokinematics, which may then require progressive range-of-motion and strengthening exercises to restore normal arthrokinematics. Normal arthrokinematics were reviewed and the principles of joint mobilization for rehabilitation were described.

Normal Arthrokinematics.—There are 5 joints involved in ankle motion. In the tibiofibular joint, the fibula glides superiorly and rotates laterally during foot dorsiflexion and glides inferiorly and rotates toward the tibia during plantar flexion. In the talocrural joint, the talus describes a helical movement, gliding posteromedially on the tibia during dorsiflexion and gliding anterolaterally during plantar flexion. Only calcaneal movement is involved in non–weight-bearing subtalar joint motion. How-

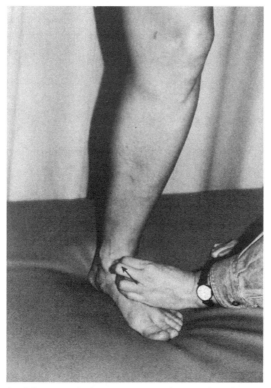

FIGURE 13.—Talar glide in a weight-bearing position. (Courtesy of Loudon JK, Bell SL: The foot and ankle: An overview of arthrokinematics and selected joint techniques. *J Athletic Train* 31:173–178, 1996.)

ever, calcaneal eversion, talar adduction, talar plantar flexion, and tibio-fibular internal rotation occur during weight-bearing pronation, with complementary events occurring in the subtalar joint during weight-bearing supination. The midtarsal joint becomes locked, via an inferior and medial glide of the navicular on the talar head during supination and becomes unlocked during pronation.

Joint Mobilization.—Sustained stretch techniques, using sustained glide force on the gliding component of each joint motion can stretch a tight joint capsule, restore normal arthrokinematics, and improve ankle mobility (Fig 13). Joint mobilization techniques can be graded by either the Maitland method, indicating the degrees of oscillations within the degrees of tissue resistance, or by the Kaltenborn method, which grades sustained translatory techniques. However, these techniques should not be applied to any hypermobile planes in an unstable joint.

Conclusions.—Focus on the components of normal joint motion has identified mobilization techniques that can restore normal biomechanics in joints with a reduced range of motion after injury and immobilization.

▶ After an ankle injury, all the accessory movements of the foot and ankle must be restored before the athlete returns to participation. Various joint and soft-tissue mobilization techniques are described in this article. In many instances, ligamentous laxity is associated with ankle injuries. The authors state that these techniques should not be used in hypermobile planes. To increase ankle dorsiflexion a technique pictured in Figure 13 may be used. The athlete stands with the knee slightly bent, and pressure is applied to the anterior talus in a posterior glide direction as the athlete flexes the knee and dorsiflexes the foot.

F.J. George, A.T.C., P.T.

The Effect of Nontraumatic Immobilization on Ankle Dorsiflexion Stiffness in Rats
Reynolds CA, Cummings GS, Andrew PD, et al (Peachtree Physical Therapy, Norcross, Ga; Georgia State Univ, Atlanta; Hiroshima Univ, Japan; et al)
J Orthop Sports Phys Ther 23:27–33, 1996   4–69

Background.—Animal studies have shown that limbs that are directly traumatized or exposed to traumatic exudate will develop contractures if subjected to 6 or more weeks of immobilization. However, it is unknown whether contractures will develop with immobilization alone, in the absence of trauma. This question was examined in a study of rats.

Methods.—Eight Sprague-Dawley rats had their right hindlimbs immobilized in a plaster cast for either 2 or 6 weeks. The rats were then killed and the limbs removed for testing on a potentiometer to determine changes in dorsiflexion in response to progressively increasing torque. The nonimmobilized left limbs were studied as controls, together with a group of 4 rats with neither limb immobilized.

Results.—The degree of dorsiflexion and joint compliance were both reduced in limbs that were immobilized for 6 weeks. The amount of torque required to achieve end range was elevated 5 times in this group, and ankle dorsiflexion in response to a fixed torque of 3.57 mNm was reduced by 70%. The other limbs tested had no significant changes in ankle dorsiflexion.

Conclusion.—Immobilization without trauma of the rat hindlimb significantly increases ankle dorsiflexion stiffness. The reduced ankle motion results from remodeling of dense connective tissue. Two weeks of casting produces biomechanical or morphological changes, but no increase in joint stiffness.

▶ It is known that prolonged immobilization causes loss of joint range of motion as the tissues of the joint lose their elasticity. There is some question regarding the length of immobilization required before there are significant losses in joint mobility. This study attempted to examine the differences between immobilization of the rat ankle joint at 2 weeks and at 6 weeks. The authors reported that there was some increased stiffness after 2 weeks but no prolonged loss in range of motion; however, after 6 weeks, there was a significant loss of range of motion in the immobilized limbs. The authors noted that there was some tissue weakening after 2 weeks, but after 6 weeks tissue adhesions formed that decreased joint mobility and increased the torque required to move the ankle joint.

The message to clinicians is that immobilized tissue shows changes after 2 weeks and that after 6 weeks, the tissues are markedly weakened and stiffer. The decision to immobilize tissue must be weighed against the resulting mechanical changes, which increased markedly with time.

M.J.L. Alexander, Ph.D.

Ankle Taping Improves Proprioception Before and After Exercise in Young Men
Robbins S, Waked E, Rappel R (Concordia Univ, Montreal; Montreal Gen Hosp)
Br J Sports Med 29:242–247, 1995   4–70

Introduction.—The most commonly reported injuries in sports are ankle sprains. A primary cause of these injuries is thought to be inadequate foot position awareness. It is possible that ankle taping improves kinesthetic sense because taping the skin of the foot with the leg may give cutaneous sensory cues of plantar surface position and orientation through traction of the tape. Poor tape adherence to the skin after exercise probably diminishes this benefit. The effect of ankle taping on foot position has never been tested. A randomized, crossover, controlled comparison was made to determine whether ankle taping improves foot position before and after exercise.

Methods.—Twenty-four healthy young volunteers participated in testing sessions before and after 30 minutes of basketball and running. Twelve volunteers had their ankles taped and 12 remained untaped. Participants wore their own athletic shoes. Foot position sense testing was performed with volunteers blindfolded. They were asked to perceive slope direction and estimate slope amplitude when bearing full body weight and standing on a series of blocks. The top slope of the blocks varied between 0 degrees and 25-degrees in 2.5 degree increments. This was done to orient the plantar surface with respect to the leg toward pronation, supination, plantar flexion, and dorsiflexion relative to its position on a flat surface.

Results.—Untaped research subjects were unable to distinguish between a flat surface and a surface slope of 20 degrees while wearing modern athletic shoes. Taped volunteers were able to detect slope surfaces greater than 10 degrees. The absolute mean estimate error overall was 3.95 degrees before exercise and 4.81 degrees after exercise in taped and untaped research subjects, respectively. Before exercise, the higher range absolute position error was significantly higher in taped than in untaped volunteers (4.23 degrees and 5.53 degrees, respectively). After exercise, these numbers were 2.5% worse in taped volunteers and 35.5% worse in untaped volunteers.

Ankle taping improved proprioception before and after exercise. Ankle taping appears to counter underestimation of foot position angle caused by modern athletic footwear. Footwear use has a significant role in ankle injury. Footwear needs to be identified and redesigned to optimize proprioceptive sense to reduce the incidence of injury in all sports.

▶ The authors state, "The inescapable conclusion is that footwear use is ultimately responsible for ankle injury" and that "taping counters underestimation of foot position angle caused by modern athletic footwear." (See abstract 4–73). There may be different factors contributing to ankle sprains, proprioception, and kinesthetic awareness that should certainly be considered and addressed in any preventive or rehabilitation program. Footwear may be a major contributing factor to ankle sprains. If athletic footwear can be designed to increase rather than decrease proprioception and kinesthetic awareness, we may see a reduction in the frequency of sprained ankles. This study indicates that one benefit of ankle taping may be an increase in proprioception and kinesthetic awareness.

F.J. George, A.T.C., P.T.

The Effect of Solid Ankle-Foot Orthoses on Movement Patterns Used in a Supine-to-Stand Rising Task
King LA, VanSant AF (Temple Univ, Philadelphia)
Phys Ther 75:952–964, 1995   4–71

Background.—In dynamic pattern theory, ankle motion can be seen as a control variable and solid ankle-foot orthoses (SAFOs) as a constraint to that variable. The effect of SAFOs on patterns of motion while rising from the supine position to an erect stance was investigated.

Methods.—Thirty-nine healthy adults aged 20–28 years were included. Each participant performed 10 trials in each of 4 conditions: without SAFOs, with a right SAFO, then with a left SAFO, then with bilateral SAFOs.

Findings.—In the no-SAFO condition, the subjects most commonly rose with a push and reach pattern of the upper extremities, a forward with rotation pattern in the trunk, and an asymmetrical squat in the lower extremities. The incidence of movement patterns was changed in all the SAFO conditions. More asymmetry of movement occurred, especially in the axial region.

Conclusion.—Solid ankle-foot orthoses constrain ankle motion during rising from a supine to a standing position, being most apparent when weight is transferred from the buttocks to the feet during rising. When ankle motion is restricted, compensatory strategies emerge to achieve weight transfer. Increased asymmetry in all 3 movement components occurs when SAFOs are worn on 1 or both legs. The axial region is most sensitive to ankle constraint.

▶ Most movement patterns are altered by the use of joint constraints such as knee braces, ankle orthoses, or plaster casts. This study attempted to describe the major alterations in movement patterns of normal subjects with the addition of SAFOs during a supine-to-stand task. Movement patterns were examined using 2 video cameras that filmed 4 conditions of ankle joint restraint.

Significant changes were found in movement patterns between the no SAFO, left SAFO, right SAFO and bilateral SAFO conditions. The major change was found to be in weight transfer from the buttocks to the feet, which normally required ankle plantar flexion that was not possible with the SAFOs. This was compensated for with a wide-based, medially rotated squat, followed by a tendency for subjects to hop to regain their balance after reaching a standing position. Restrained ankle joint movement produced increased asymmetry in the body movements required to attain standing, suggesting that similar adjustments are required for any injury-related joint constraint.

M.J.L. Alexander, Ph.D.

Evaluation of Kinesthetic Deficits Indicative of Balance Control in Gymnasts With Unilateral Chronic Ankle Sprains

Forkin DM, Koczur C, Battle R, et al (Frankford Hosp, Philadelphia; Thomas Jefferson Univ, Philadelphia; Maryview Health Care Ctr, Chesapeake, Va; et al)

J Orthop Sports Phys Ther 23:245–250, 1996   4–72

Introduction.—Seventeen percent of all injuries in college-level gymnasts are ankle injuries. Recurring injuries can result in an unstable ankle

and potentially decreased balance ability. It is possible that balance instability after recurrent ankle injuries may be a result of the disruption
between neurologic and biomechanical factors at the ankle joint. Active
college-level gymnasts with a history of unilateral, multiple ankle sprains
were evaluated for their ability to detect passive plantar flexion motion in
the injured ankle joints, compared with the uninjured side, and to determine balance deficits.

Methods.—Two male and 9 female gymnasts between the ages of 16 and
22 years underwent 30 passive movement trials performed randomly on
injured and uninjured ankles. A kinesthesiometer was used to administer
15 movement and 15 nonmovement trials. A 30-second 1-legged balance
task with eyes open and eyes closed was used to test kinesthetic sense. Two
independent observers evaluated balance ability, and gymnasts were questioned regarding their perception of balance ability.

Results.—Gymnasts were more capable of detecting movement in their
uninjured than injured ankles. Balance was better and gymnasts perceived
balance to be better in uninjured compared with injured ankles. No
gymnasts were judged by either observer to have equal balance ability
bilaterally with eyes open or closed.

Conclusion.—Gymnasts in this series had a higher incidence of balance
and kinesthetic deficits in their injured leg, compared with the contralateral uninjured leg. Findings emphasize the need for clinicians to assess
balance and kinesthetic deficits in patients with 1 or more ankle sprains. A
focus on correcting causal elements is preferred to treating signs and
symptoms of ankle injuries.

▶ This study indicates that, "injuries occurring at the ankle account for 17%
of all injuries for college-level gymnasts." Female gymnasts tend to perform
barefoot, and males wear a small slipper or sock for many events. Because
of this, factors other than the shoe must be considered when treating and
preventing ankle sprains. (Please read abstract 4–70 and my comments).
Ligament laxity, range of motion, Achilles tendon flexibility, strength, proprioception, kinesthetic awareness, taping, bracing, and footwear are all
factors that must be taken into account.

F.J. George, A.T.C., P.T.

**The Effect of Exercise, Prewrap, and Athletic Tape on the Maximal
Active and Passive Ankle Resistance to Ankle Inversion**
Manfroy PP, Ashton-Miller JA, Wojtys EM (Univ of Michigan, Ann Arbor)
Am J Sports Med 25:156–163, 1997   4–73

Objective.—Ankle injury is one of the most common athletic injuries.
Whether taping decreases ankle injury and severity is controversial, and
taping can cause significant skin irritation. Maximal active and passive
resistance to inversion developed in a weight-bearing ankle at 15 degrees
of inversion with and without the presence of prophylactic adhesive ath-

letic tape, a nonadhesive layer of prewrap under the tape, or 40 minutes of vigorous exercise was investigated.

Methods.—Maximal ankle resistance measurements during unipedal weight-bearing conditions were taken in 20 individuals (10 men), average age 25 years, randomly allocated to wear tape applied over prewrap or tape applied directly to skin after baseline without tape measurements of ankle resistance to 15 degrees of inversion. Tests were performed before and after a 40-minute exercise session. Normalized mean total moments resisting ankle inversion were compared by sex.

Results.—Men and women resisted a mean inversion moment of 52.9 newton meters and 28.3 newton meters, respectively, without tape support. At baseline before exercise, individuals with taped ankles resisted significantly larger moments that did individuals without taped ankles. Men generated significantly larger moments than women. Individuals with ankles taped over prewrap had significantly larger (11.5%) moments than did individuals without taped ankles. According to secondary analysis of variance, individuals with taped ankles after 40 minutes of vigorous exercise did not resist significantly larger moments than before it. After exercise, the untaped ankle could resist an inversion moment 5% larger than before exercise.

Conclusion.—Whereas taped ankles resisted a significantly larger inversion moment than untaped ankles, 40 minutes of exercise reduced the maximum inversion moment generated to a value similar to that of the untaped ankle. There was no significant difference between support provided by tape alone or tape over prewrap. After exercise, the untaped ankle could resist 5% larger inversion moment than before exercise.

▶ Athletic trainers generally agree that activity reduces the effectiveness of ankle taping. To combat this problem, many athletic trainers recommend that ankle braces be worn over taped ankles. This appears to improve the effect of the tape and increases the amount of time that the tape provides protection. To my knowledge, there have been no studies examining the effectiveness of the combination of taping and bracing an ankle.

F.J. George, A.T.C., P.T.

What Best Protects the Inverted Weightbearing Ankle Against Further Inversion?
Ashton-Miller JA, Ottaviani RA, Hutchinson C, et al (Univ of Michigan, Ann Arbor)
Am J Sports Med 24:800–809, 1996   4–74

Background.—Ankle injuries account for up to 25% of all time lost in sports competition. Most ankle injuries are of the inversion type. In an attempt to reduce the risk of injury, several forms of ankle protection have been developed, including high-top athletic shoes, athletic taping, and orthotic devices.

Methods.—Twenty young men participated in a study assessing the protective ability of these devices. Maximal isometric eversion moment under full weight-bearing was measured with the ankles in 15 degrees of inversion. Measurements were obtained at 0 and 32 degrees of ankle plantar flexion in low- and three-quarter–top shoes with and without adhesive athletic tape or proprietary ankle orthoses.

Findings.—At 0 degrees of ankle plantar flexion, the mean maximal voluntary resistance of the unprotected ankle to an inversion moment was 50 newton-meters; this increased by a mean of 12% with a three-quarter–top basketball shoe. The maximal voluntary resistances to inversion moments did not increase significantly with the ankles further protected by athletic tape or orthoses. Calculations suggested that, at 15 degrees of inversion, the fully active ankle evertor muscles isometrically developed a moment up to 6 times larger than that developed passively with tape or an orthosis inside a three-quarter-top shoe.

Conclusion.—Fully active evertor muscles acting isometrically in the adult male ankle at 15 degrees of inversion can provide more than 3 times more protection against an ankle inversion injury than tape or an orthosis inside a three-quarter–top shoe. Thus, the most effective form of ankle protection at footstrike is precontracted and strong evertor muscles.

▶ The importance of ankle evertor muscle strength in the prevention of ankle sprains is proven by this study. All too often, reliance is placed on adhesive tape and ankle braces, and strengthening exercise may be neglected. Everter muscle strengthening exercises should be part of preseason conditioning programs and all ankle rehabilitation programs. Athletes with ankle problems or those who participate in sports with a high incidence of ankle injuries should heed the authors' advice and be taught to co-contract their ankle muscles and flex their knee when they anticipate that the instant of retouching the ground will be unpredictable.

F.J. George, A.T.C., P.T.

Traumatic Peroneal Tendon Instability
Mason RB, Henderson IJP (Mercy Private Hosp, East Melbourne, Australia)
Am J Sports Med 24:652–658, 1996   4–75

Objective.—Traumatic peroneal tendon instability is often misdiagnosed as a sprained ankle. The causes of peroneal tendon instability, pathologic changes associated with such injury, and treatment outcomes after injury are reviewed.

Methods.—Between 1986 and 1994 10 patients (2 women), aged 16 to 48, with 11 dislocations were operated for 5 acute injuries and 6 chronic injuries.

Technique.—The detached retinaculum is exposed by means of a curved longitudinal incision anterior to the lateral malleolus and opened longitudinally. A tenosynovectomy is performed if necessary. An osteotomy is formed by creating a teardrop-shaped segment of the distal fibula and is used to stabilize the relocated peroneal tendons. The retinaculum is reattached to the posterolateral margin of the fibula. The wound is closed. The patient wears a below-the-knee plaster cast for 6 weeks with weight bearing permitted at 2 weeks.

Results.—Excellent clinical and functional results were achieved in 9 ankles. Patients involved in competitive sports returned to their preinjury levels after 3 months. Complications included persistent subluxation in 1 patient that was treated with repeat surgery; recurrent infection in 1 patient that was treated by debridement, screw removal, sural nerve neurolysis, and 6 weeks of antibiotic therapy; and 1 patient with ipsilateral deep vein thrombosis that was treated with anticoagulant therapy. At operation, all patients had grade I lesions, and 5 had significant synovitis. Subjectively, 2 patients had mild pain and tenderness in the area of the screws. All patients except the 1 with recurrent infection rated their satisfaction between 8 and 10 on a 10-point scale. Objectively, no patient had ankle stiffness. Eversion power was normal. One patient with recurrent infection had sural paresthesia. All patients had significant pes planus that was correctable.

Conclusion.—Treatment of both acute and chronic peroneal tendon instability using the superior peroneal retinacular repair with or without fibular rotational osteotomy yields successful results.

▶ I fully agree with the authors' conclusion that superior peroneal retinacular repair with or without fibular rotational osteotomy is a successful technique in treating both acute and recurrent peroneal tendon instability. It is also worth noting that all of the patients with acute peroneal tendon dislocation were treated surgically and no patient underwent a trial of nonoperative treatment. That is, there are no nonoperative controls.

J.S. Torg, M.D.

5 Biomechanics, Training, and Physiotherapy

Muscle Function in Movement and Sports
Herzog W (Univ of Calgary, Alberta, Canada)
Am J Sports Med 24:S14–S19, 1996   5–1

Background.—Relatively few studies have looked at the functional roles of muscles during sports and movement or sought to identify adaptations of the mechanical properties of muscles to exercise. The most important mechanical properties of skeletal muscles for optimizing movement are the force-length and force-power properties. These properties are reviewed, along with the functional roles of muscles during movement and sports.

Force-Length Relationship.—The force-length relationship refers to the fact that the maximal isometric force exerted by a muscle depends on its length. It is generally not possible to determine the force-length properties of individual human muscles in vivo, and there are few data on the submaximal force-length properties of muscles. Comparative studies of cyclists and runners suggest that the number of sarcomeres in rectus femoris muscle fibers can adapt to the everyday requirements of activity. The rectus femoris muscles of cyclists operate only on the descending limb of the force-length relationship if the sarcomere number in series is relatively small. Thus the average sarcomere length of cyclists is relatively larger than that of runners, and vice versa. This suggests that cycling and running are not good cross-training for each other.

Force-Power-Velocity Relationship.—Speed of contraction determines the maximal force exerted by a muscle at optimal length. Multiplying the force and velocity values of the force-velocity relationship will produce the power-velocity relationship. To measure muscle power, one must directly measure muscle force and speed of contraction. Studies of frogs showed that the muscle length during jumping was around the optimal muscle length, and that speed of shortening was kept constant so as to produce peak power throughout the jump. Power is maximized if a muscle contracts at optimal length and shortens at about 30% of maximal speed. In applying this principle to a study of cyclists, it was found that the overall optimal movement resulted not from maximal power produced throughout movement but from a combination of suboptimal muscle performances.

Functional Role of the Muscles.—To optimize performance, one needs to know the function of muscles during sports activity. The exact function of a muscle during movement is not always clear. Muscles in an agonistic group may have differing functional roles. In the absence of force measurements of individual muscles during human movement and sports, good insights may be gained by evaluating the net effects of muscle contributions. A training concept with intuitive appeal may prove to be incorrect on more careful analysis.

Summary.—Current knowledge on muscle function in human movement and sports is reviewed, including the force-length relationship, the force-power-velocity relationship, and the functional role of muscles. With further development, the study of muscle mechanics in sports could play a key role in sports movement analysis and performance optimization.

▶ This article is an excellent comprehensive review of the subject matter. The original article is recommended reading for the sports medicine practitioner.

J.S. Torg, M.D.

Muscle Fatigue: The Cellular Aspects
Fitts RH (Marquette Univ, Milwaukee, Wis)
Am J Sports Med 24:S9–S13, 1996   5–2

Purpose.—In muscle fatigue, reductions in peak tension and power output lead to reduced work capacity. Central fatigue relates to neural inputs to the higher brain center, whereas peripheral fatigue involves the cellular aspects in the muscle cell. The mechanisms and functional changes in the fatigued muscle cell are reviewed, along with the causes of the dysfunctions.

Mechanical and Functional Changes.—Fatigue is associated with a rapid drop in twitch tension and a slowing of contraction and relaxation time. The slowing of relaxation time may be related to inhibition of calcium reuptake by the sarcoplasmic reticulum. Recovery from fatigue takes place in 2 phases: a rapid recovery during 2 minutes, followed by a slower recovery to the prefatigue level, which may take an hour or more. Fatigue caused by endurance exercise differs from that caused by high-intensity exercise.

The mechanisms of peripheral fatigue involve the neuromuscular junction; excitation-contraction coupling, which involves surface membrane activation, propagation of that activation down the T-tubules, and calcium release; and activation of contractile elements. High-intensity contractile activity leads to a rapid decline in peak tension or force, reduction of shortening velocity, decline in power, prolongation of twitch duration, reduced amplitude, and a conduction velocity that can lead to conduction block. Reduced amplitude and prolonged duration are consequences of the calcium transient.

In high-intensity exercise, hydrogen may act as a direct inhibitor of the rate of force development and calcium binding to the regulatory protein troponin C, which activates myosin binding to actin, generating force and shortening. Hydrogen also inhibits cross-bridge transition from the low-force to high-force state and inhibits velocity of the cross-bridge cycle rate. By these means, hydrogen reduces power and prolongs calcium reuptake by inhibiting the sarcoplasmic reticulum calcium ATPase pump. Tension is inhibited by phosphate through reversal of the cross-bridge transition from low force to high force. However, because phosphate does not affect cycle rate, it does not affect velocity. Phosphate may decrease the free energy of ATP hydrolysis, providing less energy, and may inhibit calcium reuptake by the sarcoplasmic reticulum.

Clinical Implications.—This information on the mechanisms of fatigue has uncertain implications for the prevention of fatigue. Athletes should have a varied training program—if he or she performs only 1 type of exercise, other factors will lead to fatigue. Diet, warmup, and fluid replacement will also influence peak performance.

▶ This article is an excellent comprehensive review of the subject matter. The original article is recommended reading for the sports medicine practitioner.

J.S. Torg, M.D.

The Effects of Muscle Fatigue on Neuromuscular Function and Anterior Tibial Translation in Healthy Knees
Wojtys EM, Wylie BB, Huston LJ (Univ of Michigan, Ann Arbor)
Am J Sports Med 24:615–621, 1996   5–3

Background.—The relationship among knee joint laxity, muscle fatigue, and knee joint injury is not clear. The effect of quadriceps and hamstring muscle fatigue on anterior tibial translation and muscle reaction time was investigated in 10 healthy individuals.

Methods.—The subjects were 6 men and 4 women, aged a mean 21.3 years. None had any known knee problems. The subjects underwent a knee examination, arthrometer measures of tibial translation, subjective functional evaluation, and an anterior tibial translation stress test before and after quadriceps and hamstring muscle-fatiguing exercise.

Findings.—The lower extremity muscle recruitment order did not change with fatigue in response to anterior tibial translation. However, there was a mean 32.5% increase in anterior tibial translation after muscle fatigue. Significant slowing was observed in the muscle responses of the gastrocnemius, hamstring, and quadriceps originating at the spinal cord and cortical level. In some subjects, there was no activity after quadriceps and hamstring muscle fatigue. The increased displacement after fatigue was strongly correlated with a delay in cortical-level activity.

Conclusions.—Muscle fatigue apparently affects the dynamic stability of the knee and changes the neuromuscular response to anterior tibial translation. Thus fatigue may have an important role in the pathomechanics of knee injury during sports.

▶ This is an excellent paper and represents a long overdue attempt to identify etiologic factors responsible for the pathomechanics of knee injuries. Muscle fatigue, changes in the viscoelastic property of the collagenous tissue, and increased muscle reaction time are all clearly suspect. Clinical correlation of noncontact knee injuries with duration of participation in physically demanding activities would be most helpful.

J.S. Torg, M.D.

Muscle Strain Injuries
Garrett WE Jr (Duke Univ, Durham, NC)
Am J Sports Med 24:S2–S8, 1996   5–4

Objective.—Muscle strains are characterized by disruption of the muscle-tendon unit, with localized pain and general muscle weakness on attempted activity. Although muscle strains are extremely common, relatively little is known about their pathophysiology, treatment, and recovery. The mechanisms, treatment, and prevention of muscle strain injury are reviewed.

Mechanisms.—The authors have developed a rabbit hindlimb model to demonstrate in the laboratory 2 mechanisms of muscle strain: passive and active stretch. With both types of injuries, the site of stretch-induced injury was near the muscle-tendon junction. The model also showed ultrastructural damage in the absence of complete disruption of the muscle-tendon unit. This tissue damage significantly affects the ability of the muscle to develop tension. In addition to flexibility, warmup, and pre-exercise stretching, viscoelasticity is an important consideration. The authors' model showed that much of the muscle change induced by stretching is the result of inherent muscle-tendon viscoelasticity with neural influence.

Clinical Applications.—Imaging studies in athletes with muscle strain injuries also show that the injury is localized to the muscle-tendon junction. Both CT and MRI are useful in demonstrating muscle strain injuries. Two-joint or complex muscles are most susceptible to strain injury. Disruptions do not occur in the midsubstance of muscle fibers, but injury to the muscle-tendon unit can occur within the tendon or at the tendon-bone junction. As suggested by basic science studies, eccentric activation seems to be the main mechanism of injury.

Prevention.—Studies in the rabbit model suggest that cyclic stretching is beneficial. Stretching that produces forces greater than 70% of failure force make the muscle less vulnerable to injury. Experiments also suggested that warmup allows the muscle to stretch more before failure and to produce greater force. Further studies showed that previous minor injury predisposes to more serious injury. Early return to activity or aggressive rehabilitation could add to this problem. Also, fatigued muscle is more prone to injury because it cannot adsorb energy before reaching the point of injury-producing stretch. Experimental studies suggest that nonsteroidal anti-inflammatory drugs can help reduce pain and improve function after muscle strains, although there is some evidence of delayed histologic repair.

Conclusions.—Key issues related to muscle strain injury are reviewed. Basic science research supports the benefits of warmup, temperature, and stretching in terms of preventing muscle strains. More research is needed to clarify the process of repair and recovery after muscle strains, focusing on the recovery of function and the susceptibility to repeated injury.

▶ This article is an excellent comprehensive review of muscle strain injuries. The original article is recommended reading for the sports medicine practitioner.

J.S. Torg, M.D.

Biomechanics of Iliotibial Band Friction Syndrome in Runners
Orchard JW, Fricker PA, Abud AT, et al (Australian Inst of Sport, Canberra)
Am J Sports Med 24:375–379, 1996   5–5

Background.—Iliotibial band friction syndrome (ITBFS) may occur in long-distance runners or cyclists. This condition is generally thought to result from extrinsic factors, such as training errors and downhill running, combined with intrinsic factors, such as tightness of the iliotibial band and abnormal foot biomechanics. Several factors have been linked to the development of ITBFS, including increased leg-length discrepancy, increased forefoot varus, and increased knee Q angles. However, few of these features are significantly correlated with ITBFS. Through cadaver and dynamic studies, the authors have developed a pathogenic model of ITBFS in runners.

Model.—The findings suggested that friction of the iliotibial band occurred between the posterior edge of the band and the lateral femoral condyle underneath. The friction occurred near footstrike, mainly in the foot contact phase. Knee flexion averaged 30 degrees at the time of friction. Iliotibial band width varied substantially in cadaver studies. Downhill running reduces the knee flexion angle at footstrike, thus favoring the development of ITBFS. Friction is less likely to occur during sprinting or faster running on level ground. Using a heel raise to increase the knee angle at footstrike does not always have the desired effect.

Conclusions.—Iliotibial band friction syndrome appears to result from repetitive knee movement through an impingement zone, with impingement occurring during the foot contact phase of gait. In contrast to previous recommendations of total rest, patients can resume faster running or multidirectional sports after the initial inflammation has subsided. Slow jogging is delayed until the patient has returned to faster running. The patient should train on flat terrain, avoiding downhill running, which reduces knee flexion angle at footstrike.

▶ This study does have implications with regard to the clinical management of patients with ITBFS. Specifically, resumption of activity after resolution of the inflammatory phase should include activities that involve a faster running pace rather than slow jogging, which is the opposite of what is normally recommended after injury. Also, downhill running is to be discouraged and runners should be advised to train on flat terrain to prevent recurrence. Of note, this study considered the mechanics of the disorder in only the sagittal plane, not considering the mechanics of iliotibial band tightness in coronal plane or rotation of the tibia in the transverse plane.

J.S. Torg, M.D.

Support for a Linear Length–Tension Relation of the Torso Extensor Muscles: An Investigation of the Length and Velocity EMG–Force Relationships
Raschke U, Chaffin DB (Univ of Michigan, Ann Arbor)
J Biomech 29:1597–1604, 1996   5–6

Introduction.—For the investigation of low back pain, computerized biomechanical models of the torso continue to be developed. The torso extensor muscle length-tension and force-velocity relationships in vivo were studied. The hypothesis was that the length-tension relation of the torso erectors would be linear and would mirror the observed linear increase in extension strength capability toward full flexion. Concentric velocity-tension mismodeling was also investigated to provide data with which to compare the currently used technique.

Methods.—During controlled sagittal plane extension motions of 5 men, a myoelectric-based approach was used with a dynamic biomechanical model that incorporated active and passive tissue characteristics to provide muscle kinematic estimates. The 5 men had no history of back pain, had a mean age of 29.6 years, a mean height of 179.6 cm, and a mean weight of 73.7 kg. To find the length-tension and force-velocity relations, 3 zones of torso flexion were used (Fig 1). Sagittal plane lifts were performed beginning in a stooped posture and ending in a neutral upright posture. Muscle tension estimates were made using a double linear optimization formulation from the literature.

Results.—The hypothesis of a linear length-tension relation toward full flexion for the erector spinae and latissimus muscles was supported. Predictions of exponential relations agreed with velocity trends, and the linear trends agreed with the data as well. When the length modulator was

Zones of Analysis

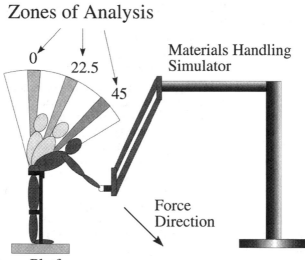

FIGURE 1.—Three zones of torso flexion used to find the length-tension and force-velocity relationships. Analysis of data from 3 zones minimized possible confounding from mismodeled length-tension relationships during the development of the force-velocity relationships. The minimal effect of the electromyograph motion artifact was confirmed by comparing relationships developed using data from each of the zones. (Courtesy of Raschke U, Chaffin DB: Support for a linear length–tension relation of the torso extensor muscles: An investigation of the length and velocity EMG–force relationships. Reprinted from the *Journal of Biomechanics* 29:1597–1604, copyright 1996, with kind permission from Elsevier Science Ltd, The Boulevard, Langford Lane, Kidlington OX5 1GB UK.)

included, the analysis of the length-tension and velocity-force modulator effects on the myoelectric to muscle tension relationship substantially improved. The additional inclusion of the velocity modulator had a lesser, but significant, improvement as well.

Conclusion.—While lifting in fully flexed postures, individuals can experience tissue strain, which may possibly cause low back pain injury, according to the muscle tension estimation in biomechanical torso modeling.

▶ It has been previously reported that trunk extensor torques increase with increased forward trunk flexion; this study examined this relationship and confirmed that strength increased toward full flexion. This finding is not in agreement with the length-tension relationship for muscle, which suggests that muscle force output is greatest close to resting length. The present finding was likely a result of fiber-type composition variability and muscle architectural variability between research subjects. The authors hypothesized that muscles that produce maximal tension when stretched to maximal lengths may produce injury to the muscle aponeurosis, which would cause back pain. This type of muscle injury may be 1 of the many causes of the high incidence of low back pain. This study has implications for increased accuracy in biomechanical models of the muscles of the lumbar spine.

M.J.L. Alexander, Ph.D.

Development and Evaluation of a Scalable and Deformable Geometric Model of the Human Torso

Nussbaum MA, Chaffin DB (Univ of Michigan, Ann Arbor)
Clin Biomech 11:25–34, 1996   5–7

Objective.—Models are sometimes constructed to simulate the behavior of biological units and to aid in understanding their function under varying conditions. Previous models of the torso have mainly considered the bony elements as rigid bodies; they have differed mainly in the number of elements included and the extent of detail. A geometric model of the human torso was developed and evaluated.

Methods.—The model represented an extension of a previously reported mathematical model, which considered the thoracic and lumbar spine, sternum, rib cage, and sacrum as rigid bodies interconnected by a set of spring and beam elements (Fig 3). The modified model was designed to permit scaling with standard anthropometric measures, deformation to specific 3-dimensional postures using surface markers, and inclusion of muscle length–tension and motion segment passive bending properties. The accuracy of the model's postural predictions was analyzed in a series of evaluative studies.

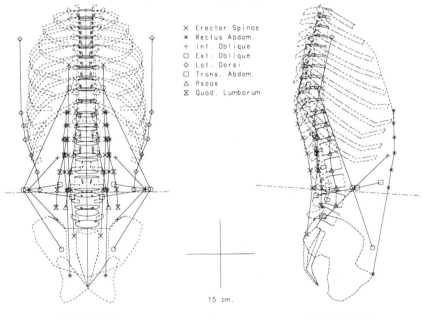

X   Erector Spinae
＊   Rectus Abdom.
+   Int. Oblique
O   Ext. Oblique
◇   Lat. Dorsi
□   Trans. Abdom.
△   Psoas
X   Quad. Lumborum

15 cm.

POSTERIOR VIEW   RIGHT-SIDE VIEW

FIGURE 3.—Muscle geometry illustrated for a 50th percentile male. Muscles are treated as pointwise connections from origin to insertion. An imaginary cutting plane that bisects the L3–L4 motion segment is also shown. (Reprinted from Nussbaum MA, Chaffin DB: Development and evaluation of a scalable and deformable geometric model of the human torso. *Clin Biomech* 11:25–34, copyright 1996, with kind permission from Elsevier Science Ltd, The Boulevard, Langford Lane, Kidlington OX5 1GB UK.)

Results.—Surface marker displacement analyses suggested that only minimal deformation of the thoracic spine occurred across a range of flexion, extension, and lateral bending. Thus, when low-weight lifting over the range of passive flexibility was considered, the thoracic spine could be treated as an essentially rigid structure. The model accurately reproduced the locations of bony landmarks, with mean errors of 2.9–6.8 mm. Likewise, measurements of several body areas were reproducible, with mean differences of 2.6–15.4 mm. On comparison with a human subject, the model predicted 84% of the passive reactive moments required to balance body segment weight moments in lateral bending and 96% in flexion.

Conclusions.—This geometric model provides a quantitative depiction of torso geometry, including the effects of anthropometry and extreme postures. Models of this type are crucial to our understanding of the physical effects of exertion in human beings. They provide accurate descriptions of spinal deformation in extreme postures, thus permitting more accurate biomechanical modeling of tissue loads. Such models should be included in future evaluations of spinal loading.

▶ Injuries to the lower back during workplace activities require closer examination to determine postures and loads that are beyond threshold levels. The use of a scaled geometric model of the spine and torso is a safe and effective way of modeling these tasks and the resulting loads on the spine. The development of an accurate 3-dimensional model is difficult because of the anatomical complexity of the bones and muscles found in the torso. This model was a refinement of an earlier model, with the addition of more accurate measurements of muscle size and location and bony landmarks. The ability of a model of this type to estimate trunk muscle forces in different positions of the trunk is a useful contribution in determining positions and loads to be avoided.

M.J.L. Alexander, Ph.D.

Determination of Fascicle Length and Pennation in a Contracting Human Muscle In Vivo
Fukunaga T, Ichinose Y, Ito M, et al (Univ of Tokyo)
J Appl Physiol 82:354–358, 1997   5–8

Introduction.—Before it appears at the joint as moments, the force exerted by muscle fibers is modified by geometric arrangement, structures of the joint, and the angle and location of the tendon with respect to the bone. The architecture of a human muscle at rest and during contractions was determined by using real-time US that visualized fascicles in vivo. The investigation included the relationship between knee joint angles and fascicle lengths as well as angles of pennation for the vastus lateralis muscle.

Methods.—Ultrasonography was used to develop a technique to determine fascicle length in human vastus lateralis muscle in vivo with 6 healthy men, aged 25 ± 1 year. They were measured while seated on a test bench of an electric dynamometer, which was visually aligned with the estimated center of the knee joint. Ultrasonic measurement was performed as the knee joint angles were changed every 10 degrees from full extension to flexion at 110 degrees. Measurements were also taken when muscles were tensed.

Results.—The fascicle length decreased from 133 to 97 mm on average when the men had the knee fully extended passively from a position of 110

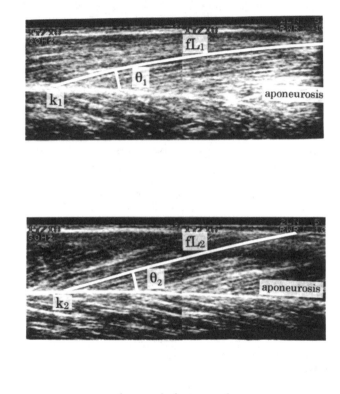

relaxed

tensed

knee joint angle

50 deg

FIGURE 1.—Ultrasonic longitudinal image of the vastus lateralis muscle. Ultrasonic transducer was placed on the skin over the muscle at 50% distance from the greater trochanter to the lateral epicondyle of the femur. Fascicle length (*fl*) was determined as the length of a line drawn along the ultrasonic echo parallel to the fascicle. Fascicle angle (θ) was determined as the angle between echoes obtained from the fascicles and deep aponeurosis in the ultrasonic image. *Abbreviation: k*, distal end of a fascicle. (Courtesy of Fukunaga T, Ichinose Y, Ito M, et al: Determination of fascicle length and pennation in a contracting human muscle in vivo. *J Appl Physiol* 82:354–358, 1997.)

degrees flexion (relaxed condition). Fascicle shortening was more pronounced (from 126 to 67 mm), especially when the knee was closer to full extension during static contractions at 10% of maximal voluntary contraction strength (tensed condition). The angle of pennation increased from 14 to 18 degrees relaxed and from 14 to 21 degrees tensed as the knee was extended. When the knee was close to extension, there was a greater increase in the pennation angle observed in the tensed than in the relaxed condition. Echoes reflected from fascicles were seen in the ultrasonic image obtained from vastus lateralis muscle tissue (Fig 1).

Conclusion.—When the muscle is in a relaxed and isometrically tensed condition, there are differences in fascicle lengths and pennation angles, and the differences are affected by joint angles, at least at the submaximal contraction level.

▶ Muscle architecture, or the geometric arrangement of muscle fibers, is an important determinant of the transmission of muscle force to the tendons and bones. Although muscle pennation angle and fascicle length are of some interest, they are difficult to study in vivo. This study used US to visualize the vastus lateralis muscle fascicles at rest and during contraction, from which length and pennation angles could be determined. Contracting the knee extensors decreased fascicle length from 133 to 97 mm on average. Contraction of the muscle also produced an increase in pennation angle, which produced a reduction in isometric force development because of the decrease in the rotational component of the muscle contractile force. However, the largest fascicle angle is 21 degrees in the contracted position and 17 degrees in the relaxed position, which produces an average loss of force of 4% to 7%. The authors concluded that the effect of pennation angles on force transmission between the contracted and relaxed conditions would not be significant here, but the contraction was only 10% of the maximal voluntary contraction strength. More study is required to determine the effects of the pennation angle on the force output at higher contractile levels of the muscle.

M.J.L. Alexander, Ph.D.

Resistance to Crack Growth in Human Cortical Bone Is Greater in Shear Than in Tension
Norman TL, Nivargikar SV, Burr DB (West Virginia Univ, Morgantown; Indiana Univ, Indianapolis)
J Biomech 29:1023–1031, 1996   5–9

Introduction.—Previous studies suggest that human bone tends to sustain microdamage in shear regions and thus may not be adapted to prevent crack growth under shear loading. However, similarities between bone and other fiber-reinforced composites that are tough indicate that human bone may have good fatigue and impact properties. Investigators hypothesized on the basis of these similarities that the resistance of bone to longitudinal crack growth under shear loading is greater than that under tensile loading. Also tested was the hypothesis that bone from older individuals and women would have less resistance to longitudinal crack growth under shear and tension loading.

Methods.—Fresh human tibias were obtained from 9 men aged 55–89 years and 6 women aged 61–89 year. Using compact shear and compact tension specimens, the critical strain energy release rate of human bone was measured for longitudinally oriented cracks under tension and shear. Specimens were randomly taken from the lateral and medial cortices of the mid-diaphysis. Donor differences were analyzed with the variability among donors divided into 3 components: age, sex, and other.

Results.—The average tensile fracture toughness of male and female human bone was 339 Nm^{-1}; average shear fracture toughness over the same range was 4,200 Nm^{-1}. Shear toughness was found to be approximately 13 times greater than tensile toughness, consistent with other fibrous composite materials. Although fracture toughness decreased with age, the fits were weak and were significant for shear loading only. There was no relationship between a patient's sex and tension and shear toughness.

Discussion.—As previously observed with other fibrous composite materials, the fracture toughness of human bone under shear is greater than fracture toughness under tension. Shear toughness was approximately 13 times that of tensile toughness. Findings support the study hypothesis and suggest that cracks are more likely to grow in tension than in shear. Bone does become less resistant to longitudinal crack growth in tension and shear with aging, but relationships were significant only for shear. Fracture toughness did not differ significantly between men and women.

▶ The mechanics of human bone fracture in older individuals is of increasing interest as the population ages and fractures are more prevalent in this older population. Bones are primarily resistant to compression forces but are also subject to bending, shear, and tensile forces during daily activities. In testing a sample of human tibiae, it was found that these bones had less resistance to crack growth under shear than under tensile forces, with these specimens having 13 times more resistance to shear.

The study also reported that bone toughness is equivalent in men and in women, a finding that was somewhat unexpected because clinical results indicate that older women are at greater risk for fractures than are older men. As bone ages and some bone mass is lost, it becomes less resistant to fracture in shear; a notable site of high shear forces and a high fracture rate is the femoral neck. Knowledge of bone fracture characteristics by loading mode, sex, and age is important to the clinicians' understanding of the fractures experienced by their older patients.

M.J.L. Alexander, Ph.D.

The Influence of Subject and Test Design on Dynamometric Measurements of Extremity Muscles

Keating JL, Matyas TA (La Trobe Univ, Bundoora, Victoria, Australia)
Phys Ther 76:866–889, 1996   5–10

Background.—Previous reports have suggested that various factors—including subject factors and test procedures—could affect clinical dynamometry measurements. However, these factors have never been specifically analyzed. The literature was reviewed to identify the effects of subject factors and test procedures on the results of clinical dynamometry.

Findings.—A detailed review of more than 200 reports identified many subject factors affecting dynamometry measurements, including age, sex, weight, athletic background, disability, and limb dominance. Certain test conditions had an important impact as well, including the range of movement in which the measurements were obtained and the type of contraction or movement performed, such as concentric, eccentric, isokinetic, isometric, or isotonic. Many different pretest procedures had an effect, including warm-up and gravity-correction procedures, starting position, stabilization, axes alignment, lever arm length, preload and damp/ramp settings. The test conditions of speed, test sequence, rest intervals, and feedback influenced the measurements obtained, as did the type of data selected and the way in which they were analyzed. Most studies using clinical dynamometry did not provide the level of detail needed to replicate the measurements or to compare them with other studies.

Recommendations.—Many different factors can affect the measurements obtained by clinical dynamometry, and these should be stated whenever such measurements are reported. Data on subject and testing variables are needed to develop normative data, to come up with ratios, to compare the results of different studies, and to correlate the dynamometric measurements with functional data. These factors also affect the clinical applicability of the results obtained.

▶ This paper provides an extensive and timely review of protocols in dynamometric measurements of limb muscles. The authors discuss such important factors as age, weight, sex, and activity background of the subjects when examining muscle group strength values. They noted that although differences have been found between these groups, often true differences are confounded by measurement error, weight-related differences, or comparison between subject groups that are not homogeneous. They further note the uncertainty that exists regarding the magnitude of difference between measurements which constitutes a significant difference between groups of different ages or sex, for example. They further discuss testing protocols such as warm-up, range of motion, subject stabilization, and testing speeds, and how these might affect results. They concluded that few studies of limb strength measurement can be reproduced, and the results should be interpreted with caution. Although there is a large body of literature in the area of muscle force measurement, no standardization of testing has occurred to date, and should be carefully considered in future strength testing protocols.

M.J.L. Alexander, Ph.D.

Resistive Eccentric Exercise: Effects of Visual Feedback on Maximum Moment of Knee Extensors and Flexors
Kellis E, Baltzopoulos V (Univ of Liverpool, England; Manchester Metropolitan Univ, Alsager, England)
J Orthop Sports Phys Ther 23:120–124, 1996   5–11

Objective.—Isokinetic dynamometry is a useful tool for assessing muscular function. Although visual feedback (VF) has an effect on isokinetic parameters during maximum exertion, its influence on maximum moment output of knee flexors and extensors at fast angular velocities has not been determined. Results of a study examining the effects of VF on maximum moments during resisted eccentric knee extension and flexion at slow and fast angular velocities were presented.

Methods.—After warm-up, 25 male volunteers (average age, 22 years) performed 5 maximal reciprocal repetitions of knee extensors and flexors at angular velocities of 30 and 150 degrees/sec, with and without VF, throughout an 80-degree range of motion with 5-minute rest periods

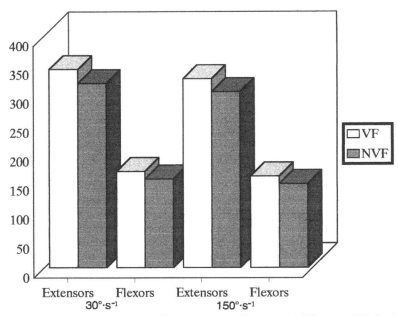

FIGURE.—Maximum moment (Nm) of knee extensors and flexors under different visual feedback and angular velocity conditions (N = 25). *Abbreviations: VF,* visual feedback; *NVF,* nonvisual feedback). (Courtesy of Kellis E, Baltzopoulos V: Resistive eccentric exercise: Effects of visual feedback on maximum moment of knee extensors and flexors. *J Orthop Sports Phys Ther* 23(2):120–124, 1996.)

between each of 4 tests. The gravitational moment was computer calculated. Visual feedback was provided as a real time display of moment output. One week later, 13 volunteers were retested to confirm measurements. A 3-factor analysis of variance test was used to evaluate the differences between VF and non-VF results.

Results.—Maximum moments for flexors and extensors at both speeds were significantly higher with VF than without NVF (Figure). With VF, extension moments at 30 and 150 degrees/sec were about 7.2% and 6.4% higher than with non-VF. Flexor moments at 30 and 150 degrees/sec were about 8.7% and 9% higher than with non-VF.

Conclusion.—Visual feedback can significantly increase maximum eccentric output and should be provided when testing strength with an isokinetic dynamometer.

▶ Isokinetic dynamometers are now almost exclusively used in evaluation of muscle strength. They are used over a wide range of speeds, for many muscle groups and for both eccentric and concentric contractions. Factors that may affect these maximal torque outputs include the effects of knowledge of strength scores and VF (torque scores) during the test. Visual feedback was found to increase torque output during eccentric testing, as the result of increased CNS response to the visual stimulus. Because CNS response time was reported to be 160–180 milliseconds and the test took from 750 milliseconds to 2.7 seconds depending on testing speed used, there was enough time for the subjects to respond to visual stimuli and improve their performance. To ensure reliability and validity, isokinetic test scores should be reported based on whether VF was given to the participants during the test.

M.J.L. Alexander, Ph.D.

EMG Activities of the Quadratus Lumborum and Erector Spinae Muscles During Flexion-Relaxation and Other Motor Tasks

Andersson EA, Oddsson LIE, Grundström H, et al (Karolinska Inst, Stockholm; Danderyds Hosp, Stockholm)
Clin Biomech 11:392–400, 1996   5–12

Background.—A complex network of muscles with various fiber directions and depths surrounds the lumbar spine. With electromyography (EMG), the actual involvement of muscles in different situations can be verified. The EMG activities of the quadratus lumborum (QL) and erector spinae muscles during flexion-relaxation and other motor tasks were reported.

Methods and Findings.—Fine-wire electrodes were inserted into 7 healthy volunteers under ultrasonographic needle guidance. The greatest activity for QL and deep lateral erector spinae was noted in ipsilateral trunk flexion in a side-lying position and for superficial medial erector spinae during bilateral leg lift in a prone position. When the flexion-

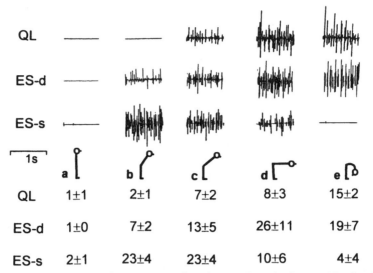

QL	1±1	2±1	7±2	8±3	15±2
ES-d	1±0	7±2	13±5	26±11	19±7
ES-s	2±1	23±4	23±4	10±6	4±4

FIGURE 2.—Electromyographic (*EMG*) recordings from quadratus lumborum (*QL*), deep lateral (*ES-d*) and superficial medial erector spinae (*ES-s*) from 1 representative subject in (*a*) normal standing, and standing with (*b*) 30, (*c*) 60, and (*d*) 90 degrees of hip flexion with the whole trunk held straight, and (*e*) with the trunk relaxed, kyphotic, at the 90-degree hip angle. Average values (± standard deviation, *n* = 7) of the normalized EMG levels, expressed as percentage of the highest activity observed, are given below. (Reprinted from *Clinical Biomechanics*, Courtesy of Andersson EA, Oddsson LIE, Grundström H, et al: EMG activities of the quadratus lumborum and erector spinae muscles during flexion-relaxation and other motor tasks. *Clin Biomech* 11:392–400, copyright 1996, with kind permission from Elsevier Science Ltd, The Boulevard, Langford Lane, Kidlington OX5 1GB, UK.)

relaxation phenomenon was present for superficial medial erector spinae, QL and deep lateral erector spinae were activated (Fig 2).

Conclusion.—The activation of the muscles investigated showed a high degree of task specificity in which activation of a certain muscle could not always be predicted from its anatomical arrangement and mechanical advantage. These data will be useful for improving biomechanical models of the lumbar spine, designing tests and training programs for the trunk musculature in rehabilitation and sports, and assessing factors causing low back pain.

▶ The QL muscle has not been extensively studied in the past, probably because of the need for inserting fine-wire electrodes into the muscle to collect EMG recordings. This study examined both the QL and the deep and superficial parts of the erector spinae group during several trunk exercises. One interesting finding was that during forward trunk flexion, the QL increases in activity until full flexion is reached, whereas the superficial erector spinae has no activity in full flexion. The highest activity for the QL and the deep erector spinae occurred in trunk flexion in a side-lying position and during bilateral leg lift in a prone position. These data have some importance in designing training programs for the trunk musculature to focus on rehabilitation of specific trunk muscle weaknesses.

M.J.L. Alexander, Ph.D.

Effects of Concentric and Eccentric Training on Muscle Strength, Cross-sectional Area, and Neural Activation

Higbie EJ, Cureton KJ, Warren GL III, et al (Univ of Georgia, Athens)
J Appl Physiol 81:2173–2181, 1996   5–13

Background.—The primary stimulus for increasing strength is the repeated development of force by skeletal muscles at levels greater than that occurring in everyday activities. Greater maximum force can be developed during maximal eccentric (Ecc) muscle actions than concentric (Con) or isometric muscle actions. Thus, heavy-resistance training using Ecc muscle actions may be more effective than training using Con or isometric muscle actions in increasing strength. The effects of Con and Ecc isokinetic training on quadriceps muscle strength, cross-sectional area, and neural activation were investigated.

Methods.—Women with a mean age of 20 years were assigned randomly to 1 of 3 groups. Sixteen were assigned to Con training, 19 to Ecc training, and 19 to a control group. The women were tested before and after 10 weeks of unilateral Con or Ecc knee-extension training.

Findings.—The mean torque measured during Con and Ecc maximal voluntary knee extensions increased 18.4% and 12.8%, respectively, in the Con group; 6.8% and 36.2%, repsectively, in the Ecc group; and 4.7% and −1.7%, repetively, in the control group. The increases in the Con and Ecc groups were significantly greater than in the control group. Quadriceps cross-sectional area, as determined by MRI, increased by 6.6% in the Ecc group and by 5% in the Con group (Fig 1).

Conclusion.—Eccentric isokinetic training is more effective than Con training for the development of strength in Ecc isokinetic muscle actions; Con is more effective than Ecc isokinetic training in the development of

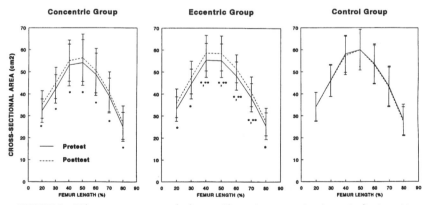

FIGURE 1.—Values are means ± standard error. Change in cross-sectional area (cm²) of quadriceps muscle measured from MRI scans at 7 levels at pretest and posttest in concentric (**A**), eccentric (**B**), and control (**C**) groups. *Asterisk* indicates values significantly greater compared with control group at $P \leq 0.05$ *Double asterisk* indicates significant difference compared with concentric group at $P \leq 0.05$. (Courtesy of Higbie EJ, Cureton KJ, Warren GL III, et al: Effects of concentric and eccentric training on muscle strength, cross-sectional area, and neural activation. *J Appl Physiol* 81:2173–2181, 1996.)

strength in Con isokinetic muscle actions. Strength increases from Con and Ecc training depend greatly on the muscle action used for training and testing. Muscle hypertrophy and neural adaptations contribute to the increases in strength consequent to Con and Ecc training.

▶ This is a unique strength training study in that it compares the effects of 2 strength training protocols, including Ecc training, on strength-related outcomes in young women. As in related studies on male subjects, it is assumed that the effects on the strength gains seen in the 2 are similar. There is an increasing interest in Ecc strength training among those interested in improving muscle strength, even though the risks of muscle injury and delayed muscle soreness are increased in Ecc programs.

After a 10-week training program, the Ecc training group improved their average knee torque by 36% when tested eccentrically, suggesting the greater efficacy of Ecc isokinetic training compared with Con training. Muscle hypertrophy and neural adaptation measured by electromyography during strength testing were also increased more with Ecc than with Con training. Prescription of a strength training regimen for healthy subjects should include a substantial amount of Ecc exercise, but this must be prescribed gradually because of the greater potential for muscle-tendon injury in Ecc training.

M.J.L. Alexander, Ph.D.

Adaptive Responses to Muscle Lengthening and Shortening in Humans
Hortobágyi T, Hill JP, Houmard JA, et al (East Carolina Univ, Greenville)
J Appl Physiol 80:765–772, 1996   5–14

Background.—Concentric contraction of a skeletal muscle or active shortening produces less force and mechanical stimulus than a lengthening or eccentric contraction. Whether maximal eccentric exercise training produces greater neuromuscular adaptations and muscle fiber hypertrophy than maximal concentric exercise training was examined.

Methods.—The study group consisted of 21 sedentary male volunteers, who were free of lower-extremity orthopedic problems and were randomly assigned to eccentric training, concentric training, or control—no training. The subjects underwent initial testing to verify the reliability of the electromyographic measurements. They were then retested once at week 6 during training and once after 12 weeks of training. A dynamometer was used to test unilateral maximal voluntary isometric and isokinetic eccentric and concentric strength of the left knee extensors and flexors. Muscle biopsy specimens were taken from both thighs before and after training. Blood samples were obtained during the pretests and at weeks 2, 4, 6, 8, 10, and 12. Subjects rated muscle soreness on a weekly basis. The training regimen was composed of 12 weeks of isokinetic eccentric or concentric quadriceps strengthening of the left leg at 1.05 rad/sec.

Results.—Eccentric training increased eccentric strength 3.5 times more than concentric training increased concentric strength (Fig 4). Eccentric

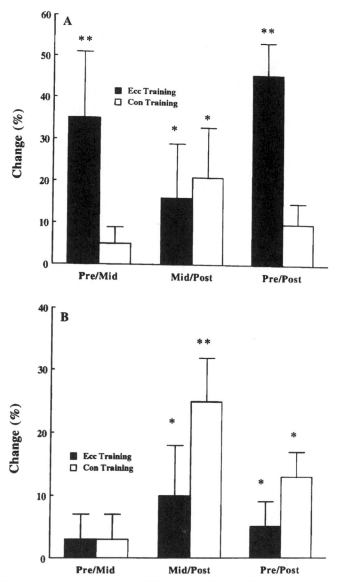

FIGURE 4.—Percent change in eccentric (1.05 rad/sec)-to-isometric (**A**) and concentric (1.05 rad.sec) -to-isometric (**B**) force ratio at pre/mid, mid/post, and pre/post in eccentrically trained and concentrically trained exercise groups. For clarity, control group's data are omitted. *Significant ($P < 0.05$) change; **significantly ($P < 0.05$) more change than opposite group. (Courtesy of Hortobágyi T, Hill JP, Houmard JA, et al: Adaptive responses to muscle lengthening and shortening in humans. *J Appl Physiol* 80:765–772, 1996.)

training increased concentric strength by about the same amount that concentric training increased eccentric strength. Eccentric training increased electromyographic (EMG) activity during eccentric testing activity 7 times more than concentric training increased EMG activity during concentric testing. Eccentric training increased the EMG activity during concentric testing by about the same amount that concentric training increased EMG activity during eccentric testing. Type I fiber areas were not significantly affected by training. Type IIa fibers significantly increased and type IIb fibers significantly decreased during both types of training. The type II fiber area increased approximately 10-fold more in the eccentric training group than in the concentric training group.

Conclusions.—Eccentric muscle training of sedentary men produced muscular adaptations that were specific to eccentric muscle action. Eccentric muscle training was associated with greater neural adaptation and muscle hypertrophy than concentric muscle training.

▶ Comparisons of strength gains between concentric and eccentric muscle contractions are a common topic for muscle researchers, and often eccentric contractions are found to be more effective. This study also reported that eccentric strength training increased eccentric and concentric strength scores more than concentric training. Eccentric training also increased EMG activity during eccentric testing more than concentric testing, suggesting an increased neural drive during eccentric exercise. Type II fibers were found to be selectively recruited during eccentric action, producing selective hypertrophy of these fibers. The authors suggested that the greater strength gains with eccentric training were probably mediated by learning to recruit more of the available type II fibers after training. The findings suggest that more emphasis should be placed on eccentric muscle actions when training in the recreational settings and in the rehabilitation of patients with musculoskeletal injuries.

M.J.L. Alexander, Ph.D.

Biomechanical Assessment of the Healing Response of the Rabbit Patellar Tendon After Removal of Its Central Third
Beynnon BD, Proffer D, Drez DJ, et al (Univ of Vermont, Burlington; Vann Atlantic Orthopaedic Specialists, Virginia Beach, Va; Knee and Shoulder Sports Medicine Ctr, Lake Charles, La)
Am J Sports Med 23:452–457, 1995   5–15

Introduction.—Autogenous patellar tendon graft is commonly used for reconstruction of anterior cruciate ligament tears. However, there are some problems with this graft, including deleterious decreases in the biomechanical properties of the patellar tendon donor site. Previous biomechanical studies of the patellar tendon donor site have yielded conflicting results. This issue was addressed in a rabbit study.

Methods.—The central third of the patellar tendon was removed from the right knees of 30 skeletally mature New Zealand White rabbits. One group of rabbits were killed at the time of surgery and their patellar tendons were prepared for failure testing. The rest were allowed to heal for 1, 2, 3, or 6 months. The results of the operated patellar tendons were compared with those of the contralateral normal tendons.

Results.—Failure strength of the operated tendons was about one third that of the nonoperated tendons. Tendons taken at the time of surgery had an ultimate failure strength of 53% of normal. In those allowed to heal for 6 months, failure strength was 72% of normal. Ultimate failure strength was significantly correlated with healing time, but the mode of failure—substance rupture vs. tibial bone fracture—was not.

Conclusion.—Rabbit patellar tendons from which the central one third has been removed have a significantly reduced failure strength. Failure load increases toward normal as healing proceeds. In humans who undergo autogenous patellar tendon grafting, the tendon may remain strong enough for normal activity, even after removal of the central one third.

▶ During much of the 1980s, the method of choice for repairing the torn anterior cruciate ligament (ACL) was to use the middle third of the patellar ligament and thread it through the proximal tibia and the distal femur while it remained attached to the tibial tubercle. For the past 5 years, this method has been used less often becaue of the reported weakening of the patellar tendon after removal of the middle third. Anterior cruciate ligament repairs are now commonly performed using the tendons of semimembranosus, semitendinosus, or iliotibial band.

This study tested the ultimate failure strength of the patellar tendons with the middle third removed, and it was much less than that of the normal patellar tendons. Even after 6 months, the rabbit patellar tendons were only at 72% of normal strength, although strength was continuing to progress toward normal. There is a greater chance of patellar tendon rupture after removal of the central one third for ACL repair because of its decreased load to failure. Alternate sites for ACL grafts should be considered by orthopedic surgeons.

M.J.L. Alexander, Ph.D.

Passive Tension in Rat Hindlimb During Suspension Unloading and Recovery: Muscle/Joint Contributions
Gillette PD, Fell RD (Univ of Louisville, Ky)
J Appl Physiol 81:724–730, 1996   5–16

Introduction.—The suspended-rat model has demonstrated that weightlessness leads to disuse and muscle/joint stiffness. Thus, conditions of weightlessness—as during a prolonged spacecraft mission—may seriously impair movement and work capacity. Rats were studied in an experimental suspended condition to develop a noninvasive model to measure hindlimb passive tension, to describe changes in passive tension during whole-body suspension and weight-bearing recovery, and to determine relative contributions of hindlimb tissues to passive tension (flexibility).

Methods.—The rats were placed in corduroy-Velcro harnesses that suspended them in a horizontal position, with the hindlimbs unable to contact a supportive surface. Their forelimbs could grasp a grid surface, allowing grooming and access to food and water. A 14-day suspension period was followed by a 14-day recovery period. The animals were anesthetized on days 0, 7, 14, 17, 21, and 28 so that hindlimb passive tension could be measured during ankle dorsiflexion.

Results.—The suspension treatment significantly reduced body weights by 10%. Passive tension was significantly increased by 7 days of suspension, and recovery of passive tension occurred by 14 days of weight-bearing. The increase in passive tension was observed at both 35- and 45-degree joint angles. The greatest recovery in hindlimb flexibility was observed within the first 3 days after return to weight-bearing. Increased passive tension in the suspended animals was caused primarily by musculotendinous units (75%) rather than by the joint (25%). Muscle atrophy was not the sole cause of passive tension increases as only 1 of the plantar flexors changed its muscle mass as a result of suspension.

Discussion.—In the suspended-rat model, passive tension significantly increased in the hindlimb after 7–14 days in the non–weight-bearing condition. These changes were reversible by a return to weight-bearing conditions. The increased passive tension in muscle may result from changes in muscle architecture, viscoelastic properties of the muscle or its connective tissue elements, or cytoskeletal protein alterations.

▶ The effects of disuse or weightlessness on flexibility in the muscle tendon unit is an important aspect of understanding mobility. Although this study used a rat model to examine the effects of a period of immobility on muscle function, the results can be applied to human movement and work capacity. The passive tension and flexibility in the muscle groups increased after a period of suspension and inactivity. The muscles studied returned to normal mobility after a period of activity, suggesting that short-term changes in passive tension of muscle are reversible.

The period of inactivity likely led to changes in muscle architecture, viscoelastic properties of muscle, or connective tissue elements—all of which were reversible after return to normal activity. A period of inactivity caused by illness or weightlessness will produce decreased flexiblity, which may lead to impaired movement or work capacity. A return to normal daily activities, including weight-bearing activity, is essential to retaining normal joint mobility.

M.J.L. Alexander, Ph.D.

Length-specific Impairment of Skeletal Muscle Contractile Function After Eccentric Muscle Actions in Man

Saxton JM, Donnelly AE (Univ of Wolverhampton, England)
Clin Sci (Colch) 90:119–125, 1996   5–17

Objective.—Repeated voluntary lengthening of forearm muscles can result in impaired contractile function and decreased range of motion of the elbow joint. Results of a study to determine whether overextension and subsequent impairment is muscle-length specific were presented.

Methods.—Muscle soreness, serum creatine kinase (CK) activity, and involuntary elbow flexion were monitored in 30 volunteers (2 women), aged 18–34 years, immediately before and 1, 2, 3, 4, 7, and 10 days after they each performed 70 maximum voluntary eccentric muscle full-range actions using forearm flexors. Forearm flexor maximum voluntary isometric contraction torque (MVC) was assessed using an isokinetic dynamometer in the isometric mode at elbow angles of 0.87, 1.57, and 2.79 rad before, immediately after, and 1, 2, 3, 4, and 10 days after exercise. Superimposed percutaneous electrical stimulation was performed during MVC tests in 8 volunteers (2 women) to test any voluntary inhibition of strength measures. Data for forearm flexor strength between joint angles, serum CK activity, relaxed and flexed elbow angle, and muscle swelling were compared statistically.

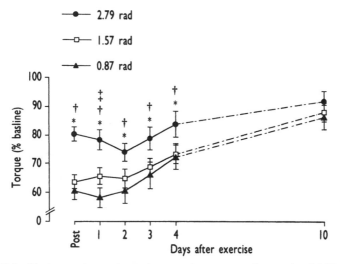

FIGURE 3.—Maximum voluntary isometric contraction torque at elbow angles of 0.87, 1.57, and 2.79 rad after 70 maximum voluntary eccentric muscle actions of the forearm flexors. Values are means with *error bars* representing standard error of the mean. Statistical significance (repeated measures analysis of variance with *t*-tests used to highlight differences between mean scores): *Asterisk* indicates $P < 0.01$ between 2.79 rad and 1.57 rad elbow angles; *dagger* indicates $P < 0.01$ between 2.79 rad and 0.57 rad elbow angles; *double dagger* indicates $P < 0.01$ between 1.57 rad and 0.57 rad elbow angles. (Courtesy of Saxton JM, Donnelly AE: Length-specific impairment of skeletal muscle contractile function after eccentric muscle actions in man. *Clin Sci [Colch]* 90:119–125, 1996.)

Results.—There were significant changes in muscle soreness, serum CK activity (66 vs. 2,196 IU/L), and relaxed elbow joint angle after exercise. Muscle soreness peaked at 3 days and serum CK values at 4 days. Flexor forearm strength decreased significantly after exercise, and relative decline differed significantly between elbow angles (Fig 3). Superimposed electric stimulation did not significantly increase torque production at any elbow angle, suggesting that loss of strength was not the result of muscle soreness. After exercise, biceps circumference at the midbelly and joint regions increased significantly. Swelling was still apparent at 10 days and was significant at 3, 4, and 7 days. Immediately after exercise, the ability to flex the elbow joint fully was significantly impaired.

Conclusion.—At short muscle length, strength was significantly impaired after repetitive eccentric exercise, probably because muscle length had increased as a result of lengthening of sarcomeres and/or elastic structures.

▶ Maximal eccentric contractions are known to elicit delayed-onset muscle soreness, a decline in joint range of motion, and prolonged loss of force production. Long-term eccentric contractions have been reported to produce a subtle increase in muscle length and a rightward shift in the length-tension relationship. This would theoretically decrease the muscle force output when the muscle is maximally shortened.

This study examined the effects of eccentric exercise of the forearm flexors on decline in muscle strength at 3 different muscle lengths (joint positions). The authors did find the expected prolonged loss of strength after severe eccentric exercise, especially at the shortest length. Using electrical muscle stimulation, they determined that the strength decreases were not caused by muscle soreness. They concluded that strength decreases were caused by sarcomere damage resulting from the eccentric work bout, including lengthened sarcomeres and disruption in the myotendinous junction. The functional significance of this study is that strenuous eccentric training will be followed by up to 7 days of decreased strength levels and, therefore, should not be undertaken before important competitions or events.

M.J.L. Alexander, Ph.D.

Effect of Resistance Training Volume on Strength and Muscle Thickness
Starkey DB, Pollock ML, Ishida Y, et al (Univ of Florida, Gainesville)
Med Sci Sports Exerc 28:1311–1320, 1996   5–18

Background.—Resistance training has become a basic part of athletic training and rehabilitation, as well as general fitness programs. The intensity, frequency, and volume of exercise must be considered before beginning a resistance training program. In an adult general fitness program, a single set of 8–12 repetitions performed to fatigue is often recommended. Multiple-set regimens take longer to perform and result in only 5% to 10% greater improvements than single-set regimens. The American College of

Sports Medicine and the American Heart Association acknowledge single-set regimens as effective for developing and maintaining muscular strength and lean body mass. There is little information in this area, however, and many authorities maintain that multiple-set programs are more beneficial. The effects of training volume on full range of motion, knee extension and flexion strength, and on muscle thickness in adults were evaluated.

Methods.—Of 59 initial subjects, 48 finished the study. All subjects were healthy, untrained adults between 18 and 50 years of age. There were 21 men and 27 women. Subjects performed 1 set or 3 sets of dynamic variable resistance exercise 3 times per week for 14 weeks. Bilateral knee extension and flexion exercise was performed to fatigue within 8–12 repetitions. Maximal isometric knee extension and knee flexion torque was measured at 6, 24, 42, 60, 78, 96, and 108 degrees of knee flexion using a knee extension/flexion ergometer. There were 10 control subjects who did not train during the study. Muscle thickness was measured with ultrasound. The length of the right thigh was measured, and sites were marked at 20%, 40%, and 60% of this distance on the anterior, lateral, and posterior faces of the thigh. Sites were also marked at the medialis lateralis muscles.

Results.—Torque output increased at most angles in both groups of training subjects (Figs 2 and 3). No differences were noted between subjects who performed 1 set or 3 sets of exercises. In the single-set group,

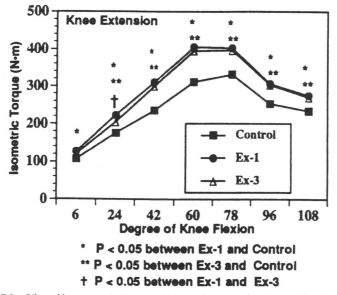

* **P < 0.05 between Ex-1 and Control**
** **P < 0.05 between Ex-3 and Control**
† **P < 0.05 between Ex-1 and Ex-3**

FIGURE 2.—Bilateral knee extension increases in isometric torque of Ex-1 ($n = 18$) and Ex-3 ($n = 20$) over the control group ($n = 10$) (analysis of covariance). Percent gains in isometric torque were 18.4% vs. 13.2% at 6 degrees, 26.7% vs. 16.3% at 24 degrees, 31.6% vs. 27.1% at 42 degrees, 30.1% vs. 26.8% at 60 degrees, 21.4% vs. 19.5% at 78 degrees, 20.9% vs. 20.0% at 96 degrees, and 17.5% vs. 15.3% at 108 degrees for the Ex-1 and Ex-3 groups, respectively. *Abbreviations: Ex-1*, 1 set of exercise, 3 times per week; *Ex-3*, 3 sets of exercise, 3 times per week. (Courtesy of Starkey DB, Pollock ML, Ishida Y, et al: Effect of resistance training volume on strength and muscle thickness. *Med Sci Sports Exerc 28:1311–1320, 1996.*)

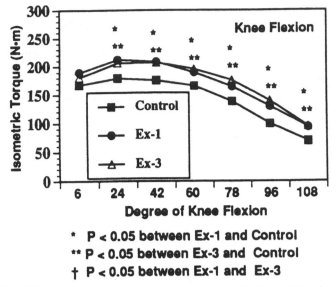

* **P < 0.05 between Ex-1 and Control**
** **P < 0.05 between Ex-3 and Control**
† **P < 0.05 between Ex-1 and Ex-3**

FIGURE 3.—Bilateral knee flexion increases in isometric torque of Ex-1 ($n = 18$) and Ex-3 ($n = 20$) over the control group ($n = 10$) (analysis of covariance). Percent gains in isometric torque were 13.0% vs. 7.8% at 6 degrees, 18.3% vs. 14.9% at 24 degrees, 18.7% vs. 17.7% at 42 degrees, 14.4% vs. 17.8% at 60 degrees, 19.0% vs. 27.0% at 78 degrees, 30.6% vs. 40.7% at 96 degrees, and 34.8% vs. 37.0% at 108 degrees for the Ex-1 and Ex-3 groups, respectively. *Abbreviation Ex-1*, 1 set of exercise, 3 times per week; *Ex-3*, 3 sets of exercise, 3 times per week. (Courtesy of Starkey DB, Pollock ML, Ishida Y, et al: Effect of resistance training volume on strength and muscle thickness. *Med Sci Sports Exerc* 28:1311–1320, 1996.)

muscle thickness increased at 60% lateral right thigh and at 40% and 60% posterior right thigh. In the multiple-set group, muscle thickness increased at the medialis muscle and at 40% and 60% posterior right thigh.

Conclusions.—In these previously untrained adults, 1 set of bilateral knee extension and flexion exercises performed to fatigue 3 times per week for 14 weeks was as effective as 3 sets for increasing isometric torque output and muscle thickness.

Clinical Significance.—One set of exercises in a resistance exercise training program is sufficient to build strength and muscle mass. Multiple-set training programs are more expensive and take more time. Overtraining may be harmful to some patients or subjects. Other training programs may be more appropriate for individuals who wish to maximize strength and power.

▶ A key question in resistance training relates to the optimal volume of training required to increase muscle strength and size. Most strength training programs suggest 2–3 sets of 8 repetitions will produce optimal strength gains; one set is thought to be inadequate. This study compared the effects of either 1 set or 3 sets of 8–12 repetitions of variable resistance exercise using the knee extensors and flexors as the muscle group being trained over 14 weeks. Groups who trained with 1 set of exercises produced the same strength gains as those who trained with 3 sets of the same exercises; there were no significant differences in the strength gains from these 2 programs. Muscle size and thickness were also found to increase at about the same rate with each of these training programs. This study has important implications for adult fitness and rehabilitation programs in which performing 1 set of exercises instead of 2 or 3 may be more cost-effective and time-efficient.

M.J.L. Alexander, Ph.D.

Weight Training Improves Walking Endurance in Healthy Elderly Persons

Ades PA, Ballor DL, Ashikaga T, et al (Univ of Vermont, Burlington; Mayo Clinic, Rochester, Minn)
Ann Intern Med 124:568–572, 1996   5–19

Background.—Many elderly individuals, even though nondisabled and community-dwelling, have substantial mobility limitations. Loss of strength in the leg muscles appears to be highly predictive for the development of disability, but some studies show that resistance training can lead to improvements in muscle size and strength and in walking endurance. A controlled trial was designed to examine the effect of a resistance-training program on walking endurance in healthy, elderly individuals.

Methods.—Study participants were 24 sedentary persons with a mean age of 70.4 years. Six men and 6 women were randomly assigned to a resistance-training group and the remaining 5 men and 7 women to a control group. None were limited in their exercise capacity by cardiopulmonary conditions or other diseases. Participants underwent endurance testing before and after the 12-week program. On 3 days per week those in the weight-training regimen performed 3 sets of 8 repetitions of 7 exercises, done 3 days per week using a Universal Gym apparatus. Resistance was increased progressively, so that participants were exercising at 80% of their single repetition maximum by week 9. Controls did not alter their usual activities.

Results.—Submaximal walking endurance in the resistance-training group increased from a mean of 25 minutes at baseline to a mean of 34 minutes at 12 weeks, a 38% increase. No change was seen in controls. Various measures of strength, such as single repetition maximums for leg extension, leg flexion, and bench press, increased in the intervention group but not in the control group (Table 1). Although fat-free mass of the leg was increased in the exercise group, neither group exhibited changes in whole-body composition or in peak aerobic capacity.

Conclusion.—A 12-week program of resistance training improved both leg strength and walking endurance in healthy, sedentary elderly individuals. The relation between change in leg strength and change in walking endurance was significant. Interventions such as resistance training can help to prevent disability in an aging population.

TABLE 1.—Resistance-Training and Control Groups at Baseline and 12 Weeks

Measure	Resistance-Training Group		Control Group		Difference Between Groups§
	Baseline	12 Weeks	Baseline	12 Weeks	
Endurance time, *min*					
Men‡	25 ± 4	32 ± 11	23 ± 6	18 ± 8	4 to 23
Women	25 ± 4	36 ± 6	18 ± 3	20 ± 12	− 9 to 26
Combined†	25 ± 4	34 ± 9	20 ± 5	19 ± 10	
Peak aerobic capacity, $mL/kg \cdot min^{-1}$*					
Men	29 ± 8	25 ± 6	29 ± 3	24 ± 3	− 1 to 6
Women	23 ± 3	23 ± 5	20 ± 4	23 ± 4	− 7 to 5
Combined	26 ± 6	25 ± 6	24 ± 6	23 ± 6	
Leg extension (single repetition maximum, *kg*)*					
Men	44 ± 14	56 ± 15	27 ± 12	40 ± 11	− 10 to 49
Women†	24 ± 3	33 ± 5	23 ± 4	21 ± 5	12 to 41
Combined‡	35 ± 15	46 ± 16	29 ± 11	29 ± 13	
Leg flex (single repetition maximum), *kg**					
Men‡	14 ± 6	20 ± 5	13 ± 4	12 ± 4	1 to 30
Women†	5 ± 1	12 ± 2	6 ± 2	6 ± 2	10 to 19
Combined‡	10 ± 6	16 ± 6	9 ± 5	9 ± 4	
Bench press (single repetition maximum), *kg**					
Men	33 ± 9	41 ± 12	29 ± 7	30 ± 7	− 5 to 34
Women†	22 ± 4	26 ± 5	20 ± 4	21 ± 3	4 to 12
Combined‡	28 ± 9	35 ± 12	24 ± 7	25 ± 7	
Body weight, *kg*					
Men	79.5 ± 12.0	80.3 ± 10.5	76.5 ± 10.0	76.6 ± 9.2	− 1.8 to 5.4
Women	70.9 ± 9.6	70.3 ± 8.5	71.9 ± 12.5	71.0 ± 12.6	− 2.4 to 2.7
Combined	75.6 ± 11.1	75.7 ± 11.4	73.8 ± 10.8	73.3 ± 11.2	
Fat mass, *kg**					
Men	21.8 ± 9.2	21.8 ± 8.4	19.2 ± 5.4	20.4 ± 5.2	− 3.0 to 2.4
Women	30.6 ± 5.0	30.3 ± 4.1	30.2 ± 8.1	30.5 ± 8.8	− 2.5 to 1.3
Combined	25.8 ± 9.2	25.6 ± 8.3	25.6 ± 9.4	26.2 ± 9.1	
Fat-free mass, *kg**					
Men	57.7 ± 5.0	58.5 ± 4.7	57.3 ± 6.7	56.2 ± 7.7	− 1.2 to 5.0
Women	40.3 ± 6.6	40.0 ± 6.1	41.7 ± 4.7	40.5 ± 4.2	− 1.3 to 2.6
Combined	49.8 ± 11.4	50.1 ± 11.1	48.2 ± 9.8	47.1 ± 10.1	
Fat-free mass of the leg, *kg**					
Men	9.3 ± 1.2	9.2 ± 1.1	9.4 ± 0.8	9.0 ± 0.9	− 0.6 to 1.1
Women‡	6.1 ± 0.6	6.4 ± 0.6	6.5 ± 0.6	6.2 ± 0.5	0.1 to 1.0
Combined‡	7.0 ± 1.2	7.1 ± 2.8	7.7 ± 1.6	7.4 ± 1.6	

*Baseline sex difference, $P < 0.05$.
†Change in the resistance group is greater than the change in the control group; $P < 0.01$.
‡Change in the resistance group is greater than the change in the control group; $P < 0.05$.
§Adjusted 12-week difference between groups, stratified by sex and expressed as a 95% confidence interval.
(Courtesy of Ades PA, Ballor DL, Ashikaga T, et al: Weight training improves walking endurance in healthy elderly persons. *Ann Intern Med* 124:568–572, 1996.)

▶ Our laboratory has long argued that weak muscles contracting at a large fraction of their peak force can develop a sufficient internal pressure to limit local perfusion.[1] Marcinik et al.[2] confirmed this hypothesis, showing that strength training substantially increased the lactate threshold. The elderly are prime candidates for problems associated with weak muscles. Fiatarone et al.[3] previously demonstrated that a strength-training program for the frail elderly enhanced their walking speed over short distances. This paper by Ades and associates illustrates how strengthening of the leg muscles by appropriate resistance exercises can dramatically enhance the performance of 70-year-olds during longer periods of submaximal walking, even though there is no significant increase in peak aerobic power. An increase of endurance from 25 to 34 minutes makes a substantial difference to what an elderly person can achieve during the activities of daily living.

R.J. Shephard, M.D.

References

1. Kay C, Shephard RJ: On muscle strength and the threshold of anaerobic work. *Int Z Angew Physiol* 27:311–328, 1969.
2. Marcinik EJ, Potts J, Schlabach G, et al: Effects of strength training on lactate threshold and endurance performance. *Med Sci Sports Exerc* 23:739–743, 1991.
3. Fiatarone MA, Marks EC, Ryan ND, et al: High-intensity strength training in nonagenarians. Effects on skeletal muscle. JAMA 263:3029–3034, 1990.

The Effect of Age, Speed, and Arm Dominance on Shoulder Function in Untrained Men

Gallagher MA, Zuckerman JD, Cuomo F, et al (Hosp for Joint Diseses, New York)
J Shoulder Elbow Surg 5:25–31, 1996 5–20

Objective.—Shoulder strength can be used to assess function in patients with shoulder disorders. Results of a study measuring bilateral shoulder motor output in older and younger populations were reported.

Peak Torque

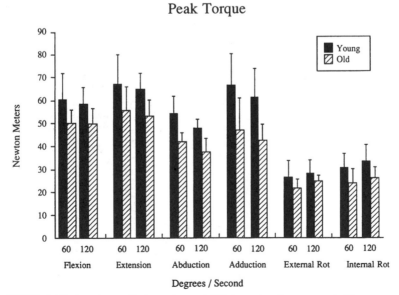

FIGURE 4.—Peak torque at 60 degrees/sec and 120 degrees/sec for young and older age groups. (Courtesy of Gallagher MA, Zuckerman JD, Cuomo F, et al: The effect of age, speed, and arm dominance on shoulder function in untrained men. *J Shoulder Elbow Surg* 5:25–31, 1996.)

Methods.—Peak torque, power, and work were measured with an iso-kinetic dynamometer in 3 axes of movement in the healthy shoulders of 40 men aged 20–30 and 50–60 years. Results were statistically compared by age, speed, and interaction of age and speed for dominant and nondominant arms.

Results.—Peak torque, work, and power for flexion, extension, abduction, adduction, external rotation, and internal rotation were significantly higher in every direction for the younger group (Fig 4). Power was directly and significantly related to speed in all directions for both groups. Dominant and nondominant measures of power motor output did not differ significantly in either group.

Conclusion.—There were significant age-related differences in shoulder strength between older and younger men. Dominant and nondominant measures of power motor output did not differ significantly in either group.

▶ Accurate assessment of shoulder function, especially in older individuals, normally requires isokinetic dynamometer testing to determine strength levels. It is assumed that these test scores are comparable between the various isokinetic dynamometers available, such as Kin Com, Cybex, and Biodex, so that data from various subjects can be compared. This study compared a number of shoulder strength variables between a group of younger and older male subjects. This was a very comprehensive testing battery, which included shoulder flexion/extension, abduction/adduction, and mediaolateral rotation at 2 speeds of movement. Also, the torque variables were combined with the displacement and time variables from the test to produce work and power values for the 3 directions of movement.

As expected, the authors found significant age-related differences in shoulder strength between the younger and older subjects, with the younger group being stronger in all variables tested. They also reported a significant decrease in peak torque and work as testing speed increased. The data reported in this study will provide a valuable base for comparison with other normal and injured subjects, assuming that the testing devices are comparable. In future, more detailed analysis of the torque-time curves and electromyography during the test would provide valuable information on the reasons for the strength deficits in older subjects.

M.J.L. Alexander, Ph.D.

Bilateral and Unilateral Neuromuscular Function and Muscle Cross-sectional Area in Middle-aged and Elderly Men and Women
Häkkinen K, Kraemer WJ, Kallinen M, et al (Univ of Jyväskylä, Finland; Pennsylvania State Univ, Philadelphia; Peurunka-Med Rehabilitation and Physical Exercise Centre, Laukaa, Finland; et al)
J Gerontol 51A:B21–B29, 1996   5–21

Background.—Human muscle strength remains relatively stable through young adulthood, peaks between the ages of 20 and 30 years, then decreases slightly until its real decline around the sixth decade of life. This change is related to declining muscle mass, mediated by a reduction in size and/or loss of individual muscle fibers, particularly fast-twitch fibers. Middle-aged and elderly men and women were studied to assess age-related differences in muscle cross-sectional area, maximal strength, and explosive strength in the knee extensor muscles.

Methods.—Four groups of 12 subjects were studied: men and women approximately 50 years of age and men and women approximately 70 years of age. All were physically active. Cross-sectional area (CSA) of the knee extensor muscles was measured by ultrasound. Dynamometric testing was performed to measure maximal voluntary bilateral and unilateral isometric peak force, force time, and relaxation time of the knee extensor muscles. Electromyographic activity and force production were also determined to seek evidence of bilateral deficit.

Results.—The middle-aged subjects of both sexes had greater maximal bilateral knee extension force and average CSA values than their elderly counterparts. The early forces in the force-time curve were also greater for the 50-year-olds than for the 70-year-olds. In all 4 groups, the CSA values for the right and left quadriceps femoris were significantly correlated with the maximal unilateral knee extension force. However, the force value in relation to the CSA of the muscle was lower in the 70-year-old women's group. The maximal voluntary bilateral force was the same as the sum of the 2 unilateral forces. There was also no difference in the maximal integrated electromyographic activity values during bilateral and unilateral contractions.

Conclusion.—The age-related decline in maximal muscle strength may be related to declining muscle CSA. However, particularly in women, multiple factors appear to be operative, possibly including decreased voluntary neural drive or qualitative changes in the muscle tissue. The age-related decline in explosive strength may be caused by a greater atrophying effect of aging on fast-twitch fibers and/or a change in the rate of neural activation.

▶ There is a well-documented decrease in muscular strength with aging in both men and women. Human muscle strength peaks between the ages of 20 and 30 years, and then decreases as the result of decreased activity and an associated loss in muscle mass. This study measured peak force in 4 groups of older men and women and found that the 50-year-old groups were significantly stronger than the 70-year-old groups and that both groups of males were stronger than both groups of females.

The decrease in maximal strength with increasing age is accompanied by a reduction in muscle mass, as well as a reduction in maximal voluntary neural input to the muscles, especially in older women. Aging also decreases the explosive strength characteristics of the neuromuscular system, as seen by the force-time curves of the contractions. This may be the result of the increased atrophying effects of age on fast-twitch fibers as compared with slow-twitch fibers because of a denervation process. The decrease in strength with aging was also substantially greater between the 2 groups of women (26%) than between the 2 groups of men (19%).

M.J.L. Alexander, Ph.D.

Measuring Functional Limitations in Rising and Sitting Down: Development of a Questionnaire
Roorda LD, Roebroeck ME, Lankhorst GJ, et al (Vrije Universiteit, Amsterdam)
Arch Phys Med Rehabil 77:663–669, 1996   5–22

Introduction.—Problems with rising and sitting down are common among the elderly and the arthritic, and this functional ability is of critical importance in maintaining independence. There is currently no comprehensive assessment instrument available for studying limitations in rising and sitting. The self-administered test for assessing perceived and actual functional limitations in the home setting was described.

Methods.—The Questionnaire Rising and Sitting Down (QR&S) was developed after a literature review and consultations with physicians, physical and occupational therapists, and sociologists. A 54-question version of the QR&S was then tested in a population of 345 outpatients with various grades of functional limitations and a variety of lower extremity orthopedic or rheumatologic disorders. The QR&S covered 5 dimensions related to various objects (high chair, low chair, toilet, bed, and car) and 1 global dimension. These dimensions were tested using Mokken scale analysis. Scale criteria included robustness, reliability, content validity, and construct validity.

Results.—The QR&S was filled out at home by 345 patients living in the Amsterdam region between 1991 and 1993. Mokken scale analysis confirmed the existence of 5 object dimensions, but 2 global dimensions were identified. Combination scale 1 comprised high chair, toilet, and bed; combination scale 2 included low chair and car. The scales were, in general, robust, and the reliability and validity were sufficient. Thirty-two items made up the final instrument.

Discussion.—The QR&S proved to be a reliable and valid self-administered questionnaire for measurement of functional limitations in rising and sitting down. It can be applied to outpatients with various grades of limitations and types of disorders. The use of combination scales is recommended when a global picture is needed; object scales can be used for a detailed assessment, as in clinical studies. The instrument contains 32 statements which are to be answered "yes" when they apply to the patients' current situation and are connected with their health. Examples are: "I always have to shift forward a little before I get up from a low chair or sofa" and "I always use 2 hands to hold on to something to get into a car."

▶ One of the critical topics in current movement analysis is evaluation of the mobility of the elderly and arthritic without the use of complex motion analysis equipment. One of the useful tools for such movement analysis is a questionnaire that can be easily administered to the population in question. The development of valid and reliable questionnaires to be used in movement analysis is an area that should receive greater attention in the future.

This paper is an excellent attempt to have patients analyze their movements by answering questions describing some of their day-to-day limitations to mobility. The questionnaire would be useful to clinicians attempting to evaluate patients' mobility in rising and sitting and to determine the degree of independence and mobility in patients living at home. Hopefully, this will be one of many questionnaires developed to analyze activities of daily living through careful and accurate questioning of the patients involved.

M.J.L. Alexander, Ph.D.

The Role of Strength in Rising From a Chair in the Functionally Impaired Elderly

Hughes MA, Myers BS, Schenkman ML (Duke Univ, Durham, NC)
J Biomech 29:1509–1513, 1996   5–23

Introduction.—Rising from a chair is a biomechanically demanding task that may determine an individual's capacity for independent living. Chair rise requires lower extremity-strength, balance, and range of motion, and can be more difficult for the elderly than either walking or stair climbing. The role of knee extensor strength in rising from a chair was determined in young healthy adults and a group of functionally impaired elderly individuals.

Methods.—The young group included 5 men and 5 women; 5 men and 6 women were recruited for the functionally impaired elderly group. Elderly participants could not descend 4 consecutive stairs step over step without using the handrail and were unable to rise from a 0.33-meter-high chair. Kinematic and ground reaction force data were collected from study participants to determine the required knee moments during rising. All were asked to rise from armless, backless chairs with their arms folded. Chair heights ranged from 0.33 to 0.58 m in 0.05-m increments. Required joint loads were calculated at 3 chair heights.

Results.—The young and elderly groups did not differ significantly in mean height or mean weight. Elderly participants were unable to rise from the lower chair heights and required 97% of their available strength to successfully rise from the lowest height chair from which they could rise. The young, in contrast, could rise from all chair heights and required only 39% of available strength to rise from the lowest chairs. Both groups required significantly greater knee moment at the lowest chair height than at the knee chair height. Although the mean maximum required knee moments were similar for the 2 groups, mean isometric strength was significantly greater in the young (276 N m vs. 103 N m).

Conclusion.—Confirming the study hypothesis, knee extensor strength was found to limit the minimum chair height from which a functionally impaired elderly individual can rise. Such elderly individuals differ from young, unimpaired adults in their statistically significantly lower strength but not in maximum required knee moment. Strengthening exercises may benefit the elderly whose independence is limited by inability to rise from a chair.

▶ The ability to rise from a chair is one of the most important skills required by older adults who wish to remain living independently. There are important questions regarding the physical abilities required to perform this task, especially rising from lower chairs. Possible limiting factors to performance could be hip joint flexibility, quadriceps strength, arm strength, or skill in moving the center of gravity over the feet. This study examined the role of strength in this important task. The researchers determined that decreases in chair height required higher strength levels. From their strength measurements, they determined that the knee strength required by the elderly subjects was 97% of the available isometric strength at the knee at the lowest height from which they could rise. Their subjects were unable to rise from lower chair heights that required strength levels above those they were able to generate with the knee extensors. It was recommended that strength training programs be undertaken for the elderly who are at risk for loss of independent living, because significant strength gains are possible for this population.

M.J.L. Alexander, Ph.D.

Measures of Paraspinal Muscle Performance Do Not Predict Initial Trunk Kinematics After Tripping

Grabiner MD, Feuerbach JW, Jahnigen DW (Cleveland Clinic Found, Ohio)
J Biomech 29:735–744, 1996   5–24

Background.—Tripping during locomotion results in postural destabilization and relatively automatic neuromuscular responses that restore stability. The ability to limit the trunk flexion associated with an anterior trip determines successful recovery and relies on the rapid detection and correction of the imposed trunk flexion in the time available. This study tested the hypothesis that individuals with greater eccentric strength of the trunk/hip extensors, faster automatic paraspinal activation latencies, larger automatic paraspinal activation levels, and faster voluntary paraspinal reaction times would also have smaller maximum trunk flexion angles during the positioning planes of recovery after tripping.

Methods and Findings.—Ten healthy young men and women volunteered for the study. Trunk extension strength, response latencies, and activation amplitudes were measured using an isokinetic protocol. Trunk kinematics during the positioning phase of recovery after an induced trip were quantified using motion analysis methods. No statistically significant or functionally meaningful relationships were found between eccentric strength of the trunk/hip extensors, voluntary reaction time, automatic reaction time, activation amplitudes, and trunk kinematics.

Conclusion.—Automatic and voluntary paraspinal muscle responses can limit trunk flexion in the positioning phase of recovery. However, this task may be accomplished through intersegmental factors or other muscular sources, such as the gluteus maximus and hamstrings.

▶ The problem of falls in the elderly is caused by aging of the neuromuscular system and failure of automatic and voluntary responses to restore postural stability. The increased number of falls in the elderly contributes significantly to injury and premature death in this population. Falls often occur after tripping, and there is a tendency to fall forward; this forward rotation may be overcome by rapid eccentric contraction of the trunk extensors.

This study examined the relationship between eccentric trunk muscle strength and reaction time of the trunk muscles to decreasing trunk flexion after tripping. The authors found there were no significant relationships between trunk strength and reaction time to ability to reposition the trunk after a tripping episode. It was suggested that repositioning of the trunk could occur by means of other muscular sources, such as the gluteus maximus and hamstrings, or by passive neuromuscular structures, such as ligaments.

M.J.L. Alexander, Ph.D.

The Effect of Hamstring Muscle Stretching on Standing Posture and on Lumbar and Hip Motions During Forward Bending
Li Y, McClure PW, Pratt N (Medical College of Pennsylvania and Hahnemann Univ, Philadelphia)
Phys Ther 76:836–849, 1996   5–25

Background.—Postural or mechanical disturbances have been reported to be the most common cause of low back pain. Changes in the normal relationship among the alignment of the spine, the position of the pelvis, and the length of the muscles attaching to the spine and pelvis are thought to contribute to the development of low back pain. However, standing lumbopelvic posture has not been clearly related to muscle length, and the effect of hamstring muscle stretching on standing lumbar and pelvic posture or the relative amounts of lumbar and hip motion during forward

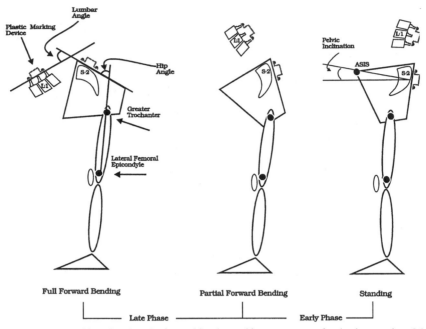

FIGURE.—Model used to describe forward bending. *Abbreviations: L-1*, first lumbar vertebra; *S-2*, second sacral vertebra (calculated as the midpoint between 2 digitized points on the sacrum); *ASIS*, anterior superior iliac spine. (Courtesy of Li Y, McClure PW, Pratt N: The effect of hamstring muscle stretching on standing posture and on lumbar and hip motions during forward bending. *Phys Ther* 76:836–849, 1996, with the permission of the American Physical Therapy Association.)

bending have not been established definitively. It was determined whether hamstring muscle stretching affects extensibility, as evidenced by straight-leg raising, lumbopelvic posture, and the relative amounts of lumbar and hip motion during forward bending.

Methods and Findings.—Thirty-nine volunteers with no known musculoskeletal impairments of the spine or lower extremities and tight hamstring muscles participated in the study. The volunteers were randomly assigned to a stretching or control group. Lumbar, pelvic, and hip positions were measured with a 3-dimensional digitizer while the subjects were in a standing position and also during partial and full forward bending (Figure). After stretching, straight leg raising and hip motion during late and total forward bending were increased. There were no changes in the standing posture or lumbar motion during forward bending.

Conclusion.—Hamstring muscle length appears to be unassociated with lumbopelvic posture. However, hamstring muscle stretching may affect motion during forward bending.

▶ The problem of hamstring tightness is often related to low back pain, although contraction of the hamstrings rotates the pelvis posteriorly, possibly resulting in a reduction in lumbar lordosis. It is likely that any abnormal position of the pelvis will produce stresses and resulting strain on the attached tissues, including the spinal structures. The healthy lower back should retain the normal lordotic curve, but excessive lumbar lordosis should be avoided. Short hamstrings may limit hip flexion range of motion, and this is also related to excessive lumbar motion to attain the fully forward flexed position.

This study examined the results of a program of hamstring stretching on standing posture and forward bending and found that increased length of the hamstrings did not alter standing lumbar and pelvic postures but did produce greater forward bending as a result of increased motion at the hips. The role of the hamstrings may be more closely related to controlling the pelvis during forward flexion than to controlling the pelvic tilt during normal standing.

M.J.L. Alexander, Ph.D.

Trunk and Hip Muscle Recruitment in Response to External Anterior Lumbosacral Shear and Moment Loads
Raschke U, Chaffin DB (Univ of Michigan, Ann Arbor)
Clin Biomech 11:145–152, 1996   5–26

Background.—Antagonistic activity has been observed in the muscles that attach to the pelvis during sagittal plane extension. The purpose of such muscle activity is not well understood. It is possible that this muscle activation is involved in the stabilization of pelvic posture. Experiments were performed to determine whether the muscles of the lumbar torso react to external shear loading on the lumbar spine or are influenced by the magnitude of the moment about the pelvis relative to the L4–L5 moment.

Methods.—The study group consisted of 5 male volunteers (average age, 29.6 years) with no history of back injury or pain and without neurologic disorder. The participants stood in a neutral, upright, and symmetric posture while their lower legs and mid-thighs were strapped to braces on a rigid frame (Fig 2). Pelvis tilt could also be constrained by an external rigid pelvic brace so that a relatively pure shear load could be applied to the lumbar region. The loading conditions consisted of 25, 112, and 230 N applied horizontally at the lower thorax and 0, 80, and 180 N applied horizontally at the level of the L4–L5 motion segment. Surface electromyography was used to monitor the activity of the erector spinae, latissimus dorsi, external oblique, rectus abdominis, gluteus maximus, and rectus femoris muscles.

Results.—Analysis of the results of muscle monitoring revealed that the use of antagonistic muscle groups was not consistent between subjects. Statistical analysis did not support the hypothesis that torso muscle activity is a response to shear loading. There was also no evidence that moments about the pelvis relative to the lumbar spine significantly influenced the recruitment of antagonistic muscle groups.

Conclusions.—The results of electromyography do not support the hypothesis that torso musculature is recruited to minimize anterior shear

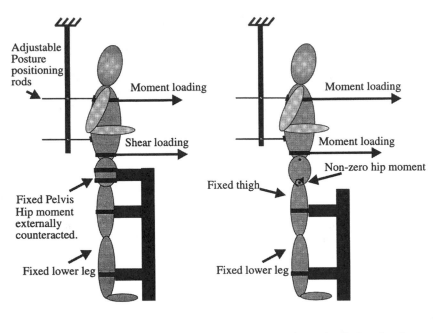

Configuration A: Shear and Moment loading of L4/L5 in the absence of Pelvic Moments.

Configuration B: Loading for L4/L5 and Pelvic Moments.

FIGURE 2.—Experimental configurations for shear and moment loading of the L4–5 (A), and moment loading across the pelvis (B). (Reprinted from Raschke U, Chaffin DB: Trunk and hip muscle recruitment in response to external anterior lumbosacral shear and moment loads. *Clin Biomech* 11:145–152, copyright 1996, with kind permission from Elsevier Science Ltd, The Boulevard, Langford Lane, Kidlington OX5 1GB UK.)

forces on the lumbar spine or that this recruitment is associated with moments about the pelvis. This indicates that in current biomechanical models of the lumbar spine, the omission of pelvic moments does not seem to be responsible for significant error in the prediction of torso muscle activity.

▶ This study examined the questions regarding the response of lumbar torso and pelvic muscles to applied shear and moment loading forces. The study was conducted to determine whether lower back lifting models should include moments caused by the pelvic muscles. It has been suggested that the abdominal oblique muscles should contract to increase the intra-abdominal pressure during lifting, but evidence is contradictory. Electromyography was used to examine the activity of the erector spinae, latissimus dorsi, external oblique, rectus abdominus, gluteus maximus, and rectus femoris. The results of this study do not support the theory that the torso musculature is recruited to minimize anterior shear forces on the lumbar spine. There was considerable muscle activity variation associated with moments about the pelvis. It was concluded that pelvic moments are not significant in flexion loading and lifting skills.

M.J.L. Alexander, Ph.D.

Why Is Countermovement Jump Height Greater Than Squat Jump Height?
Bobbert MF, Gerritsen KGM, Litjens MCA, et al (Inst for Fundamental and Clinical Movement Sciences, Amsterdam)
Med Sci Sports Exerc 28:1402–1412, 1996   5–27

Background.—It has been well established that the performance of a countermovement, a movement in the direction opposite to the goal, enhances task performance. For example, jumpers achieve greater height in a countermovement jump (CMJ), where they begin erect and make a downward movement before jumping, than in a squat jump (SJ), where they take off from a semisquat without a countermovement, even if the takeoff position is the same. The reason for the advantage of the countermovement jump was investigated.

Methods.—Six male volleyball players performed CMJ and SJ while kinematics, kinetics and muscle electric activity were monitored on 6 lower-extremity muscles. These data were used to create a model of the musculoskeletal system that calculated internal states and forces of the muscle-tendon complexes.

Results.—Even when body position at the start of push off was the same for both types of jump, jump height was an average of 3.4 cm greater with a CMJ than an SJ. Nonoptimal coordination was not a problem, as there was no sign of movement disintegration in SJ and the toe-off position was identical. The greater CMJ jump height resulted from the greater joint moments at the start of push off in CMJ. This permitted larger joint moments over the first part of the range of joint extension in CMJ, which produced more work than in SJ. According to the musculoskeletal simulator model, the important contribution of countermovement was that it allowed muscles to build up a high level of active state and force before shortening, permitting muscles to produce more work during the first part of shortening.

Conclusions.—Trained jumpers performed CMJs and SJs, and information derived from their performance was used to derive a musculoskeletal model. According to this model, the contribution of countermovement to increased jump height appeared to derive from the buildup in muscles of a high level of active state and force before the start of shortening, which increased the work produced over the first part of the shortening distance.

▶ When performing most dynamic tasks, humans typically start with a so-called countermovement, a movement in the direction opposite to the goal direction. In jumping, for example, it is well documented that subjects are able to jump higher with a CMJ than from an SJ, but the exact reasons are unclear. Some of the reasons suggested for this difference are unfamiliarity on the part of the subjects with the SJ, time needed to build up to the optimal contractile state, lack of storage of elastic energy, and triggering of the stretch reflex to facilitate muscle contraction. Six highly skilled jumpers were filmed and data collected describing the kinematics and kinetics of the jumps. The data were input into a model of the musculoskeletal system, and the simulated jumps determined that the storage of elastic energy in the muscle was not the key reason for the improvement; and that the stretch reflex could partially contribute to the increased activity of the muscle. The countermovement was found to enable the muscle to produce more work, as a result of the high level of activity in the muscles during the eccentric phase, which increased their state of readiness for concentric contraction.

M.J.L. Alexander, Ph.D.

Leg Stiffness and Stride Frequency in Human Running
Farley CT, González O (Harvard Univ, Bedford, Mass)
J Biomech 29:181–186, 1996

5–28

Background.—The body's system of muscle, tendon, and ligament springs during running behaves like a single linear spring. The mechanics of running can be well demonstrated in a simple spring-mass model (Fig 1). Force platform measures obtained from running subjects have shown that the stiffness of the leg spring remains almost the same at all speeds. The spring-mass system is adjusted for greater speeds by increasing the angle swept by the leg spring. The relative importance of changes to the leg

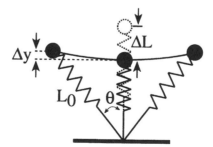

FIGURE 1.—Running is modeled as a simple spring-mass system bouncing along the ground. The model consists of a mass and a single leg spring (which connects the foot and the center of mass of the animal). This figure depicts the model at the beginning of the stance phase (**leftmost position**), at the middle of the stance phase (**leg spring is oriented vertically**), and at the end of the stance phase (**rightmost position**). The leg spring had an initial length, L_O, at the beginning of the stance phase, and its maximal compression is represented by ΔL. The dashed spring-mass model shows the length of the uncompressed leg spring. Thus, the difference between the length of the dashed leg spring and the maximally compressed leg spring represents the maximum compression of the leg spring, ΔL. The downward vertical displacement of the mass during the stance phase is represented by Δy and is substantially smaller than ΔL. Half the angle swept by the leg spring during the ground contact time is denoted by θ. (Reprinted from the Journal of Biomechanics, courtesy of Farley CT, González O: Leg stiffness and stride frequency in human running. *J Biomech* 29:181–186, copyright 1996, with kind permission from Elsevier Science Ltd, The Boulevard, Langford Lane, Kidlington OX5 1GB, UK. Courtesy of McMahon TA, Cheng GC: The mechanics of running: How does stiffness couple with speed? *J Biomech* 23 (supple 1):65–78, 1990.)

spring stiffness and angle swept by the leg spring when humans change their stride frequency at a given running frequency was investigated.

Methods and Findings.—Four young male volunteers were studied while running on a treadmill-mounted force platform at 2.5 m/sec using stride frequencies ranging from 26% below to 36% above the preferred stride frequency. Force platform measurements showed a 2.3-fold increase in the stiffness of the leg spring, from 7 to 16.3 kN/m, between the lowest and highest stride frequencies. The angle swept by the leg spring declined at higher stride frequencies, partly offsetting the effect of the increased leg spring stiffness on the mechanical behavior of the spring-mass system.

Conclusion.—Although leg spring stiffness does not change with speed in forward running, it can change more than twofold to accommodate different stride frequencies at a given speed. The adjustability of leg stiffness may be important for running on a variety of terrains. A variable leg stiffness may also be an important design parameter for spring-based prostheses for running and for robots with legs.

▶ A common analogy used to describe the behavior of the mammalian limb during running is that of a single linear spring that can store energy when stretched and return energy during recoil. The human limb modeled as a spring is stretched during initial ground contact, then maximally compressed during midcontact and stretched again before toe off. The stiffness of the spring is the ratio of the force in the spring (vertical ground forces) to the displacement of the spring (vertical displacement of the center of mass) when it is maximally compressed at midstride.

The model was tested by measuring the vertical ground reaction force of 4 trained runners at different stride frequencies. The magnitude of the vertical displacement and the vertical force decreased at higher stride frequencies, suggesting that the spring stiffness increased at the higher stride rates. As humans increase their stride frequency at a given running speed, the body adjusts by stiffening the leg spring; in fact, the stiffness of the leg spring more than doubles from lowest to highest stride frequencies. The increased leg stiffness occurs because of changes in leg muscle activiation and changes in body positions. This study may have implications for scientists interested in improving running performance by examination of optimal leg stiffness at different stride frequencies.

M.J.L. Alexander, Ph.D.

Relationship Between Maximum Aerobic Power and Resting Metabolic Rate in Young Adult Women
Smith DA, Dollman J, Withers RT, et al (Flinders Univ of South Australia, Adelaide; CSIRO Australia, Adelaide)
J Appl Physiol 82:156–163, 1997   5–29

Introduction.—The resting metabolic rate (RMR) usually accounts for 60% to 75% of daily energy expenditure. Reports are equivocal regarding the effect of aerobic fitness on RMR. The influence of aerobic fitness and body composition on the RMR was evaluated in 34 young women.

Methods.—Research subjects were healthy, non-obese nonsmokers and had a wide range of maximal aerobic power (32.3–64.8 mL/kg/min). Twelve participants each were in the high- and low-fitness groups. All participants were measured for RMR by the Douglas bag method, treadmill maximum aerobic power, and fat-free mass (FFM) using Siri's 3-compartment model.

Results.—There was a significant interclass correlation between RMR (kilojoules per hour) and maximal aerobic power (milliliters per kilogram per minute), but this relationship lost significance when RMR was indexed to FFM and when partial correlation analysis was used to control for FFM differences. Only FFM was a significant predictor of RMR (kilojoules per hour). There were significant between-group differences observed for RMR (kilojoules per kilogram per hour) and maximal aerobic power (milliliters per kilogram per minute) but not for RMR (kilojoules per hour), RMR (kilojoules per kilogram per hour) and FFM when high- and low-fitness groups were removed from the cohort on the basis of maximal aerobic power scores. There were no significant between-group differences for high- and low-fitness groups in analysis of covariance of RMR (kilojoules per hour) with FFM as the covariate.

Conclusion.—The high-fitness group expended more energy at rest, compared with the low-fitness group, but there was no indication of a positive relationship between RMR and maximal aerobic power when statistical control was exerted for the influence of FFM.

▶ The authors have carefully controlled those variables they believe have been responsible for the contradictory results from previous studies. They make a strong case for the accuracy of their techniques and the validity of their results, as well as ensuring that sample size provided a power of 0.80 to detect differences at $P = 0.05$. The result is the convincing conclusion that FFM accounts for any difference in RMR between high- and low-fitness groups of premenopausal women.

B.L. Drinkwater, Ph.D.

Changes in Aerobic Power of Women, Ages 20–64 Yr
Jackson AS, Wier LT, Ayers GW, et al (NASA/Johnson Space Ctr, Houston; Univ of Houston; Inst for Aerobics Research, Dallas)
Med Sci Sports Exerc 28:884–891, 1996   5–30

Introduction.—Factors affecting decline in aerobic power are important public health concerns, particularly regarding the aging American population. The independent effects of age, body composition, and level of physical activity on the decline in aerobic power were evaluated in 43 women.

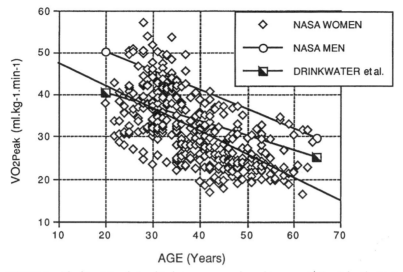

FIGURE 1.—The bivariate relationship between age and aerobic power ($\dot{V}O_{2peak}$) for the National Aeronautics and Space Administration/Johnson Space Center (NASA/JSC) women and the linear regression line that defines the cross-sectional decline in aerobic power with age. The published simple linear regression equations for NASA/JSC men (Jackson AS, Beard EF, Wier LT, et al: Changes in aerobic power of men ages 25–70 years. *Med Sci Sports Exerc* 27:113–120, 1995) and women studied by Drinkwater et al. (Drinkwater BL, Horvath SM, Wells CL: Aerobic power in females ages 10 to 68. *J Gerontol* 30:385–394, 1975) were used to define the age-$\dot{V}O_{2peak}$ trends for men and women and compare with the NASA/JSC women. The simple linear regression equation that defines the NASA/JSC women's age-aerobic power trend is: $\dot{V}O_{2peak} = 57.726 - 0.537$ (Age), SEE = 6.444. (Courtesy of Jackson AS, Wier LT, Ayers GW, et al: Changes in aerobic power of women, ages 20–64 years. *Med Sci Sports Exerc* 28(7):884–891, 1996.)

Methods.—The age range of a cross-sectional sample of 409 female employees at National Aeronautics and Space Administration (NASA)/ Johnson Space Center was 20–64 years. A longitudinal sample of 43 women was evaluated at baseline and at a mean follow-up of 3.7 years. Indirect calorimetry during a maximal treadmill test was used to calculate peak oxygen uptake. Body fat was calculated using skinfold measurements. Participants completed a self-report activity scale (SR-PA) that measured duration and intensity of weekly physical activity.

Results.—Peak aerobic power, maximum heart rate, and SR-PA declined with age and percent body fat increased. There was an average linear decrease of 0.8 units per decade in SR-PA and a linear reduction of 7.5 beats per minute in maximal heart rate. The cross-sectional, age-related reduction in aerobic power (slope) was 0.537 mL/kg/min/yr (Fig 1). Percent body fat was most highly correlated with peak aerobic power. The correlations for age and SR-PA were similar and were significantly lower than the zero-order correlation of −0.742 between peak aerobic power and percent body fat. Independent changes in percent body fat and SR-PA were responsible for changes in aerobic power when time differences between tests were controlled.

Conclusion.—When body composition and exercise habits are controlled, men and women have a similar rate in reduction of aerobic power with age.

▶ Those of us who talk to lay audiences about the importance of physical activity in maintaining good health can now assure women that physical activity can help them avoid a rapid decrease in their cardiovascular fitness level as they age—not only by a direct effect in retaining fitness but indirectly through helping maintain a lower percent body fat. This will have more meaning to the average woman if we relate "aerobic fitness" to her ability to continue activities she enjoys as she grows older and, even more importantly, to the likelihood that she can continue to live independently during the final third of her life.

B.L. Drinkwater, Ph.D.

Hospital Care in Later Life Among Former World-Class Finnish Athletes
Kujala UM, Sarna S, Kaprio J, et al (Univ of Helsinki; Univ of Turku, Finland)
JAMA 276:216–220, 1996   5–31

Introduction.—Regardless of economic status, the Finnish social security system provides appropriate hospital treatment for all citizens. Thus, hospitalization is a good measure of diseases needing special care in Finland. It is not known whether top-level athletes experience long-term benefits or adverse effects because of their high level of athletic performance. The overall effect of a physically active lifestyle on the individual and health care system usage was evaluated in Finnish athletes over a 21-year period.

Methods.—The use of hospital care was investigated in male athletes who represented Finland at the Olympic Games and other international competitions from 1920 to 1965. The Finnish hospital discharge register was used to review retrospectively the numbers of hospital days per person-years of exposure from 1970 to 1990 for 2,448 male athletes and 1,712 male controls. Former athletes were grouped by type of training: endurance sports, mixed sports, and power sports. They were also grouped according to occupation: executives, clerical staff, skilled workers, unskilled workers, and farmers. A lifestyle questionnaire was mailed to athletes who were still alive.

Results.—In the 45 to 74-year age-range, athletes spent fewer days in the hospital per person-years of exposure than controls. Hospital days were lowest among mixed sports athletes for the age range of 45–59 years and were lowest among endurance sports athletes for the age range of 60–74 years. The overall rate ratios (RRs) were significantly lower for endurance sports, then mixed sports, then power sports, compared to controls. When RRs were adjusted for age and occupational group, athletes had lower rates of cardiovascular disease, neoplasms, and diseases of the respiratory system, and digestive system, compared to controls. Athletes in all 3 sports groups had a significantly higher incidence of musculoskeletal diseases than the controls. Power lifters had significantly more ischemic heart disease, compared to controls. The RRs for ischemic heart disease in endurance athletes and respiratory diseases in mixed sports athletes were particularly low. After adjustment for age, occupation, and smoking, RRs for hospital days were lowest for former athletes who engaged in leisure-time physical activities or competitive sports, compared to those who were sedentary.

Conclusion.—Former top athletes who participated in aerobic sports used less hospital care in their later years than the controls. The RRs for hospital-days per person-years of exposure were lower by 29% in endurance athletes, 14% in mixed sports athletes, and 5% in power sports athletes, compared to controls.

▶ Although there is now general agreement that moderate physical activity is beneficial for health, there are lingering fears that high-level athletic performance can have an adverse impact upon long-term health. A 21-year follow-up of a large sample of national-level male athletes is thus of considerable interest. The overall conclusion is that after making necessary corrections for age and occupational group, the athletes required substantially fewer hospital days than control subjects. High-level competition was thus not costing health insurance plans any large expense! However, complacency should be avoided, because hospital days for musculoskeletal problems were greater for both endurance and power sports participants than for control subjects.

R.J. Shephard, M.D., Ph.D., D.P.E.

How Much Physical Activity Should We Do? The Case for Moderate Amounts and Intensities of Physical Activity
Blair SN, Connelly JC (Cooper Inst for Aerobics Research, Dallas)
Res Q Exerc Sport 67:193–205, 1996   5–32

Background.—During the past half century, numerous epidemiologic studies have documented an association between a sedentary way of life and various health problems, most notably coronary artery disease. Research on the role of exercise, usually carried out by physiologists, has centered on physical fitness as measured as maximal oxygen intake ($\dot{V}O_{2max}$). More recent investigations have combined some elements of the 2 research themes of physical activity and health and exercise training experiments on $\dot{V}O_{2max}$. The appropriate dose of activity and the recommended intensity of exercise for health and fitness outcomes have not yet been determined.

Methods.—Several recent representative studies and a few classic investigations from past years were reviewed and summarized to produce a cogent recommendation for the type and amount of physical activity required for health and function. Of particular interest was evidence

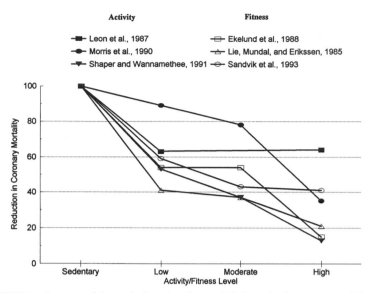

FIGURE 1.—Summary of the results from 6 studies in which fitness level was determined (3 studies) or activity level assessed by questionnaire (3 studies) in individual populations. Follow-up was generally between 7 and 9 years except that of Sandvik et al., which had a 16-year follow-up. The low-level group for each study represented was the activity and fitness level next to the least active and fit group. The high level represents the group that was the most active and fit for the particular study. If the study participants were grouped by quintile, the moderate group is the average of the third and fourth quintiles. (Courtesy of Blair SN, Connelly JC: How much physical activity should we do? The case for moderate amounts and intensities of physical activity. *Res Q Exerc Sport* 67:193–205, 1996.)

relating to the benefits of moderate amounts and intensities of physical activity. Other issues considered were the relation of physical fitness to mortality and the effect of exercise on health outcomes.

Moderate Exercise.—Several recent population-based studies have indicated that moderate and moderately vigorous activity can significantly reduce fatal and nonfatal coronary heart events compared with a sedentary way of life. Exercise test heart rate was shown to be a significant independent predictor for both coronary heart disease and all-cause mortality, even after adjustment for age, smoking, blood pressure, and serum level of cholesterol. A trend was noted for dose response, and substantial benefits were obtained when individuals changed from low to moderate physical fitness (Fig 1). Women who walked only about 1.6 km (1 mile) per day had increased bone density compared with sedentary women.

Exercise Intensity.—Early exercise training studies were limited in number of participants and duration of the exercise regimen. In addition, most participants were young men who were relatively fit at baseline. Training intensity, however, was found to have a direct impact on the amount of improvement in aerobic power. Increases in overall fitness are accompanied by reductions in body mass, lipid levels, and blood pressure.

Discussion.—In terms of risk of clinical disease, some activity is clearly better than none, and low- to moderate intensity activity is better than remaining sedentary. The least active 20% to 30% of the adult population has an increased mortality rate of at least two-fold, but their risk can be substantially reduced with even moderate activity.

▶ Blair and Connelly have argued from their own data and a number of other major epidemiologic studies that much of the health benefit associated with regular exercise is derived from modest levels of physical activity that are insufficient to augment traditional markers of fitness, such as $\dot{V}O_{2max}$. There are still well-respected investigators, such as Drs. Jeremy Morris and Ralph Paffenbarger, who do not accept this verdict, although it has been endorsed by the American College of Sports Medicine, the Centers for Disease Control, and the U.S. Surgeon General. Given government-established targets for the increase of population activity set for the Year 2000, cynics may wonder how much of the change in exercise recommendation stems from a belated recognition that the previously established goals are unlikely to be met. Certainly, the public is confused by the shifting message, and one may question the wisdom of issuing widely publicized "position statements" until the scientific community has reached a consensus on a particular issue.

R.J. Shephard, M.D., Ph.D., D.P.E.

How Much Physical Activity Is Optimal for Health? Methodological Considerations
Lee I-M, Paffenbarger RS Jr (Harvard Med School, Boston; Stanford Univ, Calif)
Res Q Exerc Sport 67:206–208, 1996   5–33

Introduction.—There is abundant evidence that regular physical activity can lower the risk of chronic diseases and enhance longevity. However, 60% of adults in the United States do not exercise regularly or do so only sporadically. Recent recommendations from the Centers for Disease Control and Prevention and the American College of Sports Medicine emphasized the need for 30 minutes or more of physical activity of moderate intensity most days of the week. Previous recommendations emphasized 30 minutes of moderately high intensity physical activity 3 times per week. Do these recommendations contradict each other? Some of the methodological problems in this area of research were discussed.

Quantity Versus Intensity.—There is consistent evidence that an inverse, dose-dependent relationship exists between physical activity and risk of morbidity or mortality from disease. The increased health benefits of higher levels of activity may result from the high total amount of energy expenditure or from the more vigorous types of activity only. Exercise of moderate intensity produces immediate short-term improvements in blood pressure, glucose tolerance, and lipoprotein profiles. There is conflicting evidence regarding the long-term health benefits of exercise of different intensities.

Assessing Physical Activities of Different Intensities.—Vigorous and nonvigorous activities may not be evaluated equally. Vigorous activities tend to be carried out on a regular basis and, therefore, may be more easily recalled by participating subjects. A lack of precision in evaluating activities of lower intensity may obscure their relative contribution to health outcomes. Questionnaires that specifically list various activities may reduce this problem.

Discussion.—Physical activity can prevent disease and improve longevity. The health benefits of exercise increase with increasing levels of activity. The best levels of intensity, frequency, and duration of exercise have not been established. The authors suggest that a practical public health message may be that "a little exercise is better than none, whereas more is better than a little." The methodological problems of absolute vs. relative intensity of physical activity were also discussed.

▶ This article highlights some of the problems associated with recent "position statements" on optimal levels of physical activity. Although the latest position papers suggest health benefit from an exercise intensity of 3–6 metabolic equivalents, Lee and Paffenbarger maintain that there is no good evidence of long-term health benefit from such low-intensity physical activity. They further emphasize the need to relate the prescribed intensity to the initial fitness of the individual, a point well recognized in previous decades of research.[1]

R.J. Shephard, M.D., Ph.D., D.P.E.

Reference

1. Shephard RJ: Intensity, duration and frequency of exercise as determinants of the response to a training regime. *Int Z Angew Physiol* 26:272–278, 1968.

Influences of Cardiorespiratory Fitness and Other Precursors on Cardiovascular Disease and All-cause Mortality in Men and Women
Blair SN, Kampert JB, Kohl HW III, et al (Cooper Inst for Aerobics Research, Dallas; Baylor College of Medicine, Houston; Univ of South Carolina, Columbia, et al)
JAMA 276:205–210, 1996   5–34

Introduction.—The relationship between physical inactivity and various health problems is well known. Physical activity is inversely correlated with death rates. The relationship of fitness and mortality with other mortality predictors has not been thoroughly explored. The relationship of fitness to risk of cardiovascular disease (CVD) mortality and all-cause mortality within strata of other predictors of early mortality was evaluated in 25,341 men and 7,080 women. The strengths of associations between fitness and other predictors of mortality were compared.

Methods.—Participants underwent history and medical examination, anthropometry and blood chemistry analysis, completed a health questionnaire, and were able to achieve at least 85% of their age-predicted maximal heart rate. Abnormalities on resting or exercise ECG were observed in 1,866 men and 350 women. A total of 4,802 men and 958 women reported a history of at least 1 chronic illness, such as myocardial infarction, stroke, hypertension, diabetes mellitus, or cancer. Participants were followed for mortality from December 6, 1970, to December 31, 1989.

Results.—Patients' ages ranged from 20 to 88 years. The average interval from baseline examination to date of death or December 31, 1989, was 8.4 years for men and 7.5 years for women. During 211,996 man-years of observation, 601 men died. Of those deaths, 226 were from CVD. In women, 21 of 89 deaths were from CVD during 52,982 woman-years of follow-up. In men, low fitness, cigarette smoking, elevated systolic blood pressure, elevated serum cholesterol level, and poor health status were significantly associated with CVD mortality and all-cause mortality. In women, low fitness and smoking were significantly correlated to all-cause mortality. Elevated fasting glucose and abnormalities on ECG were associated with CVD mortality in women. The association with low fitness was borderline. In women, smoking and elevated blood pressure had relative risks (RRs) for CVD mortality similar to those of men.

One of the strongest antecedents of mortality for both men and women was low fitness. Men were stratified into 3 fitness categories: low, moderate, and high. Men in the high fitness category had a reduced risk for all-cause mortality (cigarette smoking, systolic blood pressure, total cholesterol level, and personal health status) that was lower than men in the moderate fitness category, and men in the moderate fitness category had a reduced risk for all-cause mortality that was lower than men in the low fitness category. This inverse gradient of risk was significantly different across fitness categories. Highly fit women in each risk stratum had lower death rates, compared to women who were in moderate- or low-fitness categories. Low fitness was determined to be a precursor for CVD and all-cause mortality. Moderate and light levels of fitness seemed to provide protection against the force of combinations of other mortality predictors of death.

Conclusion.—Fit men and women with any combination of smoking, elevated blood pressure, poor health status, or elevated cholesterol level had lower adjusted death rates, compared to low-fitness participants with none of these characteristics. Moderate to high fitness levels seem to protect against the influence of the other predictors of mortality that were measured. Physicians need to encourage patients to exercise to reduce the risk of premature mortality.

▶ It is generally agreed that a low level of fitness has adverse prognostic implications, but it is less clear whether this means that we should encourage vigorous exercise in the person who will not or cannot abandon a heavy consumption of cigarettes. These data from the Cooper Clinic move us a little closer to accepting such a suggestion; indeed, among the men, fit smokers have a better prognosis than unfit nonsmokers. One potential weakness in Blair's analysis is the binary classification of recent smokers (Yes or No). Heavy exercisers are likely to be light smokers, and this confounding of data may contribute to the apparent fitness-related gradient of prognosis within the smokers.

R.J. Shephard, M.D., Ph.D., D.P.E.

Exercise Versus Heart Attack: Questioning the Consensus?
Morris JN (London School of Hygiene & Tropical Medicine)
Res Q Exerc Sport 67:216–220, 1996   5–35

Background.—Two prospective surveys of men in the executive middle-management grade of the British civil service were conducted. The researchers hypothesized that the aggregate of physical activity in the leisure time of these men with sedentary jobs would be associated with their incidence of coronary heart disease (CHD).

Methods and Findings.—The 2 surveys included 18,000 and 9,400 middle-aged men, respectively, with sedentary jobs. A total of 1,600 first myocardial infarctions occurred in 240,000 man-years of observation. Only the men engaging in substantial, regular, vigorous, dynamic aerobic exercise in sports, walking, and cycling had a markedly lower incidence of CHD through middle age and into early old age. Among the older men, entrants aged 55–64 years followed up to 73 years of age, there was found to be a somewhat lower association of CHD with lesser intensity of exercise. (Fig 1).

Conclusion.—These findings contradict the emerging view that moderate amounts and intensity of physical activity in leisure time help protect against CHD. This discrepancy may be the result of differences in the classification of activities as "moderate" or "vigorous." The populations being studied may also differ qualitatively. Most important, however, is the

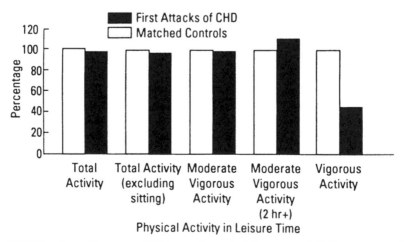

FIGURE 1.—Prospective survey of British executive-grade civil servants aged 40–64 years at entry. The first 214 clinical attacks of coronary heart disease (*CHD*), nonfatal or fatal, are compared with 428 controls. Activity was logged 5 minutes × 5 minutes on a typical Friday and Saturday. (Courtesy of Morris JN: Exercise versus heart attack: Questioning the consensus? *Res Q Exerc Sport* 67:216–220, 1996.)

possibility that what matters more in CHD prevention is not exercise per se but the health-related fitness or state of training. Generally, physical activity is a blunt proxy for fitness, because of the other powerful determinants—inherited and acquired.

▶ When the American College of Sports Medicine, the Centers for Disease Control and Prevention, the United States Surgeon General, and the American Heart Association all state categorically that moderate exercise is adequate for health, many people would quietly allow their own views to conform to this heavy weight of scientific opinion. Not so Dr. Morris. In his ninth decade of life, he vigorously reanalyzes his data in this paper, making the point that, in Britain at least, CHD is not prevented unless the exercise is vigorous (more than 31.5 kJ/min). The population he has studied (middle-grade civil servants) is very sedentary at work, but there may remain some difference in leisure activity that makes the population of the United States more susceptible to improvement by moderate activity. Dr. Morris was also very careful to classify such activities as walking according to their vigour, (a point not observed in all of the U.S. studies), and this may be a further factor contributing to the transatlantic difference in opinion.

R.J. Shephard, M.D., Ph.D., D.P.E.

The Impact of Exercise Deprivation on Well-being of Habitual Exercisers
Szabo A (Concordia Univ, Montreal)
Aust J Sci Med Sport 27:68–75, 1995   5-36

Introduction.—Many studies have investigated the effect of regular exercise on well-being, but few have focused on the effect of exercise deprivation on the well-being of those accustomed to regular exercise. Research on the effects of exercise deprivation on subjective and psychological states and well-being and the methodological problems in this area of research were reviewed and suggestions made for further studies.

Survey Research.—Survey-type methodology has been used in more than 50% of studies offering data on exercise deprivation (Table 1). Subjects were asked open-ended or structured questions about their feelings during intervals when they were unable to exercise. Most of these studies focused on runners, and only 3 studies examined other athletes. One reason that runners have been emphasized may be that exercise deprivation was studied against the background of exercise addiction, which is most commonly reported in runners. The most common symptoms reported by athletes during periods of inactivity were guilt, depression, irritability, and tension.

Cross-sectional and Experimental Research.—Cross-sectional research has examined the profiles of athletes who have been forced into abstinence because of injury. However, it is important to distinguish between the response to injury and the response to lack of exercise. Cross-sectional studies have addressed the impact of exercise deprivation on subjective

TABLE 1.—Summary of the Studies That Examined the Impact of Exercise Deprivation on Subjective Psychological States

Study	N & Sex	Age (yrs)	Type of Inquiry	Form of Exercise	Amount of Exercise	Length of* Deprivation	Instrument or Method Used	Impact of Exercise Deprivation
Acevedo et al. (1992)	112 m,f	40.2	IND/ST	Running	(?)	when not running	open-ended questions	negative feelings to 84.8% of the subjects
Anshel (1991)	60 m,f	27.8	IND/CS/ST	Mixed	50%>15h/wk 50%<5 h/wk	missing a workout	developed own QTR	related to gender & exercise volume
Baekeland (1970)	14 m	<30	DIR/EXP/WS	Mixed	3/4 times /wk (avg)	one month	developed own deprivation QTR	negative (eg anxiety & sexual tension)
Blumenthal, O'Toole & Chang (1994)	43 m, f	34/m 28/f	IND/ST	Running	<100 mi/wk	missing a run/exercise	developed own QTR	negative feelings to 72–86% of runners
Camach & Martens (1979)	315 m,f	28.8	IND/ST	Running	5.4 times /wk (avg)	missing a run	open-ended questions	negative feelings to 74% of the subjects
Chan & Grossman (1988)	60 m,f	15–50	DIR/CS/BS	Running	20 mi/wk (min.)	four wks	POMS, Zung & Rosenberg QTRs	negative feelings to the deprived subjects
Grossman et al. (1987-study I)	31 m,f	17	DIR/ST	Running	42 mi/wk (avg)	one day	anxiety & mood QTRs	related to gender & competition level
Grossman et al. (1987-study II)	20 m,f	14.3	DIR/EXP/WS (?)	Swimming	8 km/day (avg)	five days	anxiety & mood QTRs	related to gender & competition level
Gauvin (1990)	78 m,f	18–60	IND/ST	Mixed	varied	missing a workout	interview	negative to exercisers but not to dropouts
Gauvin & Szabo (1992)	21 m,f	23.6	DIR/EXP /BS/WS	Mixed	7.5 hrs/wk (avg)	seven days	well-being QTRs (4 times/day)	number of physical symptoms doubled
Harris (1981a)	411 m,f	10–71	IND/ST	Running	varied, 1 to 120 mi/wk	when stopped running	halt of running QTR	negative feelings to >80% of the subjects
Harris (1981b)	156 f	11–54	IND/ST	Running	19 mi/wk (avg)	when not running	designed own 7-point QTR	negative feelings to most of the subjects

Study	Sample	Age	Design	Type	Training volume	Deprivation	Measure	Results
Morris et al. (1990)	40 m	37	DIR/EXP/BS/WS	Running	10 mi/wk (min.)	two weeks	Zung depression & health QTRs	negative feelings to the deprived subjects
Robbins & Joseph (1985)	345 m,f	(?)	IND/ST	Running	23 mi/wk (median)	missing a run	developed own QTR	negative feelings to most of the subjects
Sachs & Pargman (1979)	12 m	23–48	IND/ST	Running	varied	when run is impossible	depth interview	negative feelings to most of the subjects
Summers et al. (1982)	363 m,f	36.1	IND/ST	Running	15–20 mVwk (minimum)	missing a run	developed own QTR	negative feelings to most of the subjects
Summers et al. (1983)	459 m,f	31.7	IND/ST	Running (avg ?)	15 mi/wk run	missing a QTR	developed own QTR	negative feelings to 83% of the subjects
Thaxton (1982)	33 m,f	36	IND/EXP/BS	Running	30 min/day (min.)	one day	POMS	negative feelings to Ss who did not run
Tooman, Harris & Mutrio (1985)	40 m,f	18–53	DIR/EXP/BS	Running	3 to 7 days/wk	two days	POMS, STAI, and EMG activity	negative feelings to induced positive effect
Wingate (1993)	102 m,f	33.2	IND/ST	Karate	3 times/wk	missing ≥2 workouts	developed own ATR & interview	negative feelings to most of the subjects
Wittig et al. (1989)	10 m	32	DIR/EXP/WS	Running	80 km/wk (avg ?)	partial† deprivation	POMS	positive changes to the POMS
Wittig et al. (1992)	10 m	(?)	DIR/EXP/WS	Running	(?)	partial‡ deprivation	POMS	negative changes to the POMS

Note: ? indicates unknown or uncertain.

*Actual or conceptualized.

†Reduced training volume by 70% for 3 weeks.

‡Reduced training volume and training intensity for 4 weeks.

Abbreviations: avg, average; *BS,* between subjects; *CS,* cross-sectional design; *DIR,* addressed the issue of exercise deprivation directly; *EXP,* experimental design; *f,* female; *hrs,* hours; *IND,* addressed the issue of exercise deprivation indirectly; *m,* male; *mi,* miles; *POMS,* Profile of Mood States questionnaire; *QTR,* questionnaire; *Ss,* subjects; *ST,* survey type; *STAI,* Spielberger's State Trait Anxiety Inventory; *wk,* week; *WS,* within subjects.

(Courtesy of Szabo, A: The impact of exercise deprivation on well-being of habitual exercisers. *Aust J Sci Med Sport* 27:68–75, 1995.)

states indirectly. Experimental studies are needed to address this issue directly. It is difficult to recruit subjects for such studies because some individuals will not stop exercising for any reason. In the few experimental studies conducted, the deprivation period was often brief. Experimental studies, however, support the findings from anecdotal reports and survey research of the negative impact of exercise deprivation on subjective states in athletes.

Discussion.—Individuals who exercise regularly and who are deprived of this exercise experience a negative effect on their subjective physical and psychological states. The specific factors that contribute to this decline in well-being have not been well defined. Future studies should examine exercise deprivation outside the concept of exercise addiction, and should include cyclists, swimmers, and other athletes in addition to runners. This article also includes a general analysis of the literature on exercise deprivation, as well as conceptual problems in this field.

▶ Many of us can recall friends who, although apparently not pathologically addicted to exercise, develop a very negative mood state when business problems or injury keep them from their regular period of physical activity. This review puts together a substantial list of papers supporting the existence of such a phenomenon. Open questions include the potential to compensate for injury by adopting more limited forms of physical activity and the parallel between exercise withdrawal and the symptoms associated with loss of other forms of relaxation, such as watching television or playing bingo.

R.J. Shephard, M.D., Ph.D., D.P.E.

Associations Between Health Behaviours and Health-Related Fitness
Shephard RJ, Bouchard C (Univ of Toronto; Laval Univ, Ste Foy, Quebec, Canada)
Br J Sports Med 30:94–101, 1996   5–37

Background.—Regular exercise or attained physical fitness has been associated with other favorable health behaviors, suggesting that multifaceted lifestyle programs would be more beneficial than simple exercise classes in enhancing industrial or community health. However, the data supporting the clustering of habitual physical activity with other positive health behaviors is not especially strong. The relationship between health behaviors and health-related fitness was further investigated.

Methods.—Three hundred fifty healthy adults completed questionnaires on physical activity and health-related behaviors. In the covariance analysis of findings, adjustments were made for the significant effects of age and socioeconomic status.

Findings.—Abstaining from cigarette smoking was correlated with a small abdominal circumference in men and a low trunk-to-extremity skinfold ratio in women. Obesity and perceived fitness were negatively associated. Perceived activity, exercise frequency, and perceived fitness influenced levels of blood glucose, cholesterol, high-density cholesterol, lipoprotein and triglycerides.

Conclusion.—Though multiphasic health promotion programs are cost effective, favorable interactions among program elements are probably very limited. Positive interactions of habitual physical activity with other health behaviors—such as abstinence from alcohol, coffee, tea, and cigarettes—are limited.

▶ This cross-sectional study of 350 healthy adults from near Quebec City explores whether the habit of physical activity clusters with other healthful habits. If such "healthy clusters" exist, then maybe, to improve public health, we should focus not just on exercise classes, but on multifaceted lifestyle programs, so that 1 healthful change will shape others. But in this study, habitual physical activity did not strongly cluster with other healthful behaviors. There was a "healthy" association between various indices of leisure activity and favorable lipid profiles. In contrast to what cigarette ads would have us believe, a link existed between smoking and greater abdominal girth in men and a "masculine" distribution of body fat in women.

Whether the use of alcohol here was healthful or not was not clear-cut, perhaps because nearly 90% of the subjects drank. After all, this is Quebec! The authors conclude that economic arguments may favor multiphasic health programs, but any positive interactions between individual program elements probably are small.

E.R. Eichner, M.D.

Sports Participation and Emotional Wellbeing in Adolescents
Steptoe A, Butler N (Univ of London; City Univ, London)
Lancet 347:1789–1792, 1996   5–38

Introduction.—Numerous studies demonstrate an association between regular physical activity and emotional well-being. Most research, however, has involved adult subjects. To investigate the relationship between sports participation and emotional health in adolescents, data were collected from a sample of 16-year-old boys and girls.

Methods.—The 1970 British Cohort Study was a longitudinal survey of all children born between April 5 and April 11, 1970, in England, Wales, and Scotland. Follow-up data were available at 16 years for 2,223 boys and 2,838 girls from the original 16,500 cohort members. The general health questionnaire (GHQ) and a modified version of the malaise inventory were used to assess emotional well-being. Respondents were asked how often they had participated in team sports, individual sports, and vigorous recreational activities during the previous year. Also recorded were the respondents' physical health status and their social class.

Results.—Girls scored significantly higher than boys on 2 malaise inventory subscales and were more likely than boys to be classified as emotionally distressed on the GHQ. Sport participation in school was similar for boys and girls, but boys pursued more out-of-school sports and vigorous recreational activities. More boys were in team sports and more girls reported individual sport activities. Psychological problems were associated with poorer physical health and lower social class, but after adjustment for these factors and for sex, there were fewer psychological symptoms among boys and girls who were more engaged in sports and vigorous activities. An independent relationship was observed between somatic symptoms and participation in nonvigorous recreational activities.

Conclusion.—For adolescents as well as for adults, emotional well-being is positively associated with regular physical activity. An unexpected finding was the higher rate of psychological and somatic symptoms among boys and girls who engaged in more nonvigorous activities, such as darts or pool. Encouragement of active lifestyles among adolescents may contribute to their improved mental health.

▶ This prospective study, based on cross-sectional analyses, supports prior randomized training programs in the conclusion that vigorous physical activity has "affective beneficience." After adjustment for gender differences in sports play and for the confounders of illness and social class, this study found that regular, vigorous activity benefits psychological health in boys and girls.

Surely this conclusion is correct, although such a study can never prove cause and effect, and other studies suggest that we cannot reach sweeping conclusions that athletic participation will always reflect or convey only positive social, educational, and personal values. To wit, another recent study—a questionnaire survey of 838 students in a New York City high school—reported that although most students participated in some athletic activity, no link was found between sports involvement and academic performance, self-esteem, or depression.[1] And in what may be the first prospective, population-based study of baseline physical activity as a predictor of adverse health behaviors, it was found that the most active or most fit adolescent females were less likely to initiate cigarette smoking, but the most active males or males who participated in competitive athletics were more apt to initiate alcohol consumption than their less active counterparts.[2] This trend toward drinking (and binge drinking) in adolescent male athletes may reflect their ebullient personality and/or their tendency to take risks. See abstract 6–10 on gender differences in drowning.

E.R. Eichner, M.D.

References

1. Fisher M, Juszczak L, Friedman SB: Sports participation in an urban high school: academic and psychologic correlates. *J Adolesc Health* 18:329–334, 1996.
2. Aaron DJ, Dearwater SR, Anderson R, et al: Physical activity and the initiation of high-risk health behaviors in adolescents. *Med Sci Sports Exerc* 27:1639–1645, 1995.

Exercise-induced Muscle Cramp: Proposed Mechanisms and Management

Bentley S (Glenleith, Dunedin, New Zealand)
Sports Med 21:409–420, 1996   5–39

Introduction.—Although exercise-induced muscle cramp is a common problem, the mechanisms involved in its pathogenesis remain uncertain. To improve understanding of the origin of muscle cramp associated with exercise and develop scientifically based management protocols, the literature was revised from a historical perspective and in relation to the neurophysiology of muscle.

Historical Research and Anecdotal Observations.—Articles on muscle cramp first appeared in the 1940s, but little new information has been produced since early electromyogram studies. Some proposed causes of exercise-induced muscle cramp, including electrolyte disturbances and calcium depletion, could not be confirmed, and studies of various drugs for relief of night cramp yielded conflicting results. A number of observations based on anecdotal reports may have relevance when considering possible mechanisms of cramp (Table 3).

Muscle Neurophysiology.—Disturbances at various levels in the CNS, peripheral nerves, and possibly muscle may result in cramp. Areas of research have included the motor unit (1 motor neuron and the muscle fibers it innervates), peripheral receptors, spinal reflexes, central control of motor activity, action potential and impulse propagation in nerves, synaptic potentials, neurotransmitters and neuromodulators, muscle contraction, and myofascial trigger points.

Mechanisms, Treatment, and Prevention of Cramp.—Multiple physiologic factors occurring simultaneously are likely to result in cramp. Among these possible factors are motor neuron excitability, muscle length, proprioceptor activity, exercise to fatigue, environmental conditions, and low extracellular Ca^{++}. Treatment is directed at reducing muscle spindle and

---

TABLE 3.—Observations on Exercise-induced Muscle Cramp

Cramp is relieved by stretching but not after prolonged exercise to fatigue
Cramp occurs in endurance events (e.g. marathon), near the end or after the race
Cramp is more common in road race events such as a half marathon or marathon
   (42.2km) than in ultradistance mountain run events
Cramp occurs during intense competition rather than in training
Athletes may on occasions 'run through' cramp
Certain individuals experience cramp, others do not
Cramp is less common in children
Massage, ice, acupuncture and TENS may relieve cramp
Cramp occurs during concentric contraction following an eccentric contraction (e.g.
   kick turn in a pool)
Twitches or fasciculations increasing in frequency may precede the occurence of
   cramp

Abbreviation: TENS, transelectric cutaneous nerve stimulation.
(Courtesy of Bentley S: Exercise-induced muscle cramp: Proposed mechanisms and management. *Sports Med* 21:409–420, 1996.)

motor neuron activity. Acute cramp may be relieved by stretching, movement (standing and walking after a race), and afferent stimulation (massage, cold spray or ice, acupuncture, and transcutaneous nerve stimulation). Possible preventive measures include aerobic fitness, stretching, correction of muscle balance and posture, strength training, nutrition, mental preparation, avoidance of drugs known to cause cramps, and plyometrics.

▶ As noted in Table 3, cramps are relieved by stretching but not after prolonged exercise to fatigue. According to the authors, "The relaxation phase of muscle contraction is prolonged in a fatigued muscle, raising the likelihood of fused summation of action potentials if motor neuron activity delivers a sustained high firing frequency." The author explains that multiple physiologic factors may occur simultaneously, thereby causing a cramp. These factors include "motor neuron excitability, muscle length, proprioceptor activity, exercise to fatigue, environmental conditions, and low extracellular Ca^{++}."

The author has presented a number of suggestions that may be beneficial in preventing muscle cramps. These methods include stretching, correcting muscle balance and posture, strength training, aerobic fitness, nutrition, mental preparation (relaxing and reducing anxiety), avoiding drugs that may precipitate cramps, and possibly plyometric training.

F.J. George, ATC, PT

Ankle and Thigh Skin Surface Temperature Changes With Repeated Ice Pack Application
Palmer JE, Knight KL (Univ of Halifax, NS, Canada; Brigham Young Univ, Provo, Utah)
J Athl Train 31:319–323, 1996   5–40

Objective.—Application and reapplication of cold to injured tissue reduces hypoxic injury, and facilitates healing and recovery. Exercise increases skin temperature. The effect of activity on rewarming of the tissue after cold application for injury was evaluated.

Methods.—Ankle and thigh skin surface temperatures on 12 volunteers (4 women) were measured on 3 separate days at least 48 hours apart. Volunteers lay supine for 15 minutes; rode an exercise bike for 15 minutes; had ice packs applied for 20, 30, or 40 minutes; simulated showering for 15 minutes; rested for 40 minutes; had ice packs applied for 20, 30, or 40 minutes; and rested for 60 minutes. Data before and after exercise were compared statistically.

Results.—There was a significant difference in temperature between thigh and ankle at all measurement points. Thigh temperature changes were significantly larger during 30- and 40-minute cold applications than during 20-minute applications. Thigh temperature changes during the second rewarming were significant. Thigh and ankle temperature changes during the first cold application and rewarming were significantly larger during the 40-minute cold application than during the 20- and 30-minute cold application. Ankle temperature changes were significantly larger during the 40-minute cold application than during the 20- and 30-minute cold application. Thigh temperature changes were significantly larger during the 30- and 40-minute cold applications than during the 20-minute cold application.

Conclusion.—Allowing 30 minutes of cold application followed by 90 minutes without it is satisfactory for an injury only if the athlete is supine or has returned home. If the athlete showers and is returning home, reapplication should occur immediately after the shower or the return home. Repeated cold application is appropriate therapy for athletic injuries immediately after activity. The time of application depends on the body part injured.

▶ It is standard procedure to apply ice to acute athletic injuries. This study helps answer the question of when the second ice pack should be applied. If the athlete is moving around, showering, dressing, and walking home, then the second ice pack should be applied as soon as the destination is reached. This abstract should be read with Abstract 5–41 regarding the benefits of applying ice over a cast.

F.J. George, A.T.C., P.T.

Effectiveness of Ice Packs in Reducing Skin Temperature Under Casts
Metzman L, Gamble JG, Rinsky LA (Stanford Univ, Palo Alto, Calif; Lucile Packard Children's Hosp, Palo Alto, Calif)
Clin Orthop 330:217–221, 1996   5–41

Objective.—Although cold application causes vasoconstriction and decreases pain and swelling, it has also been shown to cause nerve palsy. The effectiveness of cold applications in lowering skin temperature of a limb in a cast was studied.

Methods.—Thermistors were placed on the legs of 10 volunteers to measure skin temperature at 2-minute intervals before and after placement of a plaster cast to the right leg and a synthetic cast to the left leg and after 4 pounds of crushed ice was placed around the cast. Skin temperature measurements were also made on the injured legs of 3 patients with closed tibial and fibular fractures. Data were analyzed and compared statistically.

Results.—Baseline temperatures of casted and noncasted legs were 31.3°C and 31.0°C, respectively. After casting, temperatures of the plaster-casted legs averaged 34.9°C and of synthetic-casted legs averaged 35.7°C. Legs in synthetic casts reach maximum temperature significantly faster than legs in plaster casts (4.8 vs. 14.8 minutes). Baseline temperatures and maximum setting temperatures for plaster and synthetic casts were similar. After cold applications, skin temperature significantly decreased relative to baseline values. The synthetic-casted leg decreased in temperature to

19.7°C in an average of 56 minutes, whereas the plaster-casted leg decreased in temperature to 18.7°C in an average of 63.8 minutes. The rewarming period was approximately 1 hour. Results for patients were similar to those for volunteers.

Conclusion.—Application of crushed ice to a plaster or synthetic leg cast lowers the temperature an average of 10°C in approximately an hour. Rewarming takes approximately 1 hour.

▶ Application of ice over a plaster or synthetic cast for 60 minutes will lower skin temperature by approximately 10°C. All the benefits of cryotherapy, such as the reduction of swelling, the reduction of secondary hypoxic tissue damage, lower rate of metabolism, lowering the need of oxygen, and the reduction of inflammation, can all occur even with a cast in place. We should advise our patients with casts to apply ice over the injured area for 60 minutes every 3–4 hours for the first 72 hours, or longer if swelling persists. Please read this abstract with Abstract 5–40.

F.J. George, A.T.C., P.T.

Functional Performance Following an Ice Immersion to the Lower Extremity
Cross KM, Wilson RW, Perrin DH (Univ of Virginia, Charlottesville; Wilford Hall Med Ctr, Lackland Air Force Base, Tex)
J Athletic Train 31:113–116, 1996   5–42

Introduction.—Cryotherapy, widely used as a treatment for acute injuries, is gaining favor for use as a rehabilitation modality as well. Cold depresses the physiology, leading to concern over its effects on motor activity. To determine the effects of ice immersion of the lower leg on functional performance, athletes were tested.

Methods.—The study included 20 collegiate athletes with no recent injuries to the lower extremity. One group of participants did 3 trials each of 3 functional performance tests—the shuttle run, the 6-m hop test, and the single-leg vertical jump—before and after 20 minutes of ice immersion of the lower leg. The other group did the same tests with a rest period, rather than ice immersion, in between. The performance of the 2 groups was compared by analysis of variance.

Results.—Performance on the vertical jump test declined significantly after ice immersion but not after a rest period. Shuttle run times also decreased in the ice immersion group. There was no significant difference in performance in the 6-m hop test.

Conclusions.—Cold application can reduce motor performance in athletes. The conditions of this study are probably not applicable to the sports environment—cold is usually applied only to a joint and the area immediately surrounding it, not to a large muscle group. Future studies should examine the effects of more commonly used cryotherapy applications on motor performance.

▶ Functional performance was decreased immediately after ice immersion of the lower extremity. How long the effects of this ice immersion last was not addressed in this study. As the authors state, it would be very rare for athletes to immediately participate in their sport after an ice immersion. Athletes certainly should not return to participation until their balance, proprioception, strength, and agility have returned to a normal state.

F.J. George, A.T.C., P.T.

6 Environment, Drug Abuse, and Smoking

Altitude Acclimatization and Blood Volume: Effects of Exogenous Erythrocyte Volume Expansion
Sawka MN, Young AJ, Rock PB, et al (United States Army Research Inst of Environmental Medicine, Natick, Mass; Boston Univ)
J Appl Physiol 81:636–642, 1996   6–1

Background.—Increases in hemoglobin are mediated by plasma loss and/or erythrocyte volume expansion. Ascending to altitude is associated with a rapid plasma loss, followed by a gradual erythrocyte volume expansion. Rapid increases in plasma erythropoietin (EPO) are also associated with ascent to altitude, peaking after about 48 hours and declining to baseline levels during acclimatization in 5–10 days. In this study, sea-level residents were assessed during 13 days of acclimatization to determine the effects of this process on erythrocyte volume and plasma volume, whether exogenous erythrocyte volume expansion changes subsequent erythrocyte volume and plasma volume adaptations, whether an increased blood oxygen content changes EPO responses during acclimatization, and the mechanisms underlying plasma loss at altitude.

Methods and Findings.—Sixteen healthy men received a 700-mL infusion of autologous erythrocytes or saline alone 24 hours before ascent to altitude. Erythrocyte volume increased by about 10% after erythrocyte infusion. Also, blood oxygen content was 8% greater in erythrocyte-infused men than in saline-infused men initially at altitude. In the first 13 days, erythrocyte volume did not change and was unaffected by prior exogenous expansion. A modest increase in blood oxygen content did not affect EPO responses. Plasma losses were associated with vascular protein losses. Exogenous erythrocyte volume expansion coincided with transient increases in plasma loss, vascular protein loss, and mean arterial pressure rises (Fig 1).

Conclusion.—Several new findings on altitude acclimatization were reported that help define human blood volume and hematologic responses in that setting. Erythrocyte volume did not increase in the 13 days after

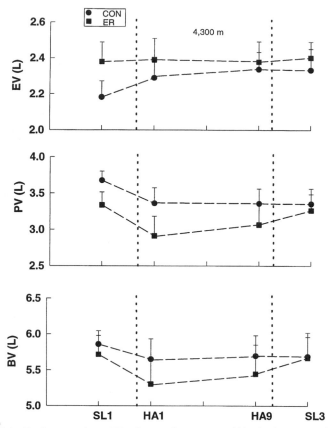

FIGURE 1.—Erythrocyte volume (*EV*), plasma volume (*PV*), and blood volume (*BV*) of erythrocyte-infused (*ER*) and control (*CON*) subjects before infusion at sea level (*SL1*) and after return from high altitude to sea level (*SL3*) and on days 1 (*HA1*) and 9 (*HA9*) during high-altitude acclimatization. Values are means ± standard error. (Courtesy of Sawka MN, Young AJ, Rock PB, et al: Altitude acclimatization and blood volume: Effects of exogenous erythrocyte volume expansion. *J Appl Physiol* 81:636–642, 1996.)

ascension to 4,300 m. The plasma volume decreases that occurred were probably mediated by protein loss that reduced vascular oncotic pressure.

▶ Although many athletes believe that altitude training benefits sea-level performance, experts are skeptical, at least regarding brief altitude training. A recent review concludes that no training strategy studied has provided unequivocal evidence that altitude training enhances sea-level performance.[1] The study abstracted here suggests 1 reason 2 weeks of training at high altitude (at the top of Pikes Peak) would not likely benefit sea-level athleticism. Although hematocrit typically increases at altitude, this study shows that this increase (at least during the first 2 weeks) does not result from an increase in red blood cell volume but from loss of plasma volume, or hemoconcentration. Plasma volume fell about 10% here, probably from intravascular protein loss because of increased capillary leak caused by hypoxia. With greater time at altitude, of course, red cell volume would increase, and other bodily adaptations to hypoxia would occur. But the question remains whether these "positive" adaptations for athletes might be offset by the loss of athletic fitness because of the inability to train hard at altitude. Thus, any "sea-level benefits" of altitude training remain in question.

E.R. Eichner, M.D.

Reference

1. Wolski LA, McKenzie DC, Wenger HA: Altitude training for improvements in sea level performance: Is there scientific evidence of benefit? *Sports Med* 22:251–263, 1996.

Energy Expenditure and Requirement While Climbing Above 6,000 m
Pulfrey SM, Jones PJH (McGill Univ, Montreal)
J Appl Physiol 81:1306–1311, 1996   6–2

Objective.—It is very difficult for humans to maintain energy balance at altitudes over 6,000 m. Weight loss is common; however, previous studies have suggested that negative energy balance in mountain climbers may be related to decreased energy intake and increased energy expenditure. Survival at these altitudes requires a complex series of metabolic adaptations, which may have high energy costs. However, there have been few studies of the effects of such extremely high altitudes on energy metabolism. Energy intake, energy expenditure, and body composition were studied in subjects climbing at a very high altitude.

Methods.—The subjects were 5 men and 1 woman attempting to climb Mt. Shisha Pangma in Tibet, which has an altitude of 8,046 m. The climbers were studied at altitudes of 5,900 to 8,046 m over 1 week. All had spent at least 3 weeks at over 5,200 m before the study and all reached at least 6,400 m. Energy intake was measured by dietary record. Energy expenditure was measured by 2 techniques—the doubly labeled water (DLW) and energy intake-balance (IB) techniques—which were compared. Body composition was assessed at the beginning and end of the study.

Results.—The mean energy intake was about 14 MJ/day. Body energy stores decreased by about 5 MJ/day, as estimated by body mass, skinfold thickness, limb circumference, and isotope dilution (Fig 2). The DLW and IB methods yielded comparable estimates of energy expenditure, with mean values of about 19 MJ/day.

Conclusion.—The difficulty of maintaining energy balance at extreme altitudes of over 6,000 m is related to an energy intake that is about 30% lower than energy expenditure. Energy expenditures at these altitudes are comparable to those observed in endurance athletes at sea level. The IB

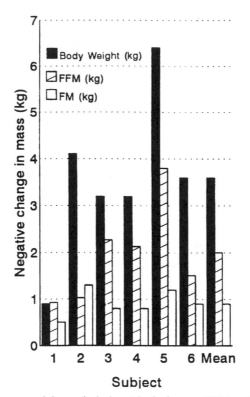

FIGURE 2.—Compartmental changes for body weight, fat-free mass (*FFM*), and fat mass (*FM*) during a 7-day period on Mt. Shisha Pangma. (Courtesy of Pulfrey SM, Jones PJH: Energy expenditure and requirement while climbing above 6,000 m. *J Appl Physiol* 81:1306–1311, 1996.)

and DLW methods provide similar estimates of energy expenditure at very high altitudes.

▶ Severe weight loss has long been recognized as an important component of high-altitude deterioration. In terms of causation, mountaineers have debated the relative importance of heavy physical work, the added energy cost of hyperventilation, and an inadequate intake of food. Pulfrey and Jones show a substantial deficit in food intake (5 MJ/day) during a mountaineering expedition. The total energy expenditure—around 19 MJ/day as measured by both the IB and DLW methods—is also at a much higher level than would be acceptable even in "heavy" occupations.

It is difficult for a climber to eat enough to meet the body's energy demands, given the limited choice of food and cooking facilities that are available at extreme altitudes. Nevertheless, it is important to try to maintain energy balance if the physical condition is not to show a progressive deterioration over the course of a climb.

R.J. Shephard, M.D., Ph.D., D.P.E.

Water Turnover and Body Composition During Long-term Exposure to High Altitude (4,900–7,600 m)
Fusch C, Gfrörer W, Koch C, et al (Univ Women's Hosp, Bern, Switzerland; Univ Children's Hosp, Tübingen, Germany; Univ Hosp, Ulm, Germany)
J Appl Physiol 80:1118–1125, 1996   6–3

Introduction.—Most studies of the effects of moderate and high altitudes on water turnover (WT) have involved a fast ascent to altitude and a short duration of exposure. To examine the changes in total body water (TBW) and WT that occur during the natural conditions of trekking and mountaineering, 13 healthy individuals were studied during a 62-day expedition in Pakistan.

Methods.—Study participants, 11 men and 2 women with a mean age of 30.2 years, were attempting an ascent of Broad Peak (8,047 m) in the Karakoram Mountains. The group stayed for 3 days at Abbottabad (1,250 m), then traveled by jeep for 5 days to reach Chongo (2,700 m). Daily trekking during days 12–20 of the expedition took the climbers to a base camp (4,750 m) where they stayed from days 21 to 51. Camps were installed during this stay at 5,800, 6,400, and 7,300 m. Because of bad weather, the maximal altitude reached during the expedition was 7,600 m. Some climbers left base camp on day 46, walked during a 2-day period to 3,600 m, and were met by helicopter; other climbers started their return on day 51, walked during a 3-day period to 2,300 m, and continued by bus. All climbers were measured on 8 occasions during the expedition for body weight (BW), TBW, and WT.

Results.—Body weight of the climbers decreased during ascent to the base camp from a mean of 73.2 to 71.7 kg, then continued to decrease until the end of base camp stay (mean 66.7 kg). The mean TBW decreased from 43.1 before arrival in Pakistan to 40.6 during the base camp stay. Water content of the body (TBW/BW) decreased significantly during the ascent, then returned to near baseline levels. The compartment of the water-free solids increased during the ascent, approached baseline value on arrival at base camp, then fell below baseline value, indicating that weight loss was a result of loss of body solid. There was an increase in WT during ascent to base camp, a further increase during the attempt to reach the summit, and an even greater increase during the climbers' descent.

Conclusion.—Body composition was stable during a 3-week period of training that preceded the trip to Pakistan. During the expedition, however, body composition showed marked changes, with various components exhibiting different effects of altitude. Initial weight loss results from dehydration, whereas later weight loss appears to reflect a loss of fat mass. Climbers seemed to have a higher degree of hydration at the end of the expedition.

▶ Sports physicians are interested in the maintenance of an appropriate fluid balance at high altitudes from 2 points of view—the athlete who competes at high altitude after only a few days of acclimatization and the person of more moderate fitness who joins a prolonged trekking expedition to ranges such as the Himalayas. The short-term effect of high-altitude exposure is a substantial and progressive dehydration, which can persist for several weeks. The athlete who spends a couple of weeks at altitude before competing may thus benefit from some increase in hemoglobin concentration, but the intended increment of cardiorespiratory performance is often largely negated by a decrease of plasma volume and a resultant reduction in cardiac preloading.

Most experimental investigations have focused on this type of scenario, with subjects transported rapidly (by helicopter, jeep, or Seilbahn) to the intended altitude. However, there have been very few studies of the typical trek, where the subject climbs to a higher altitude gradually over several weeks, as foothills are crossed. The present results suggest that although there is some trend to dehydration during the early phases of such an ascent, the final values for body water return to the normal sea-level range.

R.J. Shephard, M.D., Ph.D., D.P.E.

Acute Mountain Sickness: Increased Severity During Simulated Altitude Compared With Normobaric Hypoxia

Roach RC, Loeppky JA, Icenogle MV (Copenhagen Muscle Research Ctr; Univ of New Mexico, Albuquerque)
J Appl Physiol 81:1908–1910, 1996   6–4

Objective.—Acute mountain sickness (AMS) occurs in people who travel to altitudes above 2,500 m. Hypoxia has traditionally been considered the sole cause of AMS. However, there is evidence that hypobaria may also play a role. The effects of simulated altitude, normobaric hypoxia, and normoxic hypobaria were studied in volunteers.

Methods.—Nine healthy men were exposed to each of these conditions for 9 hours each in an environmental chamber. The experiments were performed in random order at least 1 week apart. For simulated altitude, the pressure in the chamber was reduced to 432 mm Hg, the pressure that would be encountered at an altitude of 4,564 m. For normobaric hypoxia, pressure in the chamber was normal but nitrogen was added to achieve an inspired partial pressure of oxygen (PO_2) similar to that encountered at altitude. Finally, normoxic hypobaria was achieved by lowering the pressure in the chamber while adding oxygen to produce the same inspired PO_2 as that at normal pressure. The symptoms of AMS were scored using a recent consensus scoring system.

Results.—The symptom scores were higher during simulated altitude than during normobaric hypoxia or normoxic hypobaria. Under the latter 2 conditions, scores were not significantly different from each other. Fifty-six percent of patients met the criteria for AMS during simulated altitude, compared with 11% during the other 2 conditions. Arterial oxygen saturation was 96% under normoxic hypobaria, compared with 83% under simulated altitude and normobaric hypoxia.

Conclusion.—Simulated altitude—produced by low pressure and low oxygenation in an environmental chamber—produces worse symptoms of AMS than low oxygenation with normal pressure. The way in which hypoxia and hypobaria work together to accelerate or exacerbate AMS is unknown. Further studies investigating ventilation and fluid balance and the variables governing these responses are needed.

▶ Physiologists often prefer to conduct experiments in the supposedly better controlled situation of an experimental laboratory, and it is salutory to have the occasional reminder that the behavior of the subject is not necessarily the same in an artificial environment as in the "real" world. Roach and associates here demonstrate rather nicely that chamber exposure to a simulated high altitude can induce more symptoms than either breathing a low oxygen mixture at normal atmospheric pressure or a combination of a low oxygen pressure and a low barometric pressure.

The subjects were in a decompression chamber for all 3 experiments, and test order was randomized. They should, thus, have been blinded to what they were breathing. The only potential explanation for the discrepant symptomatology seems to be a hypoventilation induced by changes in gas density.[1] One final comment: It is a little surprising that AMS developed in as little as 9 hours of exposure to the simulated 4,564 m.

Reference

1. Tucker A, Reeves JT, Robertshaw D, et al: Cardiopulmonary response to acute altitude exposure: Water loading and denitrogenation. *Respir Physiol* 54:363–380, 1983.

R.J. Shephard. M.D., Ph.D., D.P.E.

Water Balance and Acute Mountain Sickness Before and After Arrival at High Altitude of 4,350 m
Westerterp KR, Robach P, Wouters L, et al (Univ of Limburg, Maastricht, The Netherlands)
J Appl Physiol 80:1968–1972, 1996   6–5

Introduction.—Maintenance of water balance is one of the problems of high altitude. Melting snow is often the only available water. Previous studies suggested that body water loss occurs at high altitude as an adaptive mechanism that reduces acute moutain sickness, which occurs in those who retain fluid. By simultaneously measuring total water turnover and fluid loss in urine and feces, measurements were taken of insensible water loss at high altitude.

Methods.—Seven men and 3 women participated in this study in which they were transported by car and helicopter to Mont Blanc in the French Alps. During the 4-day interval before and a subsequent 4-day interval after transport to 4,350 m, measurements were taken of water intake, total water output, and water output in urine and feces. At the start and at the end of the 2 intervals, total body water and extracellular water were measured.

Results.—Between energy intake and water intake, there was a close relation, which was unchanged by the altitude intervention. Energy intake and water intake were correspondingly reduced among those in whom acute moutain sickness developed. In participants who had acute mountain sickness, there was an increase in total body water that was accompanied by a reduction in total water loss. They did not have an increased urine output. After 4 days at altitude, there was a significant increase in total body water.

Conclusion.—The biggest shifts in extracellular water relative to total body water were seen in participants with acute mountain sickness. A change in water requirements from altitude exposure is independent of fluid retention in relation to acute mountain sickness. A fluid shift of at least 1 L from the intracellular to the extracellular compartment was seen in those in whom acute mountain sickness developed.

▶ This is an interesting, well-designed and well-implemented study dealing with the phenomenon of acute mountain sickness. No attempt has been made, however, to correlate their observations regarding water balance with either the prevention or treatment of acute mountain sickness.

J.S. Torg, M.D.

Refractive Changes During 72-hour Exposure to High Altitude After Refractive Surgery
Mader TH, Blanton CL, Gilbert BN, et al (Madigan Army Med Ctr, Tacoma, Washington; Naval Med Ctr, San Diego, Calif; Cascade Eye and Skin Ctrs, PC, Tacoma, Wash)
Ophthalmology 103:1188–1195, 1996   6–6

Purpose.—In patients who have undergone radial keratotomy (RK), increasing altitude is reportedly associated with hyperopic shifts in refractive error. The mechanism of these shifts is unknown but could be related to decreased barometric pressure on the globe or the effects of hypobaric hypoxia around the incisions. Changes in refraction at altitude could have important implications for many recreational activities, including mountain climbing, hiking, and skiing. The refractive effects of high altitude in patients who have undergone RK or photorefractive keratectomy (PRK) were studied.

Methods.—The study included 6 subjects who had undergone RK, 6 who had undergone PRK, and 9 controls with myopia. Ocular examinations—including refractive measurements, keratometry, and pachymetry—were performed first at sea level. The participants then spent 3 days at an altitude of 14,100 ft; the examinations were repeated each day. Final measurements were performed 1 week after the subjects had returned to sea level.

Results.—In the RK group, spherical equivalence increased significantly and progressively during the time spent at altitude, compared with myopic controls. At the same time, keratometric values declined. No refractive changes were observed in the PRK or control groups. On pachymetry, all 4 groups had significant increases in peripheral corneal thickening during 3 days at altitude. All values returned to baseline after 1 week at sea level.

Conclusion.—In people who have undergone RK, spending 3 days at high altitude leads to a progressive but reversible hyperopic shift in refraction. A significant decrease in corneal curvature occurs as well, suggesting that the hyperopic change results from increased corneal hydration in the area of the RK incisions. No such changes occur in PRK subjects or myopic controls. The degree of the altitude-related shift may depend on the time since, and the extent of, surgery. Patients who have had RK may benefit from having multiple pairs of glasses with increasing plus power when they travel to high altitudes.

▶ Radial keratotomy seems to be an attractive option for athletes because in many sports, the use of eyeglasses is either impracticable or severely limiting. However, a number of recent reports have suggested that problems of refraction can arise when patients who have undergone such treatment reach the altitudes of many ski resorts (3,000 m and above). The optical mechanism is still debated, but it seems as though there is a reversible increase in the water content of the cornea at the sites of incision during the time the individual is at altitude. Altitude-induced disturbances of refraction diminish as the postoperative period increases. Laser keratotomy also seems to be immune to this problem, probably because the removal of corneal surface is relatively uniform in that type of operation.

R.J. Shephard, M.D., Ph.D., D.P.E.

Influence of Simulated Altitude on the Performance of Five Blood Glucose Meters
Gautier J-F, Duvallet A, Bigard AX, et al (Saint-Louis Hosp, Paris; Inst of Aerospace Medicine, Brétigny sur Orge, France)
Diabetes Care 19:1430–1433, 1996   6–7

Introduction.—Self–blood glucose monitoring plays a key role in the management of diabetes. Although various blood glucose monitors (BGMs) have tested as accurate and reliable at sea level, they may be unreliable at high altitudes because of differences in temperature, humidity, and barometric pressure. Five different BGMs were evaluated for reliability at various simulated altitudes.

Methods.—The devices studied were Accu-Chek Easy, Reflolux SF, Tracer, One Touch II, and Glucometer 3, all of which are based on the glucose oxidase-peroxidase reaction. Each device was used to measure 18 venous blood samples at 3 different ranges of blood glucose concentration: less than 5.6 mmol/L, 5.6 to 13.9 mmol/L, and greater than 13.9 mmol/L, as determined by the reference method. The tests were performed in a hypobaric chamber at simulated altitudes of up to 4,000 m, increased by intervals of 500 m. Temperature and humidity were held constant for all tests.

Results.—As barometric pressure decreased, all devices gave inaccurate readings: 4 underestimated blood glucose concentration and 1 overestimated it. From simulated altitudes of 200 to 4,000 m, the average percentage error increased from 0.26% to −28.9% with Glucometer 3, from 28.4% to 49.3% with Accu-Chek Easy, from −10.5% to 19.8% with Tracer, from −5.5% to −11.2% with Reflolux, and from 17.8% to 14.8% with One Touch. The differences were nonsignificant for Reflolux and One Touch. Reflolux was the most accurate, except for measuring high blood glucose levels at high altitudes. Agreement was good across barometric pressures and blood glucose concentrations for the One Touch II. The Glucometer 3 produced the greatest degree of underestimation.

Conclusion.—At simulated high altitudes, most BGMs underestimate blood glucose concentrations. The exception is the Accu-Chek Easy, which overestimates values. These devices may give inaccurate or inconsistent results at altitudes higher than 2,000 m. This inaccuracy is an important consideration for patients with diabetes who participate in high-altitude sports, such as skiing or trekking.

▶ Chromogen colored paper tests have greatly simplified the regulation of blood glucose in patients with diabetes, but as with any simple procedure, there are important limitations. In particular, the accuracy of such tests is adversely affected by changes in temperature, humidity, and barometric pressure.[1] The errors that many of the commercially available tests develop at altitude are large enough to be of concern to patients with diabetes. For those who spend much time at altitude, the best option may be a non–oxygen dependent hexokinase reaction.[2]

References

1. Giordano BP, Trash W, Hollenbaugh L, et al: Performance of seven glucose testing systems at high altitude. *Diabetes Educ* 15:444–448, 1989.
2. Piepmeier EH, Hammett-Stabler C, Price ME, et al: Atmospheric pressure effects on glucose monitoring devices. *Diabetes Care* 18:423–424, 1995.

R.J. Shephard, M.D., Ph.D., D.P.E.

The Effects of Heat and Exercise on Sweat Iron Loss
Waller MF, Haymes EM (Florida State Univ, Tallahassee)
Med Sci Sports Exerc 28:197–203, 1996   6–8

Background.—Iron deficiency is often seen in athletes and active individuals. There is concern about such deficiencies because iron-containing proteins have a key role in the production of energy. Loss of iron through loss of sweat may be a cause of iron deficiency. The cell-free sweat iron

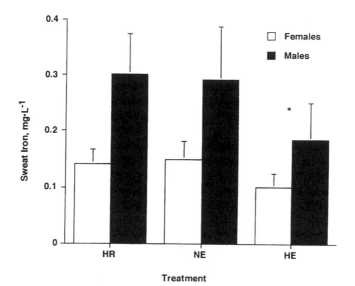

FIGURE 1.—Mean sweat iron concentration of female and male athletes during rest and exercise (50% $\dot{V}O_{2max}$) for 60 minutes in neutral and hot environments. Values are mean ± SE. *Sweat iron concentration during exercise in a hot environment was significantly lower than in a neutral environment and during rest. ($P < 0.05$). *Abbreviations: HE*, exercise in a hot environment; *HR*, rest in a hot environment; *NE*, exercise in a neutral environment. (Courtesy of Waller MF, Haymes EM: The effects of heat and exercise on sweat iron loss. *Med Sci Sports Exerc* 28:197–203, 1996.)

concentration of subjects sitting in the heat varies from 0.02 mg/L^{-1} to 0.46 mg/L^{-1}, and the sweat iron concentration of exercising subjects has been shown to vary from 0.13 mg/L^{-1} to 0.50 mg/$^{-1}$. It is unknown whether there are differences in sweat iron concentration between individuals at rest and exercising individuals. Sweat iron concentrations were examined in individuals at rest and in exercising individuals, during prolonged exercise, in neutral and hot environments, and in men and women.

Methods.—The subjects were 9 male and 9 female athletes between 23 and 34 years of age. Arm sweat was collected from subjects sitting in a hot environment and exercising at 50% maximum oxygen concentration ($\dot{V}O_{2max}$) in neutral and hot environments. Sweat iron concentrations and losses were compared. Whole-body sweat rates were calculated from weight loss every 30 minutes for 1 hour.

Results.—Sweat iron concentration during rest in a hot environment and exercising in a neutral environment was significantly higher than during exercise in a hot environment, but differences between males and females were not significant (Fig 1). Sweat iron concentration during exercise decreased significantly from 30 to 60 minutes (Fig 2). Whole-body sweat rates were significantly different across all environments. The highest whole-body sweat rate was during exercise in a hot environment and the lowest was during rest in a hot environment. During exercise, males lost significantly more sweat than females, but at rest, differences were not significant. The estimated whole-body iron loss was significantly higher

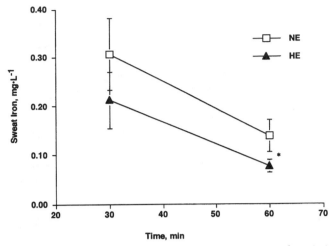

FIGURE 2.—Change in sweat iron concentration between 30 and 60 minutes of exercise in neutral and hot environments. Values are mean ± SE. *Sweat iron concentration after 60 minutes was significantly less than after 30 minutes during exercise in both neutral and hot environments. ($P < 0.05$). *Abbreviations: HE,* exercise in a hot environment; *NE,* exercise in a neutral environment. (Courtesy of Waller MF, Haymes EM: The effects of heat and exercise on sweat iron loss. *Med Sci Sports Exerc* 28:197–203, 1996.)

during exercise than at rest. The average iron loss was significantly higher in males than in females.

Discussion.—The timing of the sweat sampling is critical because different conclusions could result from the substantial differences in sweat iron concentration from the first 30 minutes to the second 30 minutes of exercise. Sweat iron concentration at rest reflects the average sweat iron of subjects exercising in a neutral or hot environment for 1 hour but may overestimate iron loss during prolonged exercise. It is unclear why sweat iron concentration decreases over time, but it may be related to the washing of cellular debris and contamination from the sweat pores into initial samples. Lower sweat iron concentration during exercise in hot environments may result from dilution because the arm sweat rate in a hot environment is double the rate in a neutral environment. There was a significant relation between sweat iron concentration and ferritin during exercise only, suggesting that iron may be conserved in individuals with low iron stores by reduced sweat iron excretion.

▶ This work probes the controversy over whether enough iron can be lost in sweat to cause iron deficiency in athletes. It shows that sweat iron concentration decreases over time, at least during the first hour of exercise. Some studies have used the concentration of iron in sweat from subjects resting in the heat to estimate iron losses during exercise. In light of the decline in sweat iron level during exercise, these studies probably overestimated sweat iron loss in athletes. This study also finds that sweat iron is lower in athletes exercising in the heat than in a neutral environment, the result in part of dilution by a greater sweat rate in the heat. Contrary to past work by one of these authors, exercising men had about twice the sweat iron loss as women, in part because of higher sweat rates in men and likely also because of greater iron stores in men. If 10% of dietary iron is absorbed, the authors calculate that 6% to 11% of the iron typically absorbed per day can be lost in sweat during 1 hour of exercise. They argue that the small amount of iron lost in sweat probably would not deplete iron stores in male athletes but might do so in female athletes whose diets are low in iron.

E.R. Eichner, M.D.

Intravenous Vs. Oral Rehydration: Effects on Subsequent Exercise-heat Stress
Castellani JW, Maresh CM, Armstrong LE, et al (Univ of Connecticut, Storrs; Texas Tech Univ, Amarillo)
J Appl Physiol 82:799–806, 1997   6–9

Background.—Direct comparisons of the effects of IV and oral fluid replacement strategies on exercise performance 1 to 2 hours after rehydration have not been published. The influence of these 2 strategies after exercise-induced dehydration during a subsequent 90-minute exercise bout was reported.

Methods.—Eight non–heat-acclimated men participated in the study. After exercise-induced dehydration to −4% body weight loss, 1 of 3 treatments was administered: IV 0.45% sodium chloride, no fluid, or oral saline. After rehydration and rest lasting a total of 2 hours, the men walked at 50% maximal oxygen consumption for up to 90 minutes at 36°C.

Findings.—The heart rate was higher in the patients receiving oral hydration than in those receiving IV hydration at 45, 60, and 75 minutes of exercise. The oral and IV groups were similar in rectal temperature, sweat rate, percentage change in plasma volume, and change in plasma osmolality. Plasma norepinephrine declined less in the men receiving oral fluids than in those receiving IV fluids at 45 minutes. The IV and oral groups had comparable changes in plasma adrenocorticotropic hormone and cortisol levels after exercise was begun. Exercise times were similar in the IV and oral groups.

Conclusion.—After exercise-induced dehydration, IV and oral fluid administrations were equally effective as rehydration treatments. Thermoregulation, change in adrenocorticotropic hormone, and change in cortisol did not differ between the 2 groups after exercise began, probably because of the similar percentage change in plasma volume and in osmolality.

▶ This study shows that, after exercise-induced dehydration, oral rehydration (oral saline) works as well as IV rehydration, as proven soon thereafter (2 hours later) by a heat-exercise trial. Another noted study in this field shows that, in boys exercising in the heat, flavoring of water (grape-flavoring) reduces voluntary dehydration, and further addition to the water of 6% carbohydrates and 18 mmol/L of sodium chloride prevents voluntary dehydration altogether.[1] Three other relevant articles show, respectively, that caffeine consumed in a carbohydrate-electrolyte solution during exercise does not cause diuresis or compromise bodily hydration status[2]; that for rehydration, sodium content and volume of ingested fluid interact[3]; and that a meal plus water can be more effective than a sports drink alone in restoring whole-body water balance.[4]

E.R. Eichner, M.D.

References

1. Wilk B, Bar-Or O: Effect of drink flavor and NaCl on voluntary drinking and hydration in boys exercising in the heat. *J Appl Physiol* 80:1112–1117, 1996.
2. Wemple RD, Lamb DR, McKeever KH: Caffeine vs caffeine-free sports drinks: Effects on urine production at rest and during prolonged exercise. *Int J Sports Med* 18:40–46, 1997.
3. Shirreffs SM, Taylor AJ, Leiper JB, et al: Post-exercise rehydration in man: Effects of volume consumed and drink sodium content. *Med Sci Sports Exerc* 28:1260–1271, 1996.
4. Maughan RJ, Leiper JB, Shirreffs SM: Restoration of fluid balance after exercise-induced dehydration: Effects of food and fluid balance. *Eur J Appl Physiol* 73:317–325, 1996.

Why Are Most Drowning Victims Men? Sex Differences in Aquatic Skills and Behaviors

Howland J, Hingson R, Mangione TW, et al (Boston Univ; JSI Research and Training Inst, Boston)
Am J Public Health 86:93–96, 1996
6–10

Background.—The rate of death from drowning is significantly higher in males than in females. Among older teens and young adults, 10 times more males than females die by drowning. Potential explanations for this difference were evaluated using data from a national survey of aquatic activities.

Methods.—The analysis used responses from a 1991 national survey of 3,042 adolescents and adults regarding their aquatic activities. The responses were used to evaluate 5 possible explanations for the differing drowning rates of men and women, i.e., exposure to aquatic environments, frequency of activities involving the potential for submersion, swimming training and ability, risk-taking behaviors in the water, and alcohol use on or near the water.

Results.—Men were more likely to report participating in aquatic activities during the last year, relative risk (RR) 1.47, though most respondents of both sexes reported some aquatic activity. Men were more likely to report activities with the potential for submersion and reported more high-exposure aquatic activity days. There was evidence that men tended to overestimate their swimming ability, particularly those who had not had swimming lessons. Men participated in more risky activities—such as swimming in natural bodies of water, swimming alone, and swimming at night—and drank more alcohol while in or near the water.

Conclusions.—Several different factors related to aquatic activities may explain the higher rates of death by drowning in men vs. women. Men have more opportunities to drown, with more high-exposure aquatic activities and more risk-taking behavior in the water. Men's alcohol use around the water may play a role, as may their tendency to overestimate their swimming abilities.

▶ This intriguing study suggests why male drowning victims outnumber females 10 to 1. Part of it is in the "denominator data." Men have greater exposure to aquatic environments than women do, so men have more "opportunity" to drown. But part of it is a difference in behavior between the sexes. Men are more apt to drink alcohol on or near the water, to take chances, and to overestimate their skills. In fact, as the authors imply, swimming lessons may initially serve to teach men that, to their surprise, they don't really know how to swim

E.R. Eichner, M.D.

Haemoconcentration in Neurological Decompression Illness
Boussuges A, Blanc P, Molenat F, et al (Hôpital Salvator, Marseilles, France; Hôpital; Font-Pre, Toulon, France)
Int J Sports Med 17:351–355, 1996   6–11

Background.—Neurologic decompression accidents in amateur divers can be permanently incapacitating. Decompression illness (DCI) is caused by bubble formation because of a decrease in ambient pressure. Circulating bubbles result in capillary leak syndrome, extravasation of plasma, and hemoconcentration. Animal experiments suggest that hemoconcentration is associated with a poor prognosis. Hematocrit levels were measured in divers with DCI, and the relationship between hematocrit level and prognosis was established.

Methods and Findings.—Fifty-eight consecutive nonprofessional divers with neurologic DCI admitted to a hyperbaric center and 16 divers without DCI were studied. The median hematocrit values of the 2 groups were 42.5% and 41.8%, respectively, the difference being nonsignificant. Divers with neurologic sequelae had a significantly greater median hematocrit level than divers without sequelae and those without DCI. A hematocrit level of 48% or greater was associated with persistent neurologic morbidity one month after the accident, although a hematocrit of less than 48% had no prognostic value (Table 4).

Conclusion.—A hematocrit level of 48% or greater in divers with DCI is associated with persistent neurologic sequelae one month after the accident, even when initial neurologic findings suggest mild disease. He-

TABLE 4.—Hematocrit of 48% or Greater and Prognosis

	Ht <48% n = 44	Ht ≥48% n = 14
Total Recovery (n = 39)	34 (77%)	5 (36%)
Sequelae (n = 19)	10 (23%)	9 (64%)

(Courtesy of Boussuges A, Blanc P, Molenat F, et al: Haemoconcentration in neurological decompression illness. *Int J Sports Med* 17:351–355, 1996.)

matocrit measures obtained on admission to the hyperbaric center may be a useful index to determine DCI severity in divers.

▶ One of my first medical appointments was as flying officer responsible for decompression tests at the Royal Air Force Institute of Aviation Medicine. I still remember the metaphoric cloud that was hanging over the Farnborough decompression chamber when I arrived. The cause was the death of a young British Airways flight attendant some 24 hours after a standard decompression test. At that time, there was no diagnostic test to identify those who might have an adverse long-term postdecompression reaction, and it was, thus, necessary to retain in the hospital for 24–48 hours all who had experienced serious symptoms during or immediately after decompression.

The hematocrit test proposed here is a useful step toward identifying those with sequelae, but, unfortunately, it is not perfect; in fact, the cut-off point of a hematocrit—<48%—identifies only 9 of 19 cases. Underlying mechanisms include the disruption of endothelial cells, the activation of leukocytes and platelets, and a release of kinins, with an extravasation of plasma that leads to hemoconcentration.[1, 2] It may be that the methods of the modern immunology laboratory will offer a more certain approach to diagnosis of this serious complication of diving and other changes in ambient pressure.

R.J. Shephard, M.D., Ph.D., D.P.E.

References

1. Levine L, Stewart S, Lunch P, et al.: Blood and blood vessel changes induced by decompression sickness in dogs. *J Appl Physiol* 50:944–949, 1981.
2. Ward CA, Koheil A, McCullough D, et al: Activation of complement at plasma air interface of rabbits. *J Appl Physiol* 60:1651–1658, 1986.

Dehydration, Hyperthermia, and Athletes: Science and Practice
Murray R (Gatorade Sports Science Inst, Barrington, Ill)
J Athletic Train 31:248–252, 1996   6–12

Background.—Dehydration can contribute to hyperthermia by decreasing the body's ability to lose heat. Even low levels of dehydration can

---

TABLE.—Physiologic Responses to Dehydration

Gastric emptying rate	Decreased
Incidence of gastrointestinal distress	Increased
Splanchnic and renal blood flow	Decreased
Plasma volume	Decreased
Plasma osmolality	Increased
Blood viscosity	Increased
Central blood volume	Decreased
Central venous pressure	Decreased
Cardiac filling pressure	Decreased
Heart rate	Increased
Stroke volume	Decreased
Cardiac output	Decreased
Sweat rate at a given core temperature	Decreased
Core temperature at which sweating begins	Increased
Maximal sweat rate	Decreased
Skin blood flow at a given core temperature	Decreased
Core temperature at which skin blood flow increases	Increased
Maximal skin blood flow	Decreased
Core temperature at a given exercise intensity	Increased
Muscle glycogen use	Increased
Endurance performance (simulated races)	Decreased
Endurance capacity (exercise to exhaustion)	Decreased

(Courtesy of Murray R: Dehydration, hyperthermia, and athletes: Science and practice. *J Athletic Train* 31:248–252, 1996.)

---

impair performance. It is important to athletes' health and performance to prevent dehydration and limit the increase in core temperature that occurs naturally during exercise.

Dehydration and Hyperthermia in Athletes.—One of the most important benefits of fluid intake during exercise is the prevention of additional increases in body temperature. Voluntarily drinking fluid during physical activity can result in wide ranges of fluid intake but generally equals only about 50% of sweat loss. Because there is no evidence that humans can adapt to chronic dehydration, drinking adequate amounts of fluid is the only way to avoid the effects of dehydration during exercise (Table). The timing of fluid ingestion is also important.

Practical Recommendations.—Increased fitness enhances an athlete's ability to train and compete in warm environments. Thus, a good base of aerobic training should be included in early season training programs. Acclimatization is also essential, necessitating at least 1–2 weeks of training in the heat. Easy access to cold fluids during training and competition is also essential. Also useful is reducing the intensity of training on warm days, extending the length of rest breaks to allow more time for cooling and for fluid and carbohydrate intake, and decreasing the intensity and duration of the warm-up to prevent body temperatures from rising too high too fast. The cooling effects of shade and electric fans are useful during breaks. The amount of equipment worn during practice, especially headgear, can be minimized.

To keep athletes hydrated, about 500 mL (17 oz) of fluid should be ingested 2 hours before exercise. On very hot days, athletes should drink another 250–500 mL of fluid 30–60 minutes before exercise. Athletes should be instructed that the goal of drinking fluids during training is to match fluid amount to sweat loss as closely as possible. For rapid and complete rehydration, athletes must ingest sodium chloride as well as fluids. When athletes are training once a day, they usually have the opportunity to consume the needed fluid and salt. Special attention is needed when athletes are training twice a day or participating in daylong bouts of competition.

Conclusion.—An aggressive fluid replacement and temperature regulation regimen is needed to prevent dehydration and hyperthermia in athletes. Athletic trainers, coaches, athletes, and support personnel need to be made aware of the benefits of sufficient fluid strategies. Also, athletes must have the opportunity to train themselves to ingest larger amounts of fluid more often.

▶ Athletes must be knowledgeable regarding the danger of dehydration and hyperthermia. Perhaps if athletes can be convinced that even low levels of dehydration will impair performance, they will heed the precautions. Hydration, rehydration, and acclimatization should be major considerations for athletes who must exercise in heat. Additional comments on this very important subject appear in the 1995 and 1996 YEAR BOOKS OF SPORTS MEDICINE.[1, 2, 3]

References

1. Lyle DM: 1995 YEAR BOOK OF SPORTS MEDICINE, pp 281–282.
2. Terrados N, Maughan RJ: 1996 YEAR BOOK OF SPORTS MEDICINE, pp 418–420.
3. Lee Chiong TL Jr, Stitt JT: 1996 YEAR BOOK OF SPORTS MEDICINE, pp. 420–421.

Postexercise Muscle Cramping Associated With Positive Malignant Hyperthermia Contracture Testing
Ogletree JW, Antognini JF, Gronert GA (Nix Sports Medicine Clinic, San Antonio, Tex; Univ of California, Davis)
Am J Sports Med 24:49–51, 1996   6–13

Background.—Malignant hyperthermia, a rare hypermetabolic disorder of skeletal muscle, usually occurs after certain anesthetic agents are administered. A young athlete in whom severe muscle cramping developed after exercise in hot, humid weather and who subsequently tested positive for malignant hyperthermia susceptibility was described.

Case Report.—Boy, 17 years, had a 3- to 4-year history of intermittent severe muscle cramping after exercising strenuously in hot, humid weather. His cramps began about 30 minutes after exercise and persisted for 30 minutes to 3 hours. The neck, back, and shoulders were affected. On physical examination, the patient was healthy. His creatine kinase level was increased to 678 U/L 1 day after playing football. His phosphorous level was low, at 3.1

mg/mL. A consulting neurologist diagnosed benign exertional cramps. However, because the patient's symptoms were more exaggerated than those of other athletes, further evaluation was done, including testing for susceptibility to malignant hyperthermia. The abnormal findings met criteria for the diagnosis of malignant hyperthermia susceptibility. The patient was instructed to limit the activities that precipitated his symptoms. Dantrolene sodium to be taken orally was prescribed to allay future episodes of muscle cramping, but no further episodes occurred. The patient was also advised to wear a MedicAlert bracelet. His family members were encouraged to have their creatine kinase levels tested, but none has done so.

Conclusions.—In this young athlete, heat and exertional muscle cramps were associated with positive malignant hyperthermia contracture testing. Although awake episodes of malignant hyperthermia may be very rare, they may be a cause of heat- and exercise-related muscle problems.

▶ The authors relate an excellent observation regarding the possible association of heat-related illnesses in malignant hyperthermia-susceptible individuals. Unfortunately, the lack of a reliable, cost-effective, noninvasive test makes screening for malignant hyperthermia difficult. However, the problem should be suspected in individuals with a family history of an anesthetic complication or death, episodic fevers of unknown origin, and history of dark urine. If for no other reason than to collect relevant data, individuals with exercise-related symptoms should be appropriately studied to determine if malignant hyperthermia, an autosomal dominant disorder muscle function, is present and if so, results should be reported to the North American Malignant Hyperthermia Registry.

J.S. Torg, M.D.

Effect of CHO Ingestion on Exercise Metabolism and Performance in Different Ambient Temperatures

Febbraio MA, Murton P, Selig SE, et al (Royal Melbourne Inst of Technology, Bundoora; Victoria Univ of Technology, Footscray; Univ of Melbourne, Australia)
Med Sci Sports Exerc 28:1380–1387, 1996   6–14

Background.—Specific requirements for carbohydrates and fluids during exercise may differ depending on ambient temperature. In hot conditions, carbohydrate ingestion may or may not improve exercise performance; fluid delivery may be relatively more important than during cool conditions. Optimal net water absorption in the heat may occur when an oral rehydration solution is slightly hypotonic. The effect of ingestion of a 7% or 14% carbohydrate solution on exercise metabolism and performance in hot and cool conditions was examined. The efficacy of ingestion of slightly hypotonic solutions (with or without carbohydrates) on exercise performance in hot weather was also examined.

Methods.—Two series of trials were performed. In the first, 12 individuals performed 3 cycling exercises to fatigue in a temperature of either 33°C (HT1) or 5°C (CT). They then ingested either a 14% carbohydrate solution (HCHO), a 7% carbohydrate solution (NCHO), or a placebo (CON1). In the second series, 6 individuals (HT2) performed the same exercises at 33°C while ingesting either NCHO, a 4.2% carbohydrate solution (LCHO), or a placebo (CON2).

Results.—In both the CT and HT1 groups, plasma glucose was highest with HCHO, lower with NCHO, and lowest with CON1. In the HT2 group, plasma glucose was lower with CON2 than with NCHO and LCHO. In both CT and HT1, the fall in plasma volume was greater with HCHO. In HT2, however, plasma volume did not differ significantly among groups. Exercise time was not different between HT1 and HT2, but in CT it was longer with NCHO compared with HCHO, and with HCHO compared with CON1.

Conclusions.—These data suggest that fatigue is related to factors other than carbohydrate availability during prolonged exercise in the heat. A 7% solution of carbohydrate appears more beneficial for exercise performance than does a 14% carbohydrate solution when exercising at 5°C. Fatigue in the cold does appear related in part to carbohydrate availability; however, ingestion of a concentrated carbohydrate solution may impair gastric emptying. Carbohydrate supplementation may not be beneficial for those who are able to maintain adequate glucose concentrations in the absence of carbohydrates. Carbohydrate ingestion also has less effect on performance when exercise lasts less than 2 hours. Fatigue with continuous exercise in the heat is likely to be related to hyperthermia rather than substrate supply. Fluid delivery may therefore be a more important factor than carbohydrate availability on endurance exercise performance in the heat. Absorption of fluids during exercise in the heat does not appear improved by slight hypotonicity of the solution.

▶ The repeated message from this study is that the data from this study, together with previous observations,[1-2] suggest that fatigue during exercise in the heat is associated with a critical level of hyperthermia. Athletes exercising in the heat should select beverages that do not impair fluid delivery. When exercising in a cool environment, athletes should select a beverage that contains a 6% carbohydrate solution. Fluid replacement for athletes exercising in the heat is a most important responsibility of the athletic trainer.

F.J. George, A.T.C., P.T.

References

1. Febbraio MA, Parkin JA, Baldwin J, et al: Metabolic indices of fatigue in prolonged exercise at different ambient temperatures. *Med Sci Sports Exerc* 28(Suppl 5):180A, 1996.

2. Nielson BJ, Hales RS, Strange S, et al: Human circulatory and thermoregulatory adaptations with the heat acclimation and exercise in a hot, dry environment. *J Physiol* 460:467–485, 1993.

Whole-body Cooling of Hyperthermic Runners: Comparison of Two Field Therapies

Armstrong LE, Crago AE, Adams R, et al (Univ of Connecticut, Storrs; Falmouth Hosp, Mass)
Am J Emerg Med 14:355–358, 1996   6–15

Introduction.—Extreme hyperthermia (rectal temperature of >40°C) in exertional heatstroke and some cases of severe heat exhaustion can be treated successfully with rapid cooling techniques and rehydration. There is some debate, however, regarding which cooling method is most effective. Two cooling therapies for hyperthermic distance runners who had completed an 11.5-km summer foot race were compared in a field study.

Methods.—In 21 distance runners (mean age, 35 years), extreme hyperthermia and either heat exhaustion or preliminary exertional heatstroke were diagnosed at completion of races. Two cooling therapies were used: ice water immersion (1–3°C) of the torso and upper legs or air exposure (24.4°C ambient) with wet towels covering the torso and upper legs. Both therapies were started 4–8 minutes after runners were admitted to the medical station. Runners were monitored for rectal temperature, blood pressure, and pulse.

Results.—The runners were treated at 3 different races, all during the month of August and under similar weather conditions. The mean ambient temperature was 24.4°C, and the mean relative humidity was 67%. The 2 treatment groups were similar in age and in weekly training distance before the race. Heart rate and systolic and diastolic blood pressure on admission to the medical station were also comparable. The initial rectal temperature of the ice water immersion group was greater than that of the air exposure group, but differences in rectal temperature were not a cause of differences in cooling rates. The water immersion technique cooled approximately twice as fast as air exposure (Table 2). Whereas air exposure required a mean of 12 minutes to reduce rectal temperature by 1°C, this same reduction was achieved in a mean of 5.6 minutes with ice water immersion.

Discussion.—Despite anecdotal evidence and logical inference, the superiority of ice water immersion for rapid body cooling has been rejected by several clinicians and physiologists. Findings of this study confirm that heat is dissipated from the body at a far greater rate during ice water immersion than during air exposure. Immediate on-site ice water immer-

TABLE 2.—Measurements of 14 Distance Runners Cooled by Ice Water Immersion

Gender	Age (yr)	T_re During Therapy			Duration (min)	Cooling Rate (°C/min)	Time to Cool T_re 1°C (min)	HR (beats/min)	BP (mm Hg)
		Pre	Post	Δ					
M	28	41.7	38.2	−3.5	15	0.23	4.4	140	120/50
M	32	41.3	39.4	−1.9	13	0.15	6.7	128	120/70
M	41	41.1	39.5	−1.6	18	0.09	11.1	—	—
M	50	43.2	38.3	−4.9	35	0.14	7.1	132	170/100
M	32	41.8	36.6	−5.2	25	0.21	4.8	132	130/40
M	26	41.1	38.8	−2.3	8	0.29	3.5	—	160/70
M	24	42.2	38.0	−4.2	29	0.14	7.1	104	80/40
M	26	41.7	38.4	−3.3	15	0.22	4.5	120	200/70
M	65	41.7	38.7	−3.0	16	0.19	5.3	100	200/70
F	41	41.9	38.9	−3.0	11	0.27	3.7	124	124/72
M	—	41.7	39.4	−2.3	19	0.12	8.3	120	150/70
M	21	41.3	38.9	−2.4	7	0.34	2.9	—	—
M	31	41.6	38.9	−2.7	10	0.27	3.7	124	130/60
M	37	41.0	39.2	−1.8	9	0.20	5.0	88	120/50
Mean (±SE)	35 (3)	41.7* (0.2)	38.7 (0.2)	−3.0* (0.3)	16 (2)	0.20* (0.02)	5.6* (0.6)	119 (5)	142/64 (±10/±5)

*Significantly different from air exposure, $P < 0.001$–0.005.

Abbreviations: M, male; F, female; T_{re}, rectal temperature; Δ, T_{re} change; HR, heart rate; BP, blood pressure.

(Courtesy of Armstrong LE, Crago AE, Adams R, et al: Whole-body cooling of hyperthermic runners: Comparison of two field therapies. *Am J Emerg Med* 14:355–358, 1996.)

sion is therefore recommended as the treatment of choice for severe exercise-induced hyperthermia or stroke.

▶ Athletic trainers often encounter athletes with exertional heat stroke and severe heat exhaustion involving extreme hyperthermia. The treatment for this emergency is rapid body cooling. This study indicates that ice water immersion (1°C to 3°C) cooled the body approximately twice as fast as air exposure. If ice water immersion is not available, then other cooling techniques, such as ice packs, ice cold wet sheets and towels, running cold water, or forced air spray, should be used. Treatment must not be delayed, and medical assistance should be sought immediately.

F.J. George, A.T.C., P.T.

Risk Factors Predicting Exertional Heat Illness in Male Marine Corps Recruits
Gardner JW, Kark JA, Karnei K, et al (Uniformed Services Univ of the Health Sciences, Bethesda, Md)
Med Sci Sports Exerc 28:939–944, 1996   6–16

Background.—Exertional heat illness can be a major problem in military training and operations. It includes disorders such as exertional dehydration, heat cramps, heat exhaustion, heat stroke, and rhabdomyolysis. Exertional heat illness occurs from elevated body core temperature and metabolic and circulatory processes. There has been substantial morbidity and mortality from exertional heat illness related to military training in hot weather in the United States. Predictive factors of exertional heat illness were studied in male Marine Corps recruits in a matched, population-based, case-control study.

Methods.—The case and control subjects were enrolled from a group of male Marine Corps recruits in basic training. There were 528 cases of exertional heat illness identified in a 4-year period. Information on demographics, anthropometrics, and physical performance was collected for case and control subjects. Risk factors for exertional heat illness were determined.

Results.—Data were obtained for 391 of the 528 case subjects who had exertional heat illness and for 1,467 control subjects. There was an increased risk for exertional heat illness with higher body mass index as measured on arrival, as well as on longer time to complete a 2.4 km (1.5-mile) run during the first week of training. Recruits with a body mass index of 22 kg/m² or more and who ran the 2.4 km in 12 minutes or more had the highest risk of exertional heat illness (Table 2); this risk was 8 times higher than that of those with a body mass index of less than 22 kg/m². Only 18% of these subjects met the criteria for high risk, but they accounted for 47% of all cases of exertional heat illness.

Discussion.—Identifying individuals at high risk for exertional heat illness can help in developing preventive measures in military training.

TABLE 2.—Matched Odds Ratios Illustrating Interaction Between 1.5-Mile Run Time and Body Mass Index in Male Marine Corps Recruits

| | 1.5-Mile PFT1 Run-Time | | |
BMI	<10 min	10–<12 min	12+ min
<22 kg · m^{-2}	1.0	1.5	3.5
	(referent)	(0.7–3.2)	(1.4–8.8)
	(10/83)	(34/247)	(15/55)
22–<26 kg · m^{-2}	1.6	2.0	8.5
	(0.6–3.8)	(0.9–4.2)	(3.8–19)
	(14/79)	(69/366)	(63/83)
26+ kg · m^{-2}	3.7	3.3	8.8
	(0.9–15)	(1.5–7.1)	(4.1–19)
	(4/9)	(48/141)	(107/133)

Note: Odds ratios (number of matched cases/number of matched controls; 95% confidence intervals) were from a physical/fitness run.
Boldface indicates high risk; italic, medium risk; lightface, low risk.
(Courtesy of Gardner JW, Kark JA, Karnei K, et al: Risk factors predicting exertional heat illness in male marine corps recruits. Med Sci Sports Exerc 28(8):939–944, 1996.)

Strengths of this study include the consistent sources of data and the ability to control the major risk factors of climate, exertion, and training conditions for exertional heat illness. These findings may not apply to other populations in other circumstances.

▶ Fatal heat illness is still too frequent a complication of "fun runs," football games, and military exercises during the summer months. It is thus helpful to review factors that predispose to exertional heat illness. This paper by Gardner and associates is much more conclusive than many scientific studies of other questions—the risk of thermal problems is increased almost ninefold in military recruits who have a body mass index of more than 26 kg/m² and a 2.4 km (1.5-mile) run time of more than 12 minutes (i.e., an aerobic power of less than 42 mL/[kg·min]. Plainly, individuals in this category should be given considerable preliminary conditioning before they are asked to undertake prolonged endurance exercise on a hot day.

R.J. Shephard, M.D., Ph.D., D.P.E.

Assessment of Chlorine Exposure in Swimmers During Training
Drobnic F, Freixa A, Casan P, et al (Instituto Nacional de Salud e Higiene en el Trabajo, Barcelona; Hosp de la Santa creu i de Sant Pau, Barcelona)
Med Sci Sports Exerc 28:271–274, 1996   6–17

Introduction.—Outside the work setting, the most common source of exposure to chlorine gas is the enclosed swimming pool. There have been reports of sudden onset of reversible airway obstruction in young swimmers, increased sensitization to aeroallergens, and a high rate of bronchial responsiveness to methacholine in swimmers. The concentration of chlorine gas in the microclimate where swimmers train was evaluated for 5 randomly chosen days in 4 different enclosed swimming pools used by the national swimming team of Spain and the autonomous team of Catalonia. For each of the 5 days, the chlorine level in the air was measured near the water (<0.1 m) on 4 sides of the pool at the same time of day.

Results.—The mean chlorine level of all 4 pools was 0.42 mg/m^{-3}, a value far below the threshold limited value (TLV) of 1.45 mg/m^{-3} for a workplace 8-hour workday. The TLV levels are based on work site chlorine exposure for a sedentary person or moderately active person. The chlorine level in the breathing zone was significantly larger with a greater number of swimmers, compared to 5 or less swimmers.

Discussion/Conclusion.—If a swimmer trains at least 2 hours per day with a ventilation of 10–12 times the resting value, the swimmer could inhale a total amount of chlorine similar to the TLV. This amount could be doubled if the training session were conducted twice daily, a common practice for competitive athletes. Frequent exposure to chlorine may cause bronchial hyperresponsiveness. Ventilation systems for enclosed pools need to be designed to maximize air exchange so chlorine concentrations can be kept at an acceptable level. Swimming is often encouraged for children with asthma because the humidity and warm ambient conditions may diminish the incidence of exercise-induced bronchoconstriction. This practice must be tempered with the understanding that high air-chlorine levels may exacerbate bronchial reactivity.

▶ Swimming is often recommended to the individual with asthma on the basis that the humid environment of a swimming pool will avoid the usual precipitant of exercise-induced bronchospasm—the inhalation of cold, dry air. However, many years ago we described the case of a swimmer whose symptoms of asthma appeared to be precipitated by the inhalation of chlorine from a swimming pool.[1] The authors of this paper make the point that although ambient chlorine concentrations in the pool area meet the usually accepted 8-hour industrial standard, they may be excessive for a swimmer who is developing a very large respiratory minute volume.

R.J. Shephard, M.D., Ph.D., D.P.E.

Reference

1. Fried T, Shephard RJ: A team approach to sports medicine. *JAMA* 216:1777–1778, 1971.

Nitrogen Dioxide Pneumonitis in Ice Hockey Players
Karlson-Stiber C, Höjer J, Sjöholm A, et al (Söder Hosp, Stockholm; Karolinska Hosp, Stockholm; Löwenströmska Hosp, Upplands Väsby, Sweden)
J Intern Med 239:451–456, 1996   6–18

Introduction.—The dangers of exposure to poisonous substances while playing ice hockey have been reported but are not well known. Carbon monoxide and nitrogen dioxide have been identified as the toxic agents and are produced by ice-resurfacing machines that use gasoline or liquefied

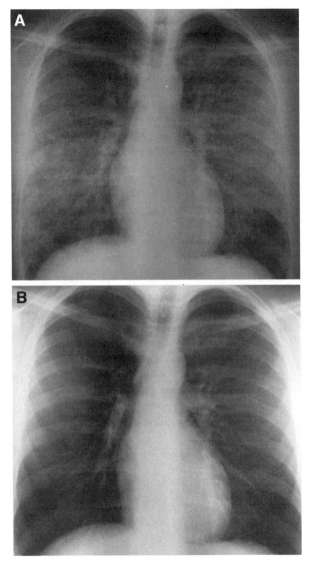

FIGURE 2.—**A,** chest radiographs of the patient taken 34 hours after exposure to nitrogen dioxide, showing widespread alveolar consolidation bilaterally, and **B,** showing normalization 7 days later. (Courtesy of Karlson-Stiber C, Höjer J, Sjöholm A, et al: Nitrogen dioxide pneumonitis in ice hockey players. *J Intern Med* 239:451–456, 1996, publisher, Blackwell Science Ltd.)

petroleum gas. Aggravating factors are inadequate ventilation, high shields around the rink, and malfunctioning machines. Symptoms include dizziness, headache, nausea, vomiting, cough, hemoptysis, dyspnea, and unconsciousness. Two individuals with delayed toxic pneumonitis and pulmonary edema were seen.

Case Report.—Boy, 17 years, was admitted to the hospital with cough, dyspnea, and hemoptysis. He had deteriorated after playing hockey the previous day. The patient's white blood cell count was elevated, but results of other routine laboratory blood tests were normal. Chest radiographs showed parenchymatous infiltrative lesions and alveolar consolidation (Fig 2). Toxic pneumonitis was suspected and the patient was given oxygen, 16 mg of IV betamethasone, and 2 mg of budesonide through an inhaler. Oral penicillin was started, but this and the systemic corticosteroid were discontinued 2 days later when the patient was discharged. Follow-up at 1 week showed normal laboratory values, blood gases, peak expiratory flow rate, and chest radiographs. Local corticosteroid therapy was continued for 4 weeks. At 1-year follow-up, the patient had no symptoms of the respiratory tract and was still playing hockey. Three other players were also admitted to the hospital but had no abnormalities on radiographs and were discharged after a few hours.

Discussion.—The symptomatology of these patients is consistent with that reported by others. During the exposure, symptoms were minor, but after several hours, relapse with hemoptysis, hypoxemia, and other severe symptoms occurred. Physicians should be aware of the possibility of delayed toxic symptoms in individuals with pulmonary symptoms within 48 hours of spending time in an indoor ice arena. It is recommended that indoor ice-resurfacing machines that use gasoline or liquified petroleum gas be replaced by machines that use electricity.

▶ Another graphic report of toxic pneumonitis from playing ice hockey in an indoor arena. The symptoms were classic: cough and diffuse chest pain early on; then a delayed, more severe illness with cough, dyspnea, hemoptysis, hypoxemia, a reduced expiratory flow rate, and infiltrates of alveolar consolidation on chest radiograph. Nitrogen dioxide is a persistent combustion emission and a hazard in indoor arenas that use fuel-driven ice-resurfacing machines. Heavier than air, nitrogen dioxide settles above the ice. Players with asthma are especially vulnerable to the toxic effects of nitrogen dioxide, as are the most active players, who have the highest minute ventilation.[1-3] A 1994 survey[4] found risky levels of nitrogen dioxide in 10% of 70 northeastern U.S. ice-skating rinks. In indoor rinks, ice-resurfacing machines should use electricity.

E.R. Eichner, M.D.

References

1. 1990 YEAR BOOK OF SPORTS MEDICINE, pp 148–149.
2. 1992 YEAR BOOK OF SPORTS MEDICINE, pp 163–164.
3. 1994 YEAR BOOK OF SPORTS MEDICINE, pp 415–417.
4. Brauer M, Spengler JD: Nitrogen dioxide exposures inside ice skating rinks. *Am J Public Health* 84:429–433, 1994.

Validity of Self-report in Identifying Anabolic Steroid Use Among Weightlifters

Ferenchick GS (Michigan State Univ, East Lansing)
J Gen Intern Med 11:554–556, 1996   6–19

Background.—Most of the original data on the physical and psychological effects of anabolic steroids have relied on self-reporting to identify users. However, the validity of self-reporting in this setting has not been established. The sensitivity and specificity of self-reporting in identifying users of anabolic steroids were investigated.

Methods.—Forty-eight weightlifters participated in the study. Self-report findings were compared with assay results of simultaneous urine samples.

Findings.—Self-reports had a sensitivity and specificity of 74% and 82%, respectively, in detecting urinary anabolic steroids. Twenty-two of the 23 participants who reported current anabolic steroid use also had at least 1 undeclared steroid in their urine. Fifteen participants said they had taken at least 1 drug that was not found in urine. In addition, 3 of the 17 subjects who said they were not users were found to have steroids in the urine (Table 1).

Conclusion.—The validity of self-reporting in identifying steroid users appears to be low. Thus, urine assays should be used in future research to determine which subjects are anabolic steroid users.

▶ Because of the ethical problems associated with the experimental administration of anabolic steroids, sports physicians have often tended to make comparisons between self-reported users and nonusers of these drugs. However, as with any health practice that is not socially sanctioned, the information provided by the patient can often be quite misleading. The study of Ferenchick illustrates that not only is there much underreporting of steroid use, users may be taking drugs other than, or in addition to, the ones they report. It then becomes very hard to draw conclusions from comparisons between supposed users and nonusers. A more valid tactic may be to make comparisons on the same subject during and between bouts of steroid use.

R.J. Shephard, M.D., Ph.D., D.P.E.

TABLE 1.—Frequency of Nonreported Drugs in Urine Assays

Drug	No. of Samples*
Nandrolone decanoate	14
Methandienone	6
Oxymetholone	3
Methyltestosterone	3
Methenolone	1

*23 samples total (some samples had more than 1 undeclared drug in the urine).
(Courtesy of Ferenchick GS: Validity of self-report in identifying anabolic steroid use among weightlifters. *J Gen Intern Med* 11:554–556, 1996, reprinted by permission of Blackwell Science, Inc.)

Plasma and Urinary Markers of Oral Testosterone Misuse by Healthy Men in Presence of Masking Epitestosterone Administration
Dehennin L, Pérès G (Fondation de Recherche en Hormonologie, Fresnes, France; Hôpital de la Pitié, Paris)
Int J Sports Med 17:315–319, 1996   6–20

Background.—The official criterion of testosterone abuse in sports is a urinary concentration ratio of testosterone glucuronide/epitestosterone glucuronide (TG/EG) of greater than 6. Complementary markers are needed to back up this criterion, especially when TG/EG is physiologically high or when joint testosterone and epitestosterone use is suspected. A search for complementary markers was undertaken.

Methods and Findings.—Seven healthy men aged 21 to 49 years volunteered for the study. All were involved in regular recreational sports activities. After a single oral dose of undecanoates of testosterone and epitestosterone (40 mg and 1.5 mg, respectively), isotope dilution–gas chromatography–mass spectrometry in plasma and urine was performed to assess testosterone, epitestosterone, and their glucuroconjugates and sulfoconjugates, 5-androstene-3β,17α-diol flucuronide, and 17-hydroxyprogesterone. The ratios of testosterone glucuronide/17-hydroxyprogesterone and testosterone glucuronide/testosterone were adequate plasma criteria for testosterone abuse. These ratios increased significantly, exceeding baseline values for up to 10 hours. This trend was also observed for the ratio of urinary glucuronides of testosterone/5-androstene-3β,17α-diol. Simultaneous administration of epitestosterone did not affect TG/EG. In one man with low basal TG/EG, none of these values responded significantly to testosterone administration (Fig 2).

Conclusion.—Even when urinary TG/EG is counteracted by epitestosterone administration, the plasma levels of testosterone glucuronide relative to unconjugated testosterone or 17-hydroxyprogesterone and the urinary concentration of testosterone glucuronide relative to 5-androstene-3β,17α-diol glucuronide may indicate oral testosterone misuse. These findings now need to be confirmed in a much larger population of athletes.

▶ Attempts to show doping by the illegal administration of androgens become ever more sophisticated as athletes adopt new ruses to avoid detection. A testosterone/epitestosterone ratio of 6 is widely accepted as providing a basis for identifying the administration of exogenous testosterone,[1] but the ratio may prove fallible if testosterone and epitestosterone are administered simultaneously. Dehennin and Pérès here identify some additional ratios that subsequent trials may show to be useful in the evaluation of doubtful cases.

R.J. Shephard, M.D., Ph.D., D.P.E.

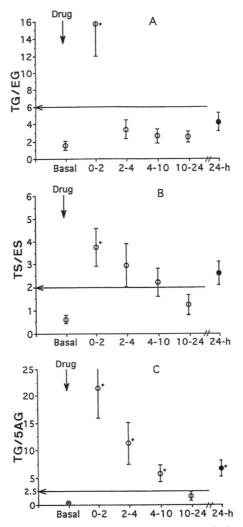

FIGURE 2.—Time course of urinary concentration ratios (mean ± standard error of the mean, N = 6) of testosterone glucuronides to epitestosterone glucuronides (*TG/EG*) (**A**), testosterone sulfates to epitestosterone (*TS/ES*) (**B**), and testosterone glucuronides to 5-androstene-3β,17α-diol (*TG/5AG*) (**C**), after oral administration of undecanoates of testosterone and epitestosterone (*Drug*) at time zero. Time intervals are in hours and 24-hour values. (*closed circles*) are concentration ratios found in the corresponding 24-hour urine collection. Basal ratios were not significantly different from each other. *Asterisk* indicates $P < 0.05$ compared with threshold values, respectively TG/EG = 6, TS/ES = 2 and TG/5AG = 2.5. For the latter 2 ratios, threshold values are yet tentative. (Dehennin L: On the origin of physiologically high ratios of testosterone to epitestosterone: Consequences for reliable detection of testosterone administration by male athletes. *J Endocrinol* 140:353–360, 1994.) (Courtesy of Dehennin L, Pérès G: Plasma and urinary markers of oral testosterone misuse by healthy men in presence of masking epitestosterone administration. *Int J Sports Med* 17:315–319, 1996.)

Reference

1. Donike M, Bärwald KR, Klostermann K, et al: Nachweis von exogenem Testosteron, in Heck H, Hollmann W, Liesen H, et al (eds): *Sport, Leistung und Gesundheit.* Köln, Deutscher Arzte-Verlag, 1983, pp 293–300.

Body Composition, Cardiovascular Risk Factors and Liver Function in Long Term Androgenic-Anabolic Steroids Using Bodybuilders Three Months After Drug Withdrawal

Hartgens F, Kuipers H, Wijnen JAG, et al (Netherlands Centre for Doping Affairs, Rotterdam; Univ of Limburg, Maastricht, The Netherlands)
Int J Sports Med 17:429–433, 1996   6–21

Purpose.—Many bodybuilders take androgenic-anabolic steroids (AAS) in an attempt to increase muscle mass. Many users of these drugs believe that taking AAS in cycles can enhance muscle mass while minimizing side effects. The effects of long-term AAS use on body composition, cardiovascular risk factors, and liver function were studied in bodybuilders who had stopped taking AAS 3 months previously.

Methods.—Two groups of experienced male bodybuilders were studied: 16 had used AAS in the past but not in the previous 3 months, and 12 had never used AAS. The 2 groups were compared as to anthropometric, muscle biopsy, blood pressure, and blood chemistry measurements.

Results.—The AAS and control groups were similar in terms of age, height, training regimen, nutrition, skinfold thicknesses, percentage fat, and fat mass. However, bodybuilders who had used steroids had heavier body mass and lean-body-mass measurements. They also had larger chests, waists, upper arms, and thighs than the control athletes. On muscle biopsy, type I muscle fibers were larger in diameter. All cholesterol, triglyceride,

TABLE 5.—Blood Pressure, Serum Lipoproteins, and Liver Enzymes in Bodybuilders With and Without Previous Androgenic-Anabolic Steroid Use

	AAS group	CO group	Reference values
Systolic blood pressure (mmHg)	127.8 ± 11.1	125.8 ± 13.8	<140
Diastolic blood pressure (mmHg)	78.9 ± 8.7	75.2 ± 12.2	< 90
Total cholesterol (mmol/l)	4.94 ± 0.91	4.69 ± 0.98	4.1–6.4
HDL-cholesterol (mmol/l)	1.02 ± 0.35	1.05 ± 0.23	0.6–1.9
Triglycerides (mmol/l)	1.28 ± 0.51	1.18 ± 0.60	0.80–1.94
Alkaline phosphatase (U/l)	58.3 ± 13.1	85.9 ± 19.7*	30–125
Gamma GT (U/l)	16.7 ± 9.3	21.1 ± 7.5	< 50

Note: Values are mean ± standard deviation.
Asterisk indicates $P < 0.05$.
Abbreviations: AAS, androgenic-anabolic steroids; *CO*, control; *HDL*, high-density lipoprotein; *GT*, glutamyl transpeptidase.
(Courtesy of Hartgens F, Kuipers H, Wijnen JAG, et al: Body composition, cardiovascular risk factors and liver function in long term androgenic-anabolic steroids using bodybuilders three months after drug withdrawal. *Int J Sports Med* 17:429–433, 1996.)

and blood pressure values were comparable between groups. Liver function tests—alkaline phosphatase and (γ)-glutamyl transpeptidase—were not significantly different (Table 5). However, alkaline phosphatase was higher in the control group.

Conclusion.—Even 3 months after drug withdrawal, long-term AAS use increases body mass, lean body mass, body circumferences, and muscle fiber type I diameters in bodybuilders. At the same time, there are no significant abnormalities in fat mass, blood pressure, blood lipoproteins, or liver enzymes.

▶ It is important that this paper not be misinterpreted! Some years ago, we documented the adverse effects of heavy steroid use on the liver.[1] Hartgens et al. argue that because values fall within the very broadly stated "normal" limits of the clinical laboratory after 3 months of abstinence from steroids, no harm has resulted. However, the clinical norms have a wide range to allow interpretation of single observations on a single patient. It is hard to "laugh off" group norms for alkaline phosphatase levels that still remain only 68% of those of controls after 3 months of abstinence from steroids.

R.J. Shephard, M.D., Ph.D., D.P.E.

Reference

1. Shephard RJ, Killinger D, Fried T: *Br J Sports Med* 11:170–173, 1977.

The Effects of Supraphysiologic Doses of Testosterone on Muscle Size and Strength in Normal Men

Bhasin S, Storer TW, Berman N, et al (Charles R Drew Univ of Medicine and Science, Los Angeles; El Camino College, Torrance, Calif; Harbor–Univ of California Med Ctr, Torrance, Calif; et al)
N Engl J Med 335:1–7, 1996   6–22

Background.—Although athletes often take androgenic steroids to increase their strength, the efficacy of this practice has not been substantiated. The value of supraphysiologic doses of testosterone, alone or combined with a standardized program of strength training, in increasing fat-free mass and muscle size and strength in normal men was studied.

Methods.—Forty-three men were assigned randomly to placebo with no exercise, testosterone with no exercise, placebo plus exercise, or testosterone plus exercise. Testosterone enanthate, 600 mg, or placebo was injected weekly for 10 weeks. Exercise involved standardized weight lifting 3 times a week.

Findings.—Among men not exercising, muscle size in the arms and legs was greater in those receiving testosterone than in those receiving placebo. The men given testosterone also had greater increases in strength in the bench press and squatting exercises. Men in the testosterone plus exercise group had greater increases in fat-free mass and muscle size than men in

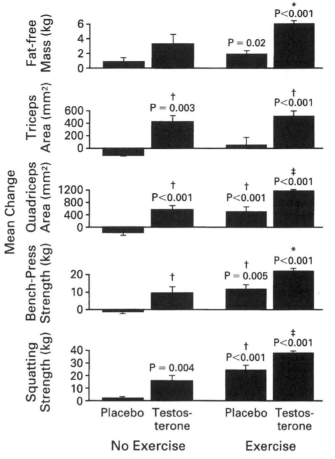

FIGURE 1.—Changes from baseline in mean (±standard error) fat-free mass, triceps, and quadriceps cross-sectional areas, and muscle strength in the bench press and squatting exercises over 10 weeks of treatment. The P values shown are for the comparison between the change indicated and a change of zero. The *asterisks* indicate $P < 0.05$ for the comparison between the change indicated and that in either no-exercise group. The *daggers* indicate $P < 0.05$ for the comparison between the change indicated and that in the group assigned to placebo with no exercise; and the *double daggers* indicate $P < 0.05$ for the comparison between the changes indicated and the changes in all 3 other groups. (Reprinted by permission of *The New England Journal of Med* from Bhasin S, Storer TW, Berman N, et al: The effects of supraphysiologic doses of testosterone on muscle size and strength in normal men. *N Engl J Med* 335:1–7, copyright 1996, Massachusetts Medical Society.)

either no-exercise group. Muscle strength increases were also greater in men exercising and taking testosterone than in either no-exercise group. No mood or behavior changes occurred in any group (Fig 1).

Conclusion.—Supraphysiologic doses of testosterone, especially when combined with strength training, increase fat-free mass, muscle size, and strength in normal men. Although the use of anabolic-androgenic steroids to increase athletic performance is not justified, short-term androgen administration may be beneficial in immobilized patients, during space travel and in patients with cancer-related cachexia, HIV disease, or other chronic wasting disorders.

▶ Physicians are increasingly taught to practice "evidence-based medicine," preferably looking at randomized, controlled trials before drawing conclusions as to an appropriate treatment. However, for ethical reasons, studies of anabolic steroids have usually relied on comparisons between self-selected abusers and drug-free athletes, with a strong possibility of biased results. There is somewhat less ethical objection to administration of massive doses of naturally occurring hormone. Now a small-scale, randomized trial has shown rather conclusively that testosterone alone augments both strength and lean mass, although gains are rather smaller than could have been obtained by strength training. Perhaps more importantly, the combination of testosterone and strength training leads to a large increase in both lean mass and strength.

R.J. Shephard, M.D., Ph.D., D.P.E.

Serious Cardiovascular Side Effects of Large Doses of Anabolic Steroids in Weight Lifters
Nieminen MS, Rämö MP, Viitasalo M, et al (Helsinki Univ; Central Military Hosp, Helsinki)
Eur Heart J 17:1576–1583, 1996   6–23

Introduction.—Anabolic steroids have been shown to increase, ventricular wall thickness, end-diastolic volume, and left ventricular mass and significantly prolong isovolumetric relaxation time in weight lifters. Anabolic steroids are considered atherogenic and have been linked to arterial occlusion in several reports. The pathologic cardiovascular manifestations in 4 young men who used high doses of anabolic steroids for several years in combination with weight training were presented.

Methods.—Patients were referred for evaluation for the following reasons: patient 1 had a long history of massive anabolic steroid use; patient 2 experienced a ventricular fibrillation during exercise; patient 3 had clinically manifest heart failure; and patient 4 had an arterial thrombus in the lower left leg. Ages ranged from 27 to 33 years. All patients gave a history, and underwent physical examination and cardiovascular evaluation.

Results.—All 4 patients had cardiac hypertrophy. Two patients who underwent endomyocardial biopsy had diffuse myocardial fibrosis. Patients 3 and 4 had signs of heart failure, patient 2 had impairment of coronary flow, and patient 3 had impairment of perfusion. A large lobular intraventricular thrombus was observed in both the left and right ventricles of patient 4 during echocardiography. Two patients had improved left ventricular function after cessation of anabolic steroids. Despite warnings, both patients restarted use of anabolic steroids.

Conclusion.—Two of the 4 weight lifters using anabolic steroids had potentially lethal side effects: malignant ventricular arrhythmia in 1 and massive intracardial thrombosis in the other. All 4 men had cardiac hypertrophy. All physicians and athletes should be warned about the serious risks involved in continuous use of large doses of anabolic steroids.

▶ Although we often think of anabolic steroids as acting only upon skeletal muscle, they also affect the heart, causing ventricular hypertrophy and depressed myocardial contractility.[1] Given also a high protein/fat diet, the stage is set for the development of a variety of cardiac disorders, as illustrated by the 4 cases presented by Nieminen et al.

R.J. Shephard, M.D., Ph.D., D.P.E.

Reference

1. Rämö P. Anabolic steroids alter the hemodynamic response of the canine left ventricle. *Acta Physiol Scand* 133:297–306, 1988.

Severe Ketoacidosis Complicated by 'Ecstasy' Ingestion and Prolonged Exercise
Seymour HR, Gilman D, Quin JD (Royal Sussex County Hosp, Brighton, England)
Diabetic Med 13:908–909, 1996   6–24

Background.—3,4-Methylenedioxymethamphetamine (MDMA, or Ecstasy) is a synthetic amphetamine derivative patented as an appetite suppressant more than 80 years ago. In the 1980s, MDMA—with its mild amphetamine-like stimulant effect associated with a happy relaxed state, mild euphoria, and low hallucinogenic potential—became a drug of misuse. Young adults tend to view MDMA as a safe recreational drug. The cases of 2 patients with insulin-dependent diabetes mellitus in whom life-threatening metabolic decompensation developed after prolonged dancing combined with MDMA use were described.

Patients.—The patients were 2 females with ketoacidosis after several hours of dancing. Both had long histories of insulin-dependent diabetes mellitus. The first patient, a 19-year-old, had a 12-hour history of vomiting and had not taken insulin for 24 hours before hospital admission. This patient was profoundly dehydrated and markedly ketotic. After 10 days of intensive therapy, she admitted to having used MDMA. The second patient, a 15-year-old, had also omitted insulin and was found to be in a state of profound dehydration and marked ketonuria. She responded promptly to treatment and eventually admitted MDMA use. Both patients recovered and remain well.

Conclusion.—Most deaths related to MDMA use are thought to be caused by hyperthermia, possibly mediated by serotonergic mechanisms. Prolonged exercise, such as dancing, may compound this effect, causing further dehydration and hyperthermia, especially in the presence of high ambient temperatures and inadequate fluid replacement. Increased educational efforts are needed to correct the misconception that MDMA is safe.

▶ These 2 young women with diabetes danced all night in an Ecstasy-fueled environment and paid the price. Ecstasy is a "designer" recreational drug, a mild amphetamine that has been touted as "safer than alcohol." It has been linked, however, to toxicity and/or death resulting from malignant hyperpyrexia, seizures, acute hepatitis, hypertension, arrhythmia, and/or exertional rhabdomyolysis and acute renal failure from "the dance of death."[1] As was the case with these 2 women, it also can lead to hyponatremia (and cerebral edema) from excessive consumption of water, perhaps to offset the heat generated by the drug and the all-night dancing in the "hot" ambience. These 2 women also neglected to take their insulin for 12 and 24 hours, respectively, which contributed to life-threatening ketoacidosis. Fortunately, they survived.

E.R. Eichner, M.D.

Reference

1. Henry JA: Ecstasy and the dance of death. *BMJ* 302:5–6, 1992.

Smoking Increases Conversion of Lactate to Glucose During Submaximal Exercise

Huie MJ, Casazza GA, Horning MA, et al (Univ of California, Berkeley)
J Appl Physiol 80:1554–1559, 1996   6–25

Background.—Previous research has shown that cigarette smoking changes whole body metabolism. Smokers have been found to have significantly greater glucose rates of appearance, disappearance, and oxidation during submaximal exercise and to reach significantly higher plasma lactate levels when they smoked before taking exercise. The effects of cigarette smoking on lactate kinetics during submaximal exercise were investigated.

Methods.—Seven male smokers and 7 nonsmokers were included in the study. A primed continuous infusion of [3-^{13}C] lactate was administered during 90 minutes of rest and 60 minutes of exercise on a cycle ergometer at 50% peak O_2 intake. The smokers were studied once after abstaining from smoking overnight and once after smoking 3 cigarettes before exercise.

Findings.—In all groups, the rates of lactate appearance and conversion to glucose were increased markedly during exercise compared with rest. When the smokers had smoked before exercise, they showed a significantly greater rate of lactate appearance than the nonsmokers and from the smokers after abstaining from smoking. The rate of lactate conversion to

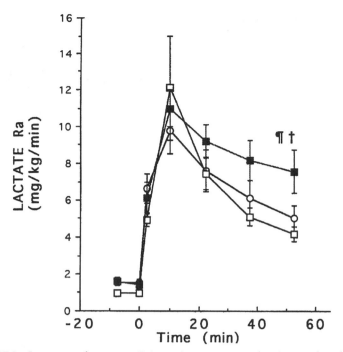

FIGURE 2.—Lactate rate of appearance (Ra) over time among nonsmokers (*open circle circle*), chronic smokers (*open square*), and acute smokers (*solid square*). *Paragraph mark* indicates significant difference from nonsmokers, $P < 0.05$. *Dagger* indicates significant difference from chronic smokers, $P < 0.05$. (Courtesy of Huie MJ, Casazza GA, Horning MA, et al: Smoking increases conversion of lactate to glucose during submaximal exercise. *J Appl Physiol* 80:1554–1559, 1996.)

glucose was similar during exercise after smoking and after abstinence in the smokers. In nonsmokers, this rate was significantly lower (Fig 2).

Conclusion.—Acute smoking increases lactate flux during exercise. Smokers have a higher rate of lactate-to-glucose conversion than non-smokers during exercise, which may indicate an increase in glucose dependence.

▶ A surprisingly large proportion of both the general population and certain classes of athletes still smoke, despite the long catalogue of ill effects from this addiction. Here, Huie and associates show that the rate of lactate appearance during exercise is greater in smokers than in nonsmokers. They suggest that this reflects an increased dependence on glucose as a source of fuel, one more factor that would impair endurance performance in the smoker.

Perhaps the most striking feature of the authors data is not the early peak of lactate appearance (which is similar for smokers and nonsmokers) but rather the continuing appearance of lactate in the smokers as the 60-minute period of exercise continued. It could be that the peripheral vascular effects of smoking are preventing the circulatory adjustments that are evidenced in the nonsmokers by a decreasing rate of lactate production. If so, the circulatory effects are acute in nature, as they are reversed by a night of abstinence from cigarettes.

R.J. Shephard, M.D., Ph.D., D.P.E.

7 Diet, Metabolism, Hormones, and Bone Density

Influence of Sleep and Meal Schedules on Performance Peaks in Competitive Sprinters
Javierre C, Calvo M, Díez A, et al (Esplugues de Llobregat, Barcelona; Universidad de Barcelona; Universitària de Bellvitge, Barcelona)
Int J Sports Med 17:404–408, 1996   7–1

Objective.—Human circadian rhythms are well documented, yet their implications for athletic performance are largely unknown. The available evidence suggests important links between exercise and circadian rhythm, some of which are modifiable by training. The impact of different sleep and meal schedules on athletic performance was studied in runners.

Methods.—The study included 8 nationally competitive short-distance runners (mean age, 21 years). Their performance in the 80-m sprint was measured several times throughout the day on 5 consecutive Saturdays. Days 1 and 4 were control days. Sleep/wake cycles and meal times were advanced for 2 hours on day 2 and delayed for 2 hours on day 3. The sleep/wake cycle was advanced for 2 hours on day 5, but meal times were the same as on control days. The effects of these changes on running performance were analyzed.

Results.—On the control days, performance increased gradually throughout the morning until 1 PM, followed by a decline at 3 PM, and then an additional improvement. The runners' best performance came at 7 PM on these days. Performance peaked at 5 PM on day 2—when sleep/wake cycles and meal times were advanced—and at 9 PM on day 3—when timetables were delayed. On both days 2 and 3, a significant improvement was noted at the time of maximum peak performance (Fig 2). On day 5—when the sleep/wake cycle was altered but meal times were not—performance was comparable to the control days.

Conclusion.—Sprinters show significant differences in athletic performance at different times during the day. The results suggest that athletes' schedules could be easily manipulated to synchronize peak performance

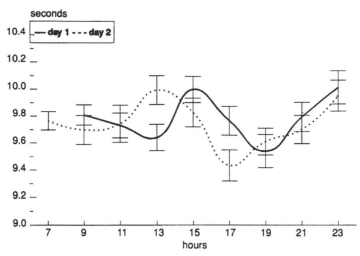

FIGURE 2.—Times registered for the 80-m race on the control day (*continuous line*) and day 2 (*dashed*). Significant improvement from 2.7% to 4.1% in performance was observed in the times registered at 5 PM as compared with the control day (*P* < 0.01). Values presented are mean ± standard error. (Courtesy of Javierre C, Calvo M, Díez, et al: Influence of sleep and meal schedules on performance peaks in competitive sprinters. *Int J Sports Med* 17:404–408, 1996.)

times with the times of competitions. Sprinting performance is better in the evening than in the morning.

▶ Performance in most types of athletic events shows an appreciable circadian rhythm. Thus, it makes sense for coaches to determine the timing of this variation in their particular charges and to manipulate the rhythm so that a competitor races when he or she is at peak form. In the example given by Javierre and co-workers, 80-m times show a 3% to 4% variation over the course of a normal day. Plainly, circadian rhythms are a major determinant of competitive standing.

R.J. Shepard, M.D., Ph.D., D.P.E.

Effect of Fluid Ingestion on Muscle Metabolism During Prolonged Exercise
Hargreaves M, Dillo P, Angus D, et al (Univ of Melbourne, Australia; Royal Melbourne Inst of Technology, Australia)
J Appl Physiol 80:363–366, 1996   7–2

Introduction.—Fluid ingestion during prolonged exercise has been shown to attenuate exercise-induced increases in heart rate and core temperature, to decrease stroke volume and cardiac output, and to improve exercise performance. An increase in glycogen utilization associated with increases in rectal and muscle temperatures and elevated plasma epinephrine levels has been observed during exercise in the heat. There are possible metabolic consequences when dehydration and hyperthermia develop subsequent to prolonged exercise without fluid replacement. The effect of fluid ingestion on muscle metabolism during prolonged exercise was evaluated.

Methods.—Five physically fit men underwent 2 trials of prolonged cycling exercise at 67 peak oxygen uptake at 20–22°C; in 1 trial they ingested no fluid (NF) and in the other they ingested a volume of distilled deionized water that prevented loss of body mass (FR). During both trials, they underwent needle biopsy from the vastus lateralis muscle; monitoring of rectal and muscle temperatures; venous blood sampling at 20, 60, 90, and 120 minutes via forearm catheter; and expired gas analysis during exercise.

Results.—Fluid ingestion prevented dehydration during prolonged exercise. There was no between-trial difference in oxygen uptake at any point of measurement. Heart rate was significantly higher during NF than FR. The respiratory exchange ratio was significantly higher during NF than FR at 60 and 120 minutes of exercise. The rectal and muscle temperatures were similar at rest for both trials. At 120 minutes of exercise, both temperatures were significantly higher in NF, compared to FR. There were no between-trial differences in rectal temperature at any other time point during exercise. Plasma glucose levels were similar at rest and during exercise for both trials. Plasma lactate was significantly higher after 30 and 120 minutes of exercise in NF, compared to FR. There were no between-trial differences in plasma epinephrine levels at rest or at 60 and 120 minutes of exercise. Plasma norepinephrine levels were similar at rest and after 60 minutes of exercise, but were significantly higher in NF, compared

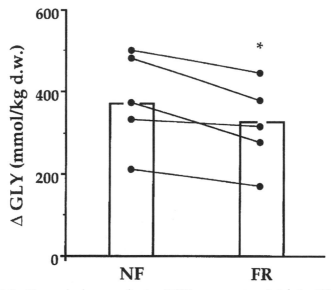

FIGURE 2.—Net muscle glycogen utilization (ΔGLY; pre- to postexercise) during 120 minutes of exercise at 67% peak 0_2 uptake FR and NF. *Abbreviations:* FR, with fluid ingestion; NF, without fluid ingestion. Mean (*open bars*) and individual data (*filled circles*) are plotted; *n* = 5 men. *Significantly different mean values from NF, *P* < 0.05. (Courtesy of Hargreaves M, Dillo P, Angus D, et al: Effect of fluid ingestion on muscle metabolism during prolonged exercise. *J Appl Physiol* 80:363–366, 1996.)

to FR at 120 minutes. Muscle adenosine triphosphate, creatine phosphate, and creatine levels were similar before and after exercise for both NF and FR. There were no between-trial differences in muscle lactate or glycogen concentrations at rest. At 120 minutes, muscle lactate was significantly lower and muscle glycogen was significantly higher in FR, compared to NF. The net muscle glycogen utilization during exercise was 16% lower with fluid ingestion, compared to no fluid ingestion (Fig 2).

Conclusion.—Fluid ingestion during prolonged exercise decreased muscle glycogen use. This may explain why fluid ingestion enchances performance during prolonged exercise.

▶ This paper reminds us of the delicate interplay between the circulation and muscle metabolism. If fluid depletion impairs muscle perfusion, the tissue becomes hypoxic, and glycogen is metabolized rather than fat. Fluid replenishment thus not only helps heat dissipation but also conserves glycogen over a prolonged run.

R.J. Shephard, M.D., Ph.D., D.P.E.

Muscle Protein Metabolism in Female Swimmers After a Combination of Resistance and Endurance Exercise
Tipton KD, Ferrando AA, Williams BD, et al (Univ of Texas, Galveston; Shriners Burns Inst, Galveston, Tex)
J Appl Physio 81:2034–2038, 1996   7–3

Introduction.—Most competitive swimmers use combined endurance and resistance training in their workouts. The response of protein synthesis (PS) or protein degradation to this training combination is not known. The acute effects of combined swimming and resistance training on protein metabolism in 7 collegiate female swimmers was quantified via direct measurement of muscle PS and whole-bone protein breakdown (WBPB).

Methods.—With a primed constant infusion of ring-$[^{13}C_6]$phenylalanine to measure the fractional synthetic rate (FSR) of the posterior deltoid and WBPB, study participants were evaluated 4 times: at rest, after a swimming workout (SW), after a resistance exercise workout with no swimming on that day (RW), and after swimming and resistance exercise combined (SR). Serum blood and muscle biopsy specimens were obtained, and patients completed 3-day diet diaries.

Results.—There were no significant between-group differences in WBPB. The FSR of the posterior deltoid was significantly increased by 81% after SR, compared to rest (Fig 3). After SW and rest, respectively, the FSR values were 35% and 41% greater, but there were no significant differences in their means. The FSR was 30% higher after SR than after SW and 73% higher than after RW, but the differences were not significant.

Conclusion.—It is not known why resistance exercise or swimming did not have a significant effect on muscle FSR in this cohort of 7 female

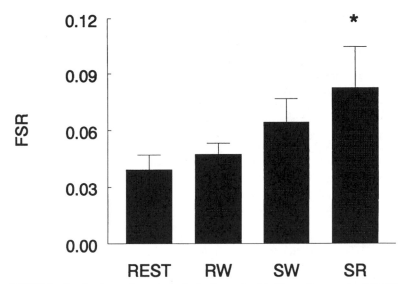

FIGURE 3.—Fractional rate of protein synthesis of posterior deltoid muscle at rest after RW, SW, and SR in 7 female swimmers. Values are means ± SE in percent per hour. *Significantly different from rest, $P < 0.05$. *Abbreviations*: RW, resistance workout; SW, swimming workout; SR, swimming and resistance workout combined; FSR, fractional rate of protein synthesis. (Courtesy of Tipton KD, Ferrando AA, Williams BD, et al: Muscle protein metabolism in female swimmers after a combination of resistance and endurance exercise. *J Appl Physiol* 81:2034–2038, 1996.)

collegiate swimmers. Findings suggest that muscle PS is increased by resistance exercise in female athletes participating in intense interval swimming.

▶ The results of this study should be interpreted strictly according to the specific purpose of the study. Does adding resistance training to swimming workouts increase PS? The effect of resistance training or swimming per se on PS cannot be determined because, as the authors point out, the total work performed in the 3 exercise sessions differed. The suggestion that gender differences might explain the lack of response to resistance training or swimming may be true, but a sample size of 7 may also account for the lack of a significant difference. Not to report the power of a statistical test when the sample size is small is a disservice to the reader.

B.L. Drinkwater, Ph.D.

Simultaneous Determination of Gastric Emptying and Intestinal Absorption During Cycle Exercise in Humans
Lambert GP, Chang RT, Joensen D, et al (Univ of Iowa, Iowa City)
Int J Sports Med 17:48–55, 1996   7–4

Introduction.—Fluid homeostasis is affected by gastric emptying rate and intestinal absorption. Although gastric emptying during exercise has been extensively tested, few studies have been conducted to measure the intestinal absorption of fluid while exercising. Intestinal absorption of a fluid that is ingested orally may not be represented by fluid absorption values derived from intestinal perfusion. Intestinal absorption was measured after oral ingestion of a beverage, with the simultaneous determination of gastric emptying during exercise.

Methods.—Under fluoroscopic guidance, 7 males positioned a nasogastric tube in the gastric antrum and a multilumen tube in the duodenum. During 85 minutes of cycle exercise at 60.6 ± 3.7% of maximum oxygen intake (x ± standard error) in a 22° environment, gastric emptying and intestinal water flux were measured. A 6% isotonic carbohydrate-electrolyte solution was ingested to equal a total of 23 mL/kg of body mass. Five minutes before exercise, the subjects drank 396 ± 34 mL. Every 10 minutes during exercise, they drank a further 198 ± 17 mL.

Results.—After the initial 35-minute equilibration period, mean stomach volume (312 ± 80 mL) and gastric emptying rate (19.7 ± 2.0 mL/min) did not change significantly. The mean intestinal water flux during perfusion of the solution directly into the duodenum (16.4 ± 1.9 mL/cm per hour) did not differ significantly from the mean intestinal water flux seen during oral ingestion of the solution (19.5 ± 2.6 mL/cm per hour) (Fig 4). There was little difference in total solute flux between drinking and infusion. There was no change in urine production between drinking and perfusion immediately following exercise.

Conclusion.—Over a prolonged period, relatively constant stomach volumes can be maintained and can produce relatively constant gastric emp-

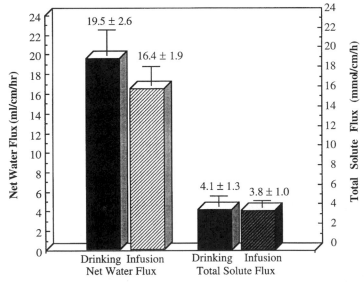

FIGURE 4.—Water and total solute flux in the duodenum under the 2 experimental conditions. (Courtesy of Lambert GP, Chang RT, Joensen D, et al: Simultaneous determination of gastric emptying and intestinal absorption during cycle exercise in humans. *Int J Sports Med* 17:48–55, 1996.)

tying rates. A modified segmental perfusion technique using ingestion rather than intestinal perfusion can accurately determine intestinal absorption of an isotonic carbohydrate-electrolyte beverage.

▶ Early studies of water balance during endurance exercise measured net changes in body mass after allowing for other forms of water exchange, such as sweating. However, critical variables from the viewpoint of maintaining tissue hydration are the bound water that is released by metabolism of glycogen (a fluid reserve of about 1.5 L[1]) and the intestinal flux of water. Investigators are measuring the latter with increasing frequency, typically by the infusion of fluid into a segment of the duodenum.

As Lambert and associates point out, this is not quite the same thing as drinking from a paper cup during a marathon. Nevertheless, the data for duodenal infusion and oral ingestion do not seem to differ significantly, provided that the rate of gastric emptying is comparable to the rate of duodenal infusion.

R.J. Shephard, M.D., Ph.D., D.P.E.

Reference

1. Kavanagh T, Shephard RJ: On the choice of fluid for the hydration of middle-aged marathon runners. *Br J Sports Med* 11: 26–35, 1977.

Gastrointestinal Permeability Following Aspirin Intake and Prolonged Running
Ryan AJ, Chang R-T, Gisolfi CV (Univ of Iowa, Iowa City)
Med Sci Sports Exerc 28:698–705, 1996   7–5

Background.—One important function of the gastrointestinal (GI) tract is to serve as a barrier against noxious substances. In conditions of severe stress, the GI barrier can break down and allow such substances to enter the body. A high incidence of GI disorders has been associated with long-distance running. The effects of exercise and aspirin on gastroduodenal and intestinal permeability were investigated.

Methods.—Seven volunteers aged a mean of 29 years were studied while resting and performing treadmill exercise. The subjects took 1.3 g of aspirin or placebo the night before and just before resting or exercising. A permeability test solution containing 10 g of lactulose, 5 g of mannitol, and 10 g of sucrose was given before resting or exercising. Intestinal permeability (lactulose/mannitol [L/M] ratio) or gastroduodenal permeability was quantified by urinary excretion rates, expressed as a percentage of ingested dose.

Findings.—Taking aspirin before running increased intestinal permeability compared with placebo in the running and resting conditions but not compared with aspirin in the resting condition. The mean values for the L/M ratio were 0.248, 0.029, 0.012, and 0.104, respectively. Gastroduodenal permeability after aspirin in the running condition was also increased compared with placebo in the running and resting conditions but not compared with aspirin in the resting condition. Gastrointestinal complaints were not associated with running or aspirin ingestion (Fig 2).

Conclusion.—Gastrointestinal permeability during running can be increased substantially by aspirin ingestion without causing subjective feel-

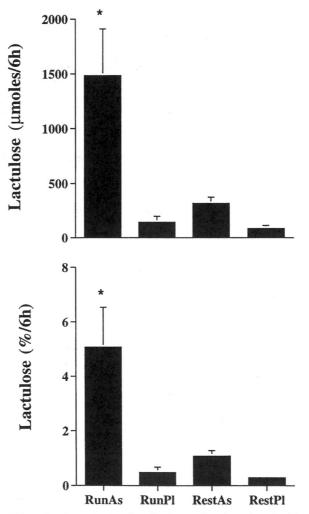

FIGURE 2.—Urinary lactulose excretion after 60 minutes of moderate-intensity (about 68% maximum oxygen consumption) treadmill running or rest, conducted with ingestion of unbuffered aspirin (2 × 1.3 g) or placebo (glucose tablets). Lactulose, a larger molecule, is almost totally excluded from the circulation under normal states, but it can permeate paracellular pathways (tight junctions) when the intestinal barrier is compromised (Travis S, Menzies I: Intestinal permeability: Functional assessment and significance. *Clin Sci* 82:471–488, 1992). Urinary lactulose excretion was greater ($P < 0.05$) after running with aspirin compared with all other conditions. Conditions were run, rest, aspirin (*As*), and placebo (*Pl*). Values are mean ± standard error (n = 7/condition). (Courtesy of Ryan AJ, Chang R-T, Gisolfi CV: Gastrointestinal permeability following aspirin intake and prolonged running. *Med Sci Sports Exerc* 28(6): 698–705, 1996.)

ings of GI distress. Nonsteroidal anti-inflammatory drug use during exercise has been associated with the occurrence of GI bleeding, food- related exercise-induced anaphylaxis, hyponatremia, and endotoxemia. The role of changes in GI barrier function in the pathogenesis of these disorders requires further study.

► Penetration of bacteria through the GI epithelium is an important factor in the development of sepsis. There have been suggestions that visceral ischemia caused by sustained vigorous physical activity can cause such an effect. However, one alternative hypothesis is that bacterial leakage is caused by a large intake of aspirin, as this drug is known to have toxic effects on the GI epithelium.[1]

The permeability of the membrane can be tested experimentally by measuring the urinary excretion of agents such as lactulose, which normally do not traverse the gut wall. Use of this approach enabled Ryan and associates to show that a combination of exercise and aspirin administration did indeed increase the permeability of the gut. Possible mechanisms include an uncoupling of oxidative phosphorylation, an inhibition of prostaglandin synthesis, and mucosal damage.

R.J. Shephard, M.D., Ph.D., D.P.E.

Reference

1. Bjarnason I, Hayllar J, MacPherson AJ, et al: Side effects of nonsteroidal anti-inflammatory drugs on the small and large intestine in humans. *Gastroenterology* 104:1832–1847, 1993.

Association Between Mild, Routine Exercise and Improved Insulin Dynamics and Glucose Control in Obese Adolescents
Kahle EB, Zipf WB, Lamb DR, et al (Ohio State Univ, Columbus; Marshall Univ, Huntington, WVA)
Int J Sports Med 17:1–6, 1996   7–6

Introduction.—Hyperinsulinemia often develops in association with obesity and carries significant health risks in childhood and adolescence. High intensity physical training may be difficult to achieve in obese adolescents, but regular exercise at mild intensity might give the same health-related benefits observed in adults. The association between mild routine exercise and glucose homeostasis, insulin dynamics, and risk factors for coronary artery disease was evaluated in obese adolescent boys.

Methods.—The mean age of 7 obese adolescent boys was 13.3 years. All ranked above the 90th percentile for weight, based on age and height. Participants took part in a 15-week program of supervised exercise conducted 3 days each week at the students' school. Participants were evaluated at baseline and program completion for blood pressure at rest; heart rate and peak oxygen uptake during a maximal graded treadmill exercise test; body composition via hydrostatic weighing; lipid profile; and plasma glucose, insulin, and C-peptide at rest and after a test meal.

Results.—No significant changes were observed from baseline to follow-up in percent body fat or body weight. Changes in the mean values for serum glucose and peptides at follow-up were −15% fasting serum glucose, −15% total serum glucose response, −51% peak insulin response, −46% total insulin response, +55% peak C-peptide response, and +53% total C-peptide response. There was no significant increase in peak oxygen uptake at follow-up, but significant and consistent reductions in systolic blood pressure and levels of low-density lipoprotein cholesterol were observed.

Conclusion.—Fifteen weeks of a mild physical activity program was associated with glucose control and reduced peripheral insulin values but no change in percent body fat or fitness level in obese adolescent boys. The increase in peripheral C-peptide concentrations may be more indicative of increased hepatic extraction of insulin rather than decreased secretion of insulin by the pancreas.

▶ This study of obese adolescent boys shows that thrice weekly calisthenics and games at school can improve glucose control and decrease insulin levels, blood pressure, and low-density lipoprotein cholesterol despite no change in body fatness or fitness. Surely, more exercise would confer even more benefit to these boys, reducing their coronary risk profile. A recent survey of 800 tenth graders found that obese adolescent males tend to ignore their health risks. Only 13% of obese boys were on a diet vs. 62% of obese girls, and obese boys (compared with girls) perceived themselves as less overweight and happier with their looks.[1] Relevant is a 55-year follow-up of 508 Bostonians first studied as adolescents. Chubby adolescent boys, whether or not they lost weight as adults, were twice as likely as their thin cohorts to die prematurely, and most premature deaths were from heart disease.[2]

E.R. Eichner, M.D.

References

1. Steen SN, Wadden TA, Foster GD, et al: Are obese adolescent boys ignoring an important health risk? *Int J Eat Disord* 20:281–286, 1996.
2. Must A, Jacques PF, Dallal GE, et al: Long-term morbidity and mortality of overweight adolescents: A follow-up of the Harvard Growth Study of 1922 to 1935. *N Engl J Med* 327:1350–1355, 1992.

The Negative Association Between Traditional Physical Activities and the Prevalence of Glucose Intolerance in Alaska Natives

Adler AI, Boyko EJ, Schraer CD, et al (Veterans Affairs Med Ctr, Seattle; Alaska Area Native Health Service, Anchorage)
Diabetic Med 13:555–560, 1996   7–7

Background.—The past 3 decades have seen a fourfold increase in the prevalence of non–insulin-dependent (type 2) diabetes mellitus (NIDDM) among Eskimos and Indians. The trend suggests that some nongenetic factor is affecting the prevalence of NIDDM in these groups. As the prevalence of NIDDM has increased, the need for a subsistence lifestyle, and the associated physical activity, have decreased. In other groups, physical activity can prevent NIDDM. The association between physical activity and glucose intolerance was evaluated in a case-control study of Eskimos and Indians.

Methods.—The study included 666 Yup'ik Eskimos and Athabaskan Indians older than 40 years of age. The subjects were drawn from 15 villages in one area of Alaska. They were surveyed regarding participation in various traditional activities, e.g., dog sledding, or their modern equivalents, e.g., riding in a motorized vehicle. Based on the intensity values assigned for each activity, the subjects were classified into low, moderate, and high physical activity groups. The "cases" for the case-control analysis were subjects with either known or newly recognized impairment of glucose tolerance. Subjects with a screening blood glucose value of 6.7 mmol/L or greater on random capillary blood glucose testing were considered newly recognized cases.

Results.—There were 37 cases of NIDDM (26 known and 11 newly recognized) and 18 cases of impairment of glucose tolerance (1 known and 17 newly recognized). The physical activity level varied according to glucose tolerance and ethnicity but not by obesity or sex (Table 1). After adjustment for age, ethnicity, body mass index, and sex, subjects in the

TABLE 1.—Physical Activity Level by Ethnicity, Sex, Body Mass, Age, and Glucose Tolerance Status

	Low activity		Moderate activity		High activity		p value*
Yup'ik Eskimo	179	35.0%	171	33.4%	162	31.6%	<0.001
Athabaskan	72	68.6%	26	24.8%	7	6.7%	
Male	109	39.2%	94	33.8%	75	27.0%	0.77
Female	142	41.9%	103	30.4%	94	27.7%	
Overweight*	109	44.0%	79	31.9%	60	24.2%	0.106
Not overweight	142	38.5%	118	32.0%	109	29.5%	
Glucose intolerance	31	62.0%	15	30.0%	4	8.0%	<0.001‡
Normal glucose tolerance	220	38.8%	182	32.1%	165	29.1%	

*National Center for Health Statistics criteria: for women, > 27.3 kg/m²; for men, > 27.8 kg/m².
†P value represents test for trend with increasing activity for difference between binary column variables.
‡Exact test.
(Courtesy of Adler AI, Boyko EJ, Schraer CD, et al: The negative association between traditional physical activities and the prevalence of glucose intolerance in Alaska natives. *Diabetic Med* 13:555–560, 1996, reprinted by permission of John Wiley & Sons, Ltd.)

moderate and high physical activity groups were significantly less likely to have glucose intolerance. Adjusted odds ratios, compared with the low physical activity group, were 0.7 for moderate physical activity and 0.2 for high physical activity.

Conclusion.—The risk of glucose intolerance among Eskimos and Indians living in Alaska becomes higher as these groups become less reliant on the traditional physical activities associated with a subsistence lifestyle. This negative association between physical activity and glucose intolerance is consistent with the results of previous prospective studies.

▶ Physicians have long regarded obesity, diabetes, and ischemic heart conditions as "diseases of civilization." A striking verification of this concept has occurred in recent years, as indigenous populations in many parts of the world have become acculturated to a sedentary "Western" style of living.[1] This study shows a striking parallel between preservation of a traditional lifestyle and the avoidance of obesity and glucose intolerance. Longitudinal studies conducted in the Inuit community of Igloolik over a 20-year period[1] provide an even more convincing documentation of the same phenomenon.

R.J. Shephard, M.D., Ph.D., D.P.E.

References

1. Rode A, Shephard RJ: The Health Consequences of 'Modernization.' London, Cambridge University Press, 1996.

Changes in Bone Mineral Content in Male Athletes: Mechanisms of Action and Intervention Effects

Klesges RC, Ward KD, Shelton ML, et al (Univ of Memphis, Tenn)
JAMA 276:226–230, 1996   7–8

Introduction.—A moderate level of physical activity leads to increased bone density. However, highly trained, amenorrheic female athletes show decreased bone mineral content (BMC), presumably because of reduced estrogen levels. There is also evidence of reduced BMC in trained male athletes, perhaps caused by calcium imbalance during training. Exercise-related changes in BMC were studied in male athletes, including the potential mechanisms and the effects of intervention.

Methods.—The subjects were 11 players on a Division I-A collegiate basketball team. During a 2-year period, the athletes underwent periodic dual-energy x-ray absorptiometry (DEXA) scans to determine their BMC. Sweat and urine samples were obtained to measure calcium loss during a training period. During the second year of the study, the athletes received calcium supplements, with the dose depending on their amount of calcium loss. Calcium supplementation started the week before training began and continued until the end of postseason play.

Results.—In the first year, the men showed a 4% increase in total body BMC from the preseason to the midseason DEXA scans. A nonsignificant

1% increase occurred during the offseason, but this was followed by another 3% loss during summer practice. The athletes lost an average of 422 mg of calcium per training session. Total BMC decreased by 6% from preseason to late summer, including a 10.5% decrease in BMC of the legs. When calcium supplementation was given in the second year, there were significant increases in BMC and lean body mass. The rate of increase during the second year was comparable to the rate of decrease in the first year.

Conclusions.—Male athletes who train intensively for an extended period may experience significant losses of BMC. Large amounts of calcium can be lost through sweat in a single training session. Calcium supplementation may be able to offset this source of calcium loss; future studies will tell if this intervention can maintain BMC and reduce the incidence of stress fractures in athletes.

▶ The danger that vigorous training may decrease rather than enhance bone mineral density has long been recognized in female athletes. Blame has been attached to suppression of estrogen levels, sometimes in association with a negative overall energy balance. The authors highlight a similar risk in male athletes and point to dermal loss of calcium as the cause. A previous report[1] suggested that the dermal loss of calcium was relatively small (40–140 mg/day), but the individuals concerned were not engaged in rigorous training. In the present study, university basketball players lost up to 600 mg of calcium in a single training session, and the associated decrease of BMC could be countered by providing calcium supplements to match this loss.

R.J. Shephard, M.D., Ph.D., D.P.E.

Reference

1. Charles P, Erikssen EF, Hashing C, et al: Dermal, intestinal and renal obligatory losses of calcium: Relation to skeletal calcium loss. *Am J Clin Nutr* 54: 266S–272S, 1991.

Effects of Endurance Exercise and Hormone Replacement Therapy on Serum Lipids in Older Women

Binder EF, Birge SJ, Kohrt WM (Washington Univ, St Louis)
J Am Geriatr Soc 44:231–236, 1996   7–9

Background.—Hormone replacement therapy (HRT) generally reduces the rate of cardiovascular disease, an effect believed to be mediated partly by the favorable effects of estrogen on plasma lipoprotein levels. Physical activity also favorably affects serum lipids and lipoproteins. The effects of 11 months of exercise training and HRT, individually and combined, on serum lipids and lipoproteins were investigated.

Methods.—Seventy-one healthy postmenopausal women aged 60–72 years were prospectively assigned to 1 of 4 groups: control, exercise alone,

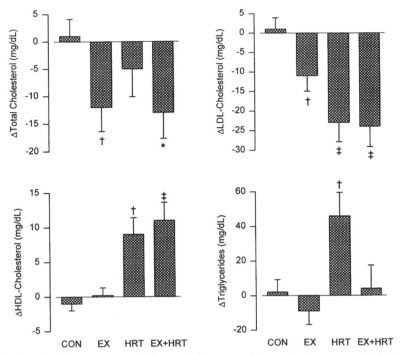

FIGURE 1.—Changes in serum lipids in control (*CON*), and in response to exercise (*EX*), hormone replacement therapy (*HRT*), and the combination of exercise and HRT (*EX + HRT*). Significantly different from initial value. *$P < 0.05$; †$P < 0.01$; ‡$P < 0.001$. *Abbreviations*: HDL, high-density lipoprotein; LDL, low-density lipoprotein. (Courtesy of Binder EF, Birge SJ, Kohrt WM: Effects of endurance exercise and hormone replacement therapy on serum lipids in older women. *J Am Geriatr Soc* 44[3]:231–236, 1996.)

HRT alone, or exercise plus HRT. Women receiving HRT took conjugated estrogens, 0.625 mg/day, and trimonthly medroxyprogesterone acetate, 5 mg/day, for 13 days. Exercise included 2 months of low-intensity training followed by 9 months of rigorous exercise for 45 min/day for 3 or more days a week at 65% to 85% of maximal heart rate.

Findings.—After 11 months, low-density lipoprotein (LDL) cholesterol was reduced in the women in the exercise group. However, high-density lipoprotein (HDL) cholesterol and triglycerides were not affected (Fig 1). Women receiving HRT alone had reduced LDL cholesterol, increased HDL cholesterol, and unchanged total cholesterol. Women in the exercise plus HRT group had reduced total cholesterol and LDL cholesterol and increased HDL cholesterol. Exercise prevented the HRT-related triglyceride increase in this group.

Conclusions.—In older postmenopausal women, exercise training and HRT apparently exert independent beneficial effects on serum lipids and lipoproteins. There are, however, disadvantages to each form of treatment. Exercise had no effect on HDL cholesterol, and HRT adversely affected triglycerides. Combining exercise and HRT seems to optimize lipid and lipoprotein response.

▶ Readers of this report by Binder and associates will be left with an important and unanswered question: Were these women randomly assigned to the 4 groups? When randomization is not specified, one generally infers self-selection, which diminishes the impact of the results. Although the changes in lipids attributed to exercise and HRT are similar to those reported in several other studies, the unique finding is that exercise appears to attenuate the HRT-mediated rise in triglycerides. However, it is premature to suggest that these changes in the lipid profile will reduce the risk of cardiovascular disease. Only the long-term, randomized clinical trial now under way can provide a definitive answer to that question.

B.L. Drinkwater, Ph.D.

Bone Mass and Subtle Abnormalities in Ovulatory Function in Healthy Women
Waller K, Reim J, Fenster L, Swan SH, et al (California Dept of Health Services, Berkeley; Veterans Affairs Med Ctr, Palo Alto, Calif; Stanford Univ, Calif; et al)
J Clin Endocrinol Metab 81:663–668, 1996   7–10

Objective.—Even a temporary cessation of menses leads to impaired bone acquisition in adolescent girls and to bone loss in young women. Amenorrheic athletes have reduced bone mineral density (BMD) even though they have high skeletal loading. The reduced bone density in these women carries a substantial risk of injury and fracture. Hormonal status throughout the menstrual period was studied to seek possible associations with BMD loss.

Methods.—The study included 53 healthy married women aged 18–39 years. All were participating in a comprehensive study of ovulatory function. The women collected and froze their first morning urine every day for 6 consecutive cycles, or until they missed 2 consecutive periods. Levels of creatinine and sex steroid hormone metabolites were measured in each sample. Metabolite excretion patterns were analyzed to assess the day of ovulation and to estimate luteal phase (LP) length. Serial bone density measurements were obtained in each subject, with areal BMD measured at the lumbar spine, right total hip, and whole body using dual-energy x-ray absorptiometry. The average follow-up was 17.5 months.

Results.—Usable data were collected on 217 cycles, an average of 4 per subject. Twenty-seven women had all normal cycles; 7 had LP abnormalities, with 1 or more anovulatory or short LP cycles; and 17 had other cycle abnormalities. These 3 groups were comparable in their baseline BMD values, although mean whole-body BMD was slightly higher than normal in the women with LP abnormalities. The trends continued in the same direction after adjustment for covariates. Loss of BMD at the lumbar spine and total hip were no greater for women with abnormalities than for those in the other groups. Women with LP abnormalities lost just 1% more whole-body BMD than did women with all normal cycles.

Conclusion.—Baseline BMD is no lower and loss of BMD is no greater than normal in women with abnormalities in the LP of the menstrual cycle. They appear to have little effect on BMD among women of the body weights and activity levels seen in the general population.

▶ A previous study by Prior et al.[1] reported that 1 or more anovulatory cycles per year or more than 1 short LP per year resulted in a significant decrease in BMD. This study by Waller et al. refutes that claim. Nevertheless, differences in protocol, study population, and technique for measuring BMD make a direct comparison of the results difficult. There is obviously a need for further investigation of the effect of LP abnormalities on BMD.

B.L. Drinkwater, Ph.D.

Reference

1. Prior JC, Vigna YM, Schechter MT, et al: Spinal bone loss and ovulatory disturbances. *N Engl J Med* 323:1221–1227, 1990.

Bone Density and Cyclic Ovarian Function in Trained Runners and Active Controls
Winters KM, Adams WC, Meredith CN, et al (Univ of California, Davis)
Med Sci Sports Exerc 28:776–785, 1996   7–11

Introduction.—Low circulating estrogen has been suggested as the cause of the association between intense training and low bone mineral density (BMD) in amenorrheic athletes. Low circulating progesterone may also reduce BMD in female athletes who are not amenorrheic but have less severe endocrine disturbances, such as a short or inadequate luteal phase (LP). Female runners with regular menstrual cycles were studied to see whether they had lower estrogen levels, altered ovulation, or shorter LP length, and how these factors were related to BMD. The effects of diet and energy balance were assessed as well.

Methods.—The study included 10 competitive distance runners and 10 moderately active controls. The controls all had a history of normal menstrual cycles; the runners also had cyclic menstruation, although the cycles varied in length. Each participant collected a daily morning urine sample for 1 complete menstrual cycle. Energy expenditure, diet, body composition, maximal aerobic power, and bone density were also assessed during that cycle. The ratio between mean baseline pregnanediol-3-glucuronide (PdG) and daily PdG from day 11 to the end of the cycle was used as an indicator of ovulation and LP function. Dual-energy x-ray absorptiometry was performed to determine lumbar and whole-body BMD. The women also completed a survey to assess eating behaviors, screen for eating disorders, and provide a complete menstrual history.

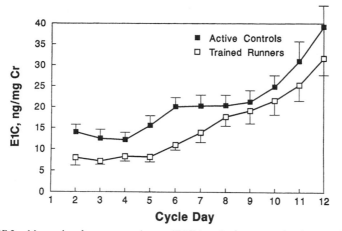

FIGURE 2.—Mean values for estrone conjugates (*E1C*) in trained runners and active controls for days 2–12, with day 1 being the beginning of menstruation (runners, *n* = 7; active controls, *n* = 8). *Bars* represent standard error of the group mean values for each day. *Abbreviation:* CR, creatinine. (Courtesy of Winters KM, Adams WC, Meredith CN, et al: Bone density and cyclic ovarian function in trained runners and active controls. *Med Sci Sports Exerc* 28(7):776–785, 1996.)

Results.—Total body BMD was similar in the 2 groups. Within the group of runners, mean whole-body BMD was similar for oligomenorrheic and eumenorrheic subjects. Lumbar spine BMD was significantly higher for the controls. On urinary metabolite analysis, ovulatory cycles were normal in 6 of the runners and 5 of the controls. Ovulation was absent in 3 runners and 2 controls; cycles of normal length but with ovulatory disturbance were found in 1 runner and 3 controls. Follicular phase length and LP length were similar in the 2 groups. From the start of follicular growth, there was no significant difference in urinary estrone conjugates from day 6 to ovulation or during the LP (Fig 2). Mean PdG from day 6 to day 10 was similar in runners and controls.

Conclusion.—The reduced lumbar BMD in female runners probably results from delayed estrogen production in the early follicular phase, rather than the amount of progesterone in the LP. Female runners with cyclic menstruation may still be at risk of osteopenia, but not as much so as amenorrheic runners. The difference in lumbar BMD is present without any systematic differences in menstrual cycle disturbances or LP characteristics when runners are compared with moderately active controls.

▶ Bone mineral density is determined by a number of variables: genetics, diet, menstrual history, etc. It is not clear whether any of the runners in this study had had amenorrheic periods in the past or whether age at menarche was related to BMD. The lack of a difference between runners and controls in progesterone during the LP appears to refute Prior's hypothesis that decreased levels of progesterone account for low BMD in cyclic runners with a short LP. [1] However, the conclusion that a delay in estrogen production in the early follicular phase can explain the lower lumbar BMD in the runners requires more supporting evidence. To conclude that women who train vigorously may be at risk for bone loss in spite of normal menstrual cycles is premature and might be used to discourage young women from participating in vigorous sports.

B.L. Drinkwater, Ph.D.

Reference

1. Prior JC, Vigna YM, Schechter MT, et al: Spinal bone loss and ovulatory disturbances. *N Engl J Med* 323:1221–1227, 1990.

Effect of Past Gymnastics Participation on Adult Bone Mass
Kirchner EM, Lewis RD, O'Connor PJ (Univ of Georgia, Athens)
J Appl Physiol 80:226–232, 1996   7–12

Introduction.—Even in athletes with a low calcium intake and a history of menstrual irregularities, there is evidence that gymnastics participation enhances bone mass in the lumbar spine. However, there are no data on what happens to bone mass after the athlete stops gymnastics. Bone mineral density (BMD) was assessed in former college gymnasts, including an analysis of how BMD is affected by physical activity, diet, and menstrual history.

Methods.—The study included 18 women aged 29–45 years who were former college gymnasts and 15 matched controls. All women underwent assessment of body composition, physical activity, diet, any symptoms of eating disorders, and menstrual history. Their athletic and reproductive histories were assessed, together with various factors that might influence bone, such as oral contraceptive use, major illnesses, and smoking. Bone mineral density in the lumbar spine, proximal femur, femoral neck, Ward's triangle, and whole body was measured by dual-energy x-ray absorptiometry. Total mass and fat and fat-free soft-tissue mass were assessed using whole-body software.

Results.—The former gymnasts began participation in that sport at an average age of 12 years, competing for an average of 7 years. The former gymnasts were currently more active than the controls; they expended more energy (2,614 vs. 2,151 kcal) and spent more time performing very hard activity (0.3 vs. 0.1 hr/day). Predictably, the former gymnasts exercised more hours per week and at higher intensity than the controls. In the 10 years before the study, the former gymnasts had exercised more hours/week and more intensively. Bone mineral density values were higher for the former gymnasts than for the controls (Fig 1). This was true even after adjustment for current and past physical activity. Within the group of former gymnasts, there were no differences in BMD for those who had a history of regular vs. interrupted menstrual periods.

Conclusion.—Women who are former gymnasts have higher BMD values than matched controls. Gymnastics may have a residual effect on bone mass that carries over into later decades. Intensive athletic training at a

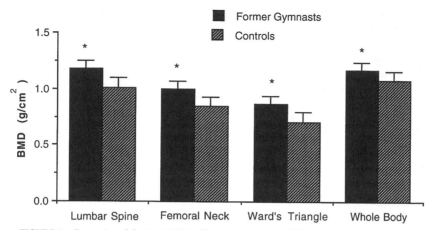

FIGURE 1.—Bone mineral density (*BMD*) of former gymnasts (*solid bars; n* = 18) and controls (*open bars; n* = 15). Values are means ± standard error. *Asterisk* indicates subject groups significantly different, *P* < 0.001. (Courtesy of Kirchner EM, Lewis RD, O'Connor PJ: Effect of past gymnastics participation on adult bone mass. *J Appl Physiol* 80:226–232, 1996.)

young age may lead to a higher peak bone mass. Bone mineral density does not appear to be compromised in women who had irregular menstrual cycles during their years of gymnastics participation.

▶ The difference in the results of this study and that of the study by Lindholm et al. (abstract 7–13) is puzzling. Both examined the effect of prior participation in elite gymnastics on the bone mass of former gymnasts and came up with very different results. In the Kirchner et al. study, former gymnasts had a higher BMD than a group of matched controls. In fact, their lumbar BMD of 1.176 g/cm² was far above the 1.047 g/cm² peak BMD for average young women.

The authors suggest several explanations for the high BMD in the former gymnasts. The most intriguing is that the high impact loading in gymnastic routines performed at an early age encouraged attainment of a higher peak bone mass in these former gymnasts. This would support the belief that there is a window of opportunity during childhood and adolescence during which physical activity can help ensure attainment of a maximal peak bone mass.

B.L. Drinkwater, Ph.D.

Bone Mineral Content of Young Female Former Gymnasts

Lindholm C, Hagenfeldt K, Ringertz H (Karolinska Hosp, Stockholm)
Acta Paediatr 84:1109–1112, 1995   7–13

Introduction.—Girls who train heavily before and during puberty may have late menarche, oligomenorrhea, and/or amenorrhea with low estrogen levels. Adolescents with low estrogen levels may be at risk for reduced bone mineral accretion, leading to decreased peak bone mass. The effects of delayed puberty and later menarche on skeletal development were studied in young female gymnasts.

Methods.—The study included 19 females who received elite training in gymnastics at a young age. They were followed up every 6 months throughout puberty. They were studied again at the age of 19–23 years. A group of 21 women of similar age, with normal age at menarche and regular menstrual periods, served as controls. Whole-body and lumbar spine bone mineral content was measured by dual-energy x-ray absorptiometry (DXA).

Results.—The mean age at menarche was 15 years for the gymnasts vs. 12 years for the controls. Most of the gymnasts were oligomenorrheic or amenorrheic for the first 2–3 years after menarche. By age 16–18 years, many were using oral contraceptives. Bone mineral areal mass (BMA) and bone mineral content were similar between groups. The exception was arm BMA, which was significantly higher in the gymnasts as a group and the subgroup of gymnasts with late menarche. Total bone calcium, fat, and lean body mass were similar between groups. Both study groups were similar in total body and spine BMA to a matched standard population.

Conclusion.—Intensive physical training during puberty does not seem to have any adverse effects on skeletal development in female gymnasts despite the late pubertal development and irregular menstruation seen in these athletes. Bone mineral areal mass is normal in young adult women who received elite gymnastics training as girls, perhaps because of "catch-up" related to reduced athletic activity, normalization of menstrual cycles, and oral contraceptive use.

▶ In contrast to the Kirchner (abstract 7–12) study, the bone mass of these former gymnasts is no different from that of matched controls or of average women in the normative database for the DXA equipment used. The authors were concerned that poor diets, late menarche, and irregular menstrual periods would have adversely affected the bone mass of these former gymnasts. Finding no difference in bone mass between the gymnasts and controls was considered a positive result. Why these former gymnasts, who also began training in their prepubertal years, did not gain the same benefit from their gymnastic routines as those in the previous study is not immediately clear.

B.L. Drinkwater, Ph.D.

Bone Mineral Density in Mother-Daughter Pairs: Relations to Lifetime Exercise, Lifetime Milk Consumption, and Calcium Supplements

Ulrich CM, Georgiou CC, Snow-Harter CM, et al (Univ of Washington, Seattle; Oregon State Univ, Corvallis)
Am J Clin Nutr 63:72–79, 1996   7–14

Introduction.—It is clear that heredity plays an important role in the development of osteoporosis. However, the relative influence of genetic and environmental factors on bone mineral density (BMD) is unclear. Therefore, the influence of lifetime calcium consumption, weight-bearing exercise, calcium supplementation, and hormone use on BMD was analyzed in mother-daughter pairs.

Methods.—Twenty-five mother-daughter pairs completed a questionnaire asking for detailed information about lifetime milk consumption, lifetime physical exercise, medical history and drug use, reproductive history, smoking history, current alcohol consumption, family history of osteoporosis, and history of hormone use. The mothers were at least 64 years of age and the daughters were premenopausal. All of the participants underwent anthropometric measurements and assessment of BMD with dual-energy x-ray absorptiometry.

Results.—Compared with the mothers, the daughters were significantly taller and had greater BMD, more lean body mass, a lower body mass index, and higher lifetime milk consumption. The mothers' age was neg-

TABLE 4.—Correlations Between Age and Anthropometric Measurements and Bone Mineral Density in Mothers and Daughters*

	Total BMD	Axial BMD†	Peripheral BMD
		g/cm^2	
Mothers (*n* = 25)			
Age	−0.49†	−0.34	−0.58†
Weight (kg)	0.64‡	0.63‡	0.64‡
Height (cm)	0.06	0.17	0.06
BMI (kg/m²)	0.58‡	0.44‡	0.59‡
Percentage body fat (%)	0.50†	0.22	0.52‡
Total fat mass (g)	0.61‡	0.40	0.62‡
Total lean mass (g)	0.31	0.55‡	0.30
Daughters (*n* = 25)			
Age	0.48†	0.32	0.45†
Weight (kg)	0.28	0.29	0.27
Height (cm)	0.03	0.08	0.11
BMI (kg/m²)	0.28	0.28	0.22
Percentage body fat (%)	−0.21	−0.25	−0.14
Total fat mass (g)	0.03	0.00	0.05
Total lean mass (g)	0.39	0.44†	0.36

*Values are Pearson correlation coefficients.
†$P < 0.05$.
‡$P < 0.01$.
Abbreviation: BMD, bone mineral density.
(Courtesy of Ulrich CM, Georgiou CC, Snow-Harter CM, et al: Bone mineral density in mother-daughter pairs: Relations to lifetime exercise, lifetime milk consumption, and calcium supplements. *Am J Clin Nutr* 63:72–79, 1996. Copyright *Am J Clin Nutr*. American Society for Clinical Nutrition.)

atively correlated with their total and peripheral BMD (Table 4). Although calcium supplementation after age 60 years was positively correlated with BMD in the mothers, the lifetime milk consumption was not significantly associated with BMD in either mothers or daughters. Lifetime weight-bearing exercise correlated positively with total and peripheral BMD in the daughters, but not in the mothers. Bone mineral density increased in association with former oral contraceptive use and current estrogen replacement therapy in the mothers, whereas BMD was not affected by oral contraceptive use in the daughters. However, the effects of estrogen replacement therapy in the mothers were not significant after adjustment for age. Bone mineral density correlations between paired mothers and daughters were not significant with analysis of the crude data, but became evident after adjustment for the age, body weight, and use of estrogen replacement therapy in the mothers and the lifetime weight-bearing exercises and peripheral BMD of the daughters.

Conclusions.—Anthropometric indexes and exogenous estrogen are the predominant influences on BMD in postmenopausal women. In both mothers and daughters, the effects on BMD of behavioral and hormonal factors were greater than the effects of heredity, suggesting the potential for interventions, including increased exercise and calcium intake and postmenopausal estrogen replacement therapy.

▶ The contribution of physical activity to *prevention* of osteoporosis in the postmenopausal years has never been quantified. There is no doubt that active premenopausal women have a higher BMD than sedentary women, but there is no evidence that activity prevents bone loss after menopause. In this study, for example, there was no relation between the mothers' BMD and their lifetime weight-bearing activity. Estrogen replacement therapy and previous use of oral contraceptives were more important predictors of current BMD. This does not negate the value of physical activity in enhancing the overall health of women but does suggest caution in overselling exercise as a means of preventing osteoporosis.

B.L. Drinkwater, Ph.D.

The Effect of Weight-bearing Exercise on Bone Mineral Density: A Study of Female Ex-elite Athletes and the General Population
Etherington J, Harris PA, Nandra D, et al (St Thomas' Hosp, London; Royal Natl Orthopaedic Hosp, Middlesex, England; Whipps Cross Hosp, London)
J Bone Miner Res 11:1333–1338, 1996   7–15

Introduction.—The positive effect of physical activity on bone mineral density (BMD) in female athletes is well known, but less is understood about the effects of exercise in the mostly sedentary general population. Changes in BMD as a consequence of exercise were retrospectively compared in female ex-elite athletes and age-matched controls.

Methods.—The age range of 83 female ex-elite athletes (67 middle and long distance runners and 16 tennis players) was 40–65 years, compared to 44–47 years for 1,003 controls. Physical activity for both groups was recorded for current activity at baseline assessment, current activity at years 5–6, and reported past levels of exercise. The BMD was measured by dual-energy X-ray absorptiometry at L1–L4, at the femoral neck (FN), and in the forearm.

Results.—Sixty percent of runners and 94% of tennis players were still active in their sports. Compared with sedentary controls, athletes and active controls had significantly greater BMDs at the FN and lumbar spine (LS). Athletes had an overall higher BMD, with a significantly higher value at the FN and a nonsignificant higher BMD at the LS than did active controls. Compared with sedentary controls, athletes had significantly higher BMDs at the FN and LS (Fig 1). Tennis players had significantly higher BMDs at the LS and higher BMDs at the FN, compared with runners.

Conclusion.—Ex-elite female athletes with a lifetime history of strenuous weight-bearing physical activity had higher levels of BMD than did sedentary controls. Higher levels of exercise activity were associated with increasing BMD in the general population. Bone mineral density of the LS

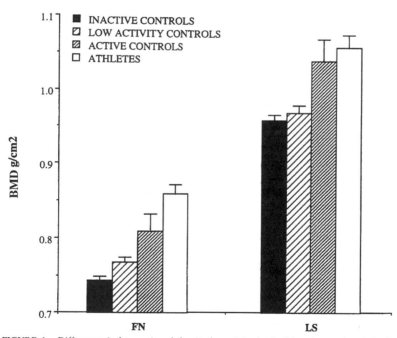

FIGURE 1.—Differences in bone mineral density by activity levels. Mean bone mineral density by activity level with standard errors, following analysis of covariance. Adjusted for age, height, weight, and smoking status. *Abbreviations*: *FN*, femoral neck; *LS*, lumbar spine, *BMD*, bone mineral density. (Reprinted by permission of Blackwell Science, Inc, from Etherington J, Harris PA, Nandra D: The effect of weight-bearing exercise on bone mineral density: A study of female ex-elite athletes and the general population. *J Bone Miner Res* 11:1333–1338, 1996.)

was higher in tennis players than runners. These findings support weight-bearing activities as an important modifiable risk factor for regulating bone mass and preventing fractures.

▶ Some of the most interesting conclusions in this article are drawn from data that are not presented. For example, much of the discussion revolves around differences in BMD between runners and tennis players at various sites, but none of the actual BMD data are shown. Twenty-seven of the runners who had given up all sporting activity had the same lumbar BMD as current runners, leading the authors to conclude that the benefit of the activity on BMD remained after training stopped. No information is provided on how long ago training stopped or whether the ex-runners are participating in other, noncompetitive activity. In any event, their spinal BMD of 1.029 g/cm² was no different from that of the active controls, 1.038 g/cm², suggesting that even moderate activity for 1 hour a week would have been sufficient to maintain BMD.

B.L. Drinkwater, Ph.D.

Effects of Unilateral Strength Training and Detraining on Bone Mineral Mass and Estimated Mechanical Characteristics of the Upper Limb Bones in Young Women
Heinonen A, Sievänen H, Kannus P, et al (UKK Inst for Health Promotion Research, Tampere, Finland)
J Bone Miner Res 11:490–501, 1996   7–16

Introduction.—Strength training investigations typically focus on bone mass changes only and may have omitted important aspects of bone strength by ignoring potential changes in bone geometry. It is possible that mechanical competence of bone may be improved through geometric changes without basic changes in bone mass. The effects of 12 months of unilateral high resistance strength training and 8 months of detraining on bone mineral content (BMC), bone mineral density (BMD), geometry, and estimated mechanical characteristics of upper limb bones were evaluated. Consequent loading-induced strains were estimated in forearm bone shafts.

Methods.—Eighteen healthy physical therapy students participated in the training group and 20 acted as nonexercising controls. Exercise training consisted of progressive left upper limb elbow flexion and extension strength training with dumbbells 5 times weekly for 1 year. An isometric arm dynamometer was used to determine maximal elbow extension and flexion strength. The BMC, areal BMD, bone width, and estimated cortical wall thickness were measured at 5 different sites.

Results.—Attendance averaged 2.8 times per week in the training group. Both groups met the recommended daily intake of calcium for females. The mean strength and isometric elbow flexion increases were 14% and 28%, respectively, in the training group (Fig 5). Corresponding increases

ELBOW FLEXION   ELBOW EXTENSION

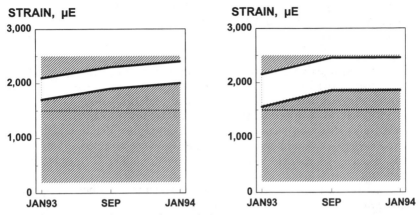

FIGURE 5.—Estimated strains in forearm shafts. *Gray area* represents mechanical usage. *Area between broken line and upper limit of gray area* represents the minimal effective strain range. *White area* represents 95% confidence interval of the estimated strains in the left forearm and extension exercises during the training period. (Courtesy of Heinonen A, Sievänen H, Kannus P, et al: Effects of unilateral strength training and detraining on bone mineral mass and estimated mechanical characteristics of the upper limb bones in young women. *J Bone Miner Res* 11(4):490–501, 1996, reprinted by permission of Blackwell Science, Inc.)

in the control group were 1% and 4%, respectively. There was a significant intergroup difference in the pretraining to posttraining change in elbow flexion and increase in elbow extension. The mean decrease in strength was 8% for elbow flexion and 7% for extension during the 8-month detraining period. There were no significant BMC changes in left or right limb in either group. There were no intergroup distinctions in BMD or BMC changes at any measured site.

Conclusion.—Despite a clear training effect on muscle strength, participants did not experience an increase in BMC or BMD or estimated mechanical characteristics at any measured site. Bone parameters were also not affected by the detraining period of 8 months.

▶ This paper provides one more example of strength training having the expected positive effect on muscular strength without producing any significant increase in BMD. However, the inclusion of biomechanical data in this study offers new insights into why strength training appears to be relatively ineffective in increasing bone mass. The authors note, for example, that the estimated mechanical strain during training was within the customary strain range for these active young women. Two other factors—the unidirectional characteristic of the loading and the slow rate at which force was applied—were identified by the authors as possibly contributing to the lack of effect on bone and should be considered in the design of future studies.

B.L. Drinkwater, Ph.D.

Effects of Resistance Training on Regional and Total Bone Mineral Density in Premenopausal Women: A Randomized Prospective Study

Lohman T, Going S, Pamenter R, et al (Univ of Arizona, Tucson)
J Bone Miner Res 10:1015–1024, 1995   7–17

Introduction.—Physical exercise has been suggested as an inexpensive and widely applicable alternative to traditional therapeutic regimens in the prevention of osteoporosis in postmenopausal women. The effects of 18 months of resistance exercise on regional and total body bone mineral density (BMD) was assessed in 106 premenopausal women.

Methods.—Women were randomly allocated into exercise (59 women) and control (47 women) groups. Both groups were assessed at baseline and at 5, 12, and 18 months for body composition BMD, muscle strength, hormonal status, urine and serum clinical chemistry, results, and diet. Twenty-two and 34 exercise and control group members, respectively, were available for 18-month follow-up. Control group members were asked to continue their sedentary lifestyle. Exercise group members participated in a program that met 3 times weekly for 1 hour. Exercises consisted of 3 sets of 8–12 repetitions for 12 free weight exercises designed to stress all major muscle groups. The exercise load was increased from 70% of maximal capacity (1 repetition maximum) at baseline to 80% by 18-month follow-up.

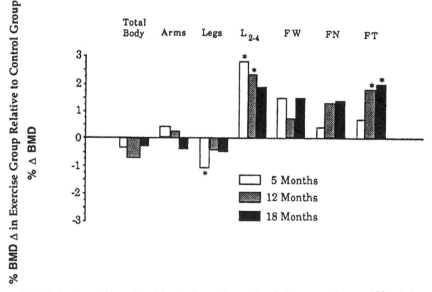

FIGURE 2.—Percent bone mineral density changes in exercise relative to control group. *Abbreviations:* BMD, bone mineral density; FW, femur wand triangle; FN, femur neck; FT, femur trocharite. (Reprinted by permission of Blackwell Science, Inc, from Lohman T, Going S, Pamenter R, et al: Effects of resistance training on regional and total bone mineral density in premenopausal women: A randomized prospective study. *Bone Miner Res* 10:1015–1024, 1995.)

Results.—The average increase in 1 repetition maximum averaged over all exercises was 28.3%, 45.2%, and 58.1% at 5, 12, and 18 months, respectively, for the exercise group. The mean increase in Cybex force production at 5, 12, and 18 months, respectively, was 9.5%, 22.3%, and 33.8%. There was a significant increase in BMD of the lumbar spine at 5, 12, and 18 months and in the trochanter at 12 and 18 months. The difference in BMD for the exercise group vs. control was 2.8%, 2.3%, and 1.9%, respectively, at 5, 12, and 18 months (Figure 2).

Conclusion.—Strength increased over time in the exercise group, but the major changes in BMD occurred in the first 5 months. Weight training is effective in increasing muscle strength, regional BMD, and total-body soft-tissue lean mass in women who are premenopausal. The effect of training on the incidence of bone fractures is not known.

▶ This is the usually carefully designed and conducted study from the Arizona group so it is particularly disappointing to find relatively small increases in BMD after 18 months of weight training. Although even small gains in BMD are preferable to any loss, the authors rightfully raise the issue as to the effect on fracture risk. Even more discouraging was the high (53%) dropout rate after 1 year of training. Will these formerly sedentary women who completed the study maintain a weight-training program or will even their slight improvement in BMD disappear as they too return to an inactive lifestyle? It would be interesting to bring these women back to the laboratory after a year, document their activity in the preceding 12 months, and remeasure their BMD. My guess is that the BMD would have reverted to the baseline values.

B.L. Drinkwater, Ph.D.

Television Viewing as a Cause of Increasing Obesity Among Children in the United States, 1986–1990
Gortmaker SL, Must A, Sobol AM, et al (Harvard School of Public Health, Boston; Tufts Univ, Boston; New England Med Ctr, Boston)
Arch Pediatr Adolesc Med 150:356–362, 1996   7–18

Background.—Studies have shown that in the past 30 years the incidence of obesity has increased in children and adolescents. In this age group, obesity is the most common nutritional disorder in the United States. Decreased activity may play a part in this rise in obesity. Today, children spend more time watching television than they do in school. Television viewing is strongly related to the onset of obesity and lack of remission in obese children. In the 1970s, television viewing and the rate of obesity were on the rise, but the energy intake of children and adolescents remained constant. Therefore, lower activity levels may be the major cause of the increase in obesity. In contrast, several studies have reported only modest associations between hours of television viewed and obesity, and other studies have shown no association. The relationship between childhood obesity and television viewing was investigated with control for various confounding factors.

Methods.—The relation between television viewing and overweight in 1990 was examined, as was the incidence and remission of overweight in 1986 and 1990 in a nationally representative sample of 746 subjects between 10 and 15 years of age. The mothers of the subjects were between 25 and 32 years of age. Subjects with a body mass index higher than the 85th percentile for their age and sex were said to be overweight.

Results.—The prevalence of overweight was 25% at baseline and 29% 4 years later. The average amount of television watched in 1990 was 4.8 hours per day, or 34 hours per week. More than 33% of the subjects watched television for more than 5 hours per day; 11% watched for 0–2 hours per day. A strong, dose-response relationship was seen between the incidence of overweight in 1990 and hours of television viewed. Subjects who watched more than 5 hours of television per day had a 4.6 times greater likelihood of being overweight than those who watched for 0–2 hours. Results were similar after adjustment for previous overweight, baseline maternal overweight, socioeconomic status, household structure, ethnicity, and maternal and child aptitude test scores. There was a significant relation between television viewing and higher incidence and lower remission of overweight. The adjusted odds of becoming overweight were 8.3 times greater for subjects who watched more than 5 hours of television per day than for those who watched 0–2 hours per day.

Discussion.—There was a positive correlation between time spent watching television and incidence of overweight and a negative correlation between time spent watching television and remission of overweight. More than 60% of overweight incidence in this population is related to time spent watching television. Time spent watching television cannot be spent on more energy-intense activities. Also, consumption of food can increase while watching television. Food advertising can also affect food choice. These findings are consistent with other reports of reductions in obesity when television viewing time was reduced as part of an activity and dietary intervention. There was no evidence that overweight causes more television viewing. The American Academy of Pediatrics recommends that children watch no more than 2 hours of television per day. This recommendation was followed by only 11% of the study population.

▶ This report makes a strong observational case for television (TV) viewing as a cause of obesity. In a 4-year follow-up of nearly 750 children (aged 10–15 years at the end of the study), those who viewed more than 5 hours of TV per day were nearly 5 times more apt to be overweight than those who viewed from 0–2 hours a day. This trend held true after adjustment for maternal overweight, socioeconomic differences, family size, and aptitude test scores. The counterhypothesis—that overweight causes TV viewing— was refuted by showing that being overweight in 1986 did not predict TV-viewing habits in 1990. It is pathetic that one third of the youths viewed more than 5 hours of TV a day, whereas only 11% watched for 0–2 hours, the limit recommended by the American Academy of Pediatrics. The editor added a suggestion that we rig TV sets to bicycle-driven generators, to guarantee that viewing would decrease or exercise would increase. An earlier study found that 1 added hour of physical activity per day notably augments the overall energy expenditure of obese children, even when the level of spontaneous physical activity does not increase.[1]

E.R. Eichner, M.D.

Reference

1. 1993 YEAR BOOK OF SPORTS MEDICINE, pp 381–382.

Validity of Skinfold Estimates of Percent Fat in High School Female Gymnasts
Housh TJ, Johnson GO, Housh DJ, et al (Univ of Nebraska, Lincoln)
Med Sci Sports Exerc 28:1331–1335, 1996   7–19

Introduction.—Emphasis on thinness and appearance has set a standard that encourages female gymnasts to engage in pathogenic weight-control behaviors. Assignment of a minimal weight based on the gymnast's percent body fat could decrease excessive weight loss and use of potentially dangerous weight-control behaviors. Success of such an approach depends on accurate and practical assessment of body composition. Eleven existing skinfold equations were evaluated on a sample of 73 female high school gymnasts.

Methods.—Body density (BD) was evaluated from underwater weighing with correction for residual lung volume (RV). The conversion constants of Brozek et al. were used to calculate percent body fat from BD. Predicted percent fat was determined using 11 skinfold equations. These skinfold sites were measured on the right side of the body: triceps, subscapular, axilla, anterior suprailium, abdominal, and thigh sites described by Jackson and Pollock. The equations were analyzed for accuracy.

Results.—Underwater weighing determined the mean percent fat to be 18.6%. The quadratic sum-of-three skinfold equation (EQ 10) of Thorland et al. met the most cross-validation criteria and may be recommended for estimating body composition in high school female gymnasts. Using the triceps, subscapular, and anterior suprailium skinfold measurements, the recommended equation is: % fat = $(457/(1.0987 - 0.00122(\times\ 14) + 0.00000263(\times\ 14^2)) - 414.2$.

Conclusion.—The EQ 10 may be used as a preseason assessment of body composition for high school female gymnasts in the absence of a laboratory procedure such as underwater weighing. Female high school athletes should not be allowed to compete without medical clearance for preseason body fat determinations less than 12%. The minimal predicted minimal body weight should be 50.9 kg when using the EQ 10.

▶ The authors express the hope that having an accurate method of estimating percent body fat will permit coaches to assign a *minimal* body weight that can be attained without resource to pathologic weight-control behaviors. However, by setting 12% body fat as the minimum fat permitted without a medical clearance for a lower percent, the authors are moving well ahead of research in this area. Some gymnasts might perform very well at 15% body fat; yet their coach will feel justified in requiring them to reach 12%. Will a gymnast who is healthy, eumenorrheic, and 10% body fat be required to gain weight? Although the purpose of this study is commendable, those of us who work with the Female Athlete Triad would prefer to see less emphasis placed on the control of an athlete's weight/body fat.

B.L. Drinkwater, Ph.D.

Morphometric and Neurodevelopmental Outcome at Age Five Years of the Offspring of Women Who Continued to Exercise Regularly Throughout Pregnancy
Clapp JF III (Case Western Reserve Univ, Cleveland, Ohio)
J Pediatr 129:856–863, 1996   7–20

Introduction.—The impact of regular, sustained, antigravitational exercise on long-term outcome for pregnant mothers and their offspring has not been clearly defined. The offspring of 20 women who voluntarily stopped all sustained exercise other than walking during pregnancy were prospectively compared with those of 20 physically active women to determine if continuous, regular, vigorous, sustained exercise throughout pregnancy adversely affected morphometric and neurodevelopmental outcome of their children at 5 years of age.

Methods.—Women who were physically active during pregnancy participated in aerobic exercise 3 or more times weekly for more than 30 minutes at an intensity greater than 55% of their maximal capacity. Controls exercised regularly before pregnancy. Women in both groups were individually matched for smoking status; socioeconomic status; education; marital stability; maternal and paternal morphometry; parity; maternal work outside the home; preconceptional fitness; and preconceptional exercise type, frequency, and duration. Postnatal variables included lactation, type of child care, regular parental exercise after birth, and maternal change in weight during the 6-year interval. Offspring were matched individually for sex, birth order, gestational age at delivery, growth and development, type of child care, and new siblings.

Results.—Between-group head circumference and length of offspring were similar at birth, but offspring of exercising women weighed less (3.4 vs. 3.64 kg) and had less fat (10.5% vs. 15.1%), compared with controls. At age 5 years, the head circumference and height were similar for both

TABLE 1.—Maternal and Paternal Physical Characteristics

Physical characteristic	Exercise group	Control group	*p*
Maternal age (yr)	31 ± 1	31 ± 1	NS
Weight (kg)	57.5 ± 1.2	57.6 ± 1.4	NS
Height (cm)	169.2 ± 2.6	168.8 ± 2.3	NS
Body fat (%)	16.6 ± 1.3	17.1 ± 1.4	NS
VO_{2max} (ml/kg/min)	54.4 ± 2.6	53.1 ± 2.9	NS
Pregnancy weight gain (kg)	12.8 ± 1.1	16.2 ± 1.4	0.01
5-Yr Δ weight (kg)	0.1 ± 1.5	0.9 ± 1.1	NS
Paternal weight (kg)	73.2 ± 2.3	70.9 ± 3.1	NS
Height (cm)	178.3 ± 3.1	176.4 ± 3.3	NS

Note: Values (except *P* values) are expressed as mean ± standard error of the mean.
Abbreviation: NS, not significant.
(Courtesy of Clapp JF III: Morphometric and neurodevelopmental outcome at age five years of the offspring of women who continued to exercise regularly throughout pregnancy. *J Pediatr* 129:856–863, 1996.)

groups, but the offspring of exercising women weighed less (18.0 kg vs. 19.5 kg) and had a lower sum of 5 site skinfolds (37 vs. 44 mm) than controls (Table 1). There were no between-group differences in motor, integrative, and academic readiness skills. Offspring of exercising women performed significantly better on the Wechsler scales and tests of oral language skills than their counterparts in the control group.

Conclusion.—There was no evidence of comparative deficit in any area measured in offspring of exercising women. Offspring of women who exercise during pregnancy have lower subcutaneous fat mass than those of women who are not physically active.

▶ For someone like myself who has found it difficult to match women in experimental and control groups on even 4 variables, the author's success in matching his exercise and nonexercise control groups on more than a dozen maternal variables and 6 offspring factors is incredible. Based on their aerobic power, neither the exercise group (maximum oxygen consumption [VO_2max] = 54.2 mL/kg/min) nor the controls (VO_2max = 53.1 mL/kg/min) could be considered a sample from a normal population of women in age from the late 20s to the early 30s. Even more amazing is the fact that women in the control group with that level of fitness would agree to stop all exercise except walking during the 9 months of their pregnancy. I would not recommend that women place too much reliance on these results in determining an activity during pregnancy.

B.L. Drinkwater, Ph.D.

Exercise and Weight Control in Sedentary Overweight Men: Effects on Clinic and Ambulatory Blood Pressure

Cox KL, Puddey IB, Morton AR, et al (Univ of Western Australia, Perth)
J Hypertens 14:779–790, 1996   7–21

Introduction.—It is unclear whether exercise without weight loss can independently reduce blood pressure. Some studies show reductions in daytime blood pressure only, whereas others report no change in ambulatory blood pressure with exercise training. A modeling approach with time series analysis was used to assess ambulatory blood pressure monitoring. The effects of vigorous exercise training, restriction of food intake or both, on blood pressure of sedentary overweight men were determined.

Methods.—Nonsmoking men, aged 20–50 years, whose body mass was 120% to 160% greater than the ideal for their height were recruited. From an initial group of 500 interviewed by telephone, 260 attended a screening visit; 60 satisfied all entry criteria. Participants had 2 blood pressure measurements; the mean was in the range of 130–160 mm Hg systolic and 80–110 mm Hg diastolic. The men were randomly assigned to 1 of 4 groups for the 16-week study. Two groups were asked to maintain normal dietary habits, and 2 received a weight reduction program. Participants were further allocated to a control light exercise group or a vigorous intensity exercise group (30-minute sessions, 3 times a week). Twenty-four–hour ambulatory blood pressure monitoring was performed at baseline and at the end of the intervention. Clinic blood pressure, body mass, and alcohol intake were also monitored.

Results.—Fifty-one men completed the study. Maximal oxygen intake was unchanged in the light exercise group but increased approximately 24% with vigorous exercise. Those whose food intake was restricted had a significant loss of body mass (mean, 9.5 kg), whereas vigorous exercise alone did not reduce weight. Time series analysis revealed that both vigorous exercise and food intake restriction were associated with lower daytime ambulatory systolic blood pressure. When vigorous exercise and the dietary program were combined, reduction in systolic blood pressure was sustained during the 24-hour period. The combined approaches resulted in additive effects (Fig 5) on the blood pressure response to exercise at a submaximal work-rate of 140 W.

Discussion.—Sedentary overweight men exhibited a reduction in ambulatory blood pressure throughout a 24-hour period when vigorous exercise was combined with a weight reduction program. Each intervention alone was associated with only lower daytime ambulatory systolic blood pressure.

▶ Debate continues as to the extent of blood pressure reduction achieved by regular exercise. Many reports suggest that mean daytime pressures are a few millimeters of mercury lower after beginning an exercise program, but there is no change in nocturnal readings. This could mean that any decrease in daytime readings is an acute response to physical activity, rather than a

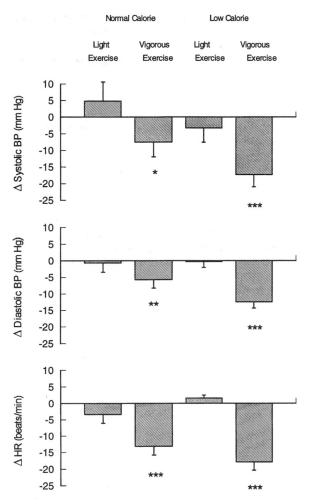

FIGURE 5.—Bar chart shows mean ± SEM changes (Δ) in the response of systolic and diastolic blood pressures *(BP)* and heart rate *(HR)* to a workload of 140 W on a bicycle ergometer during week 16 of the intervention. *Asterisk, $P < 0.05$; double asterisk, $P < 0.001$; triple asterisk, $P < 0.001$* by Student's *t*-test with Bonferroni's correction. (Courtesy of Cox KL, Puddey, IB, Morton AR, et al: Exercise and weight control in sedentary overweight men: Effects on clinic and ambulatory blood pressure. *J Hypertens* 14:779–790, 1996.)

longer term reduction in the underlying hypertension. A further possibility is that an increase in physical activity is beneficial because it reduces body mass[1, 2]; however, some studies have claimed the blood pressure reduction is independent of weight loss[3]. This report has applied the sophisticated technique of time series analysis, which allows observation of pressures at various points in the day. Using this approach, the data suggest that pressures are reduced with both exercise and weight loss, although the largest effect is seen from a combination of the 2 treatments. Pressures are reduced not only at rest, but also during exercise. The mechanisms of benefit remain unclear; in this particular study, salt intake and catecholamine excretion were unchanged, and the Profile of Mood States questionnaire showed no alteration in the state anxiety score.

R.J. Shephard, M.D., Ph.D., D.P.E.

References

1. Gilders RM, Voner C, Dudley GA: Endurance training and blood pressure in normotensive and hypertensive adults. *JAMA* 21:629–636, 1989.
2. Blumenthal JA, Siegal WC, Appelbaum M: Failure of exercise to reduce blood pressure in patients with mild hypertension. *JAMA* 266:2098–2104, 1991.
3. Meredith IT, Jennings GL, Esler MD, et al: Time course of the antihypertensive and autonomic effects of regular endurance exercise in human subjects. *J Hypertens* 8:859–866, 1990.

Influence of Menstrual Status on Fluid Replacement After Exercise Induced Dehydration in Healthy Young Women
Maughan RJ, McArthur M, Shirreffs SM (Univ Med School, Aberdeen, Scotland)
Br J Sports Med 30:41–47, 1996   7–22

Introduction.—Menstrual status affects thermoregulation, and exercise-related fluid loss varies at different times during the menstrual cycle. Thus, hormonal status may affect fluid balance, and menstrual status may influence rehydration after exercise-related fluid loss. Differences in exercise-induced fluid loss during different stages of the menstrual cycle were investigated.

Methods.—The study included 5 healthy women (mean age, 23 years). All had a normal menstrual history with regular cycles, and none were currently taking steroid contraceptives. The women were studied on 4 different occasions: twice at 2 days before the onset of menses and once at 5 and 19 days after the onset of menses. After baseline measurements, the women were subjected to a dehydration procedure, consisting of 10 minutes of immersion in hot water followed by intermittent cycle ergometer exercise in a warm room. The women exercised at about 60% of maximum oxygen uptake for up to six 10-minute sessions or until lost body mass approached 2%. After another blood sample was taken, the women were rehydrated with a fluid volume equal to 150% of the mass lost during the dehydration process. Blood and urine samples were collected up to 6 hours after the end of the rehydration period.

Results.—In all trials, mean body mass lost during the dehydration process was about 1.8%. Sweat rate and cumulative urine output were comparable at all 3 stages of the menstrual cycle. There was no significant difference in total electrolyte excretion after rehydration. Net fluid balance after rehydration—and thus the percentage of rehydration fluid retained—was no different between trials (Fig 1). At no menstrual stage was the blood or plasma volume altered between the predehydration and postde-

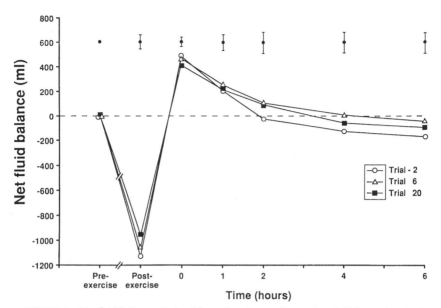

FIGURE 1.—Net fluid balance calculated from the volumes of sweat loss, fluid ingested, and urine output over the course of the experiment. The pre-exercise urine sample is not included in these calculations. The group standard error of the mean of the values for all trials at each time point is represented at that time point. (Courtesy of Maughan RJ, McArthur M, Shirreffs SM: Influence of menstrual status on fluid replacement after exercise induced dehydration in healthy young women. *Br J Sports Med* 30:41–47, 1996.)

hydration samples. Menstrual stage did not affect serum electrolyte concentration.

Conclusion.—In healthy young women, the stages of the menstrual cycle have no effect on acute replacement of exercise-induced fluid loss. Women appear to be at no disadvantage when it comes to rapid and complete restoration of exercise-induced sweat loss.

▶ The luteal phase of the menstrual cycle is associated with an increase in the thermoregulatory set-point; however, there are conflicting reports as to the practical significance of this slight elevation for women exercising in the heat. The effect of cardiovascular fitness, acclimation, and body size are among a number of factors that have a greater impact on a woman's ability to exercise in hot environments. The conclusion by Maughan et al. that cycle phase does not affect rehydration is further evidence that, although the effect of the cycle phase on thermoregulatory mechanisms is of theoretical interest, the practical effect on the trained acclimated female athlete is probably negligible.

B.L. Drinkwater, Ph.D.

Postexercise Proteinuria in Childhood and Adolescence

Poortmans JR,Geudvert C, Schorokoff K, et al (Université Libre de Bruxelles, Belgium; Institut d'Hygiène et d'Epidémiologie, Bruxelles, Belgium)
Int J Sports Med 17:448–451, 1996   7–23

Introduction.—Healthy adults are known to show a transient state of excess protein excretion in urine after strenuous exercise. Limited data are available, however, on postexercise proteinuria in children and adolescents. This lack of information on renal responses to exercise in young individuals led to an investigation in a group of boys and girls aged 6 to 18 years.

Methods.—Healthy volunteers, 93 girls and 77 boys, were recruited from elementary and secondary schools. They were divided by sex and into 4 age groups: 6 to 9 years, 10 to 12 years, 13 to 15 years, and 16 to 18 years. Urine was collected before and 30 minutes after maximal exercise (the 20-m shuttle run test).

Results.—Maximal speed increased according to age and was higher in boys than in girls. The excretion rates of creatinine at rest rose steadily with increasing age, and changes in excretion rates were more pronounced in boys than in girls. Exercise had no effect on creatinine excretion. In children aged 6 to 9 years, a difference was noted in boys and girls in postexercise proteinuria. Whereas boys enhanced the excretion of macromolecules, girls showed no increase by maximal exercise. There was a relation between the excretion rates of all protein components and the absolute intensity of exercise expressed as maximal speed. Between the ages of 9 and 18 years, high– and low–molecular weight protein excretion indicated increasing disturbances in both boys and girls.

Discussion.—A slight, gradual increase in the excretion of proteins is observed from childhood to adolescence. In the early stage of childhood (6 to 9 years), there is a slight sex difference for both high– and low–molecular weight proteins, but this difference does not exist in post-pubertal adolescents. The magnitude of protein excretion is related to the absolute intensity of exercise.

▶ It has long been known that strenuous exercise in healthy adults increases glomerular filtration permeability and saturates proximal tubular re-absorption of filtered proteins, causing a transient proteinuria of mixed, glomerular-tubular type. This study, by experts in the field, shows that the same occurs in boys and girls from 6 to 18 years of age when they undergo a maximal exercise test, the 20-m shuttle run to exhaustion. The magnitude of proteinuria was related to intensity of exercise, and the sex difference (more proteinuria in boys) from ages 6 to 9 years probably reflects only the higher speed obtained by boys during the run. Habits and patterns of exercise should be taken into account by physicians who find proteinuria in children.

E.R. Eichner, M.D.

Extrarenal Potassium Homeostasis With Maximal Exercise in End-stage Renal Disease

Clark BA, Shannon C, Brown RS, et al (Harvard Med School, Boston; Northeastern Univ, Boston)

J Am Soc Nephrol 7:1223–1227, 1996   7–24

Background.—During vigorous exercise, serum potassium concentrations increase markedly as a result of potassium release from contracting muscle cells. Erythropoietin administration increases exercise capacity in patients with end-stage renal disease (ESRD). The widespread use of this agent raises concerns about severe exertional hyperkalemia. Whether ESRD is associated with changes in potassium and the neurohumoral mediators of extrarenal potassium disposal with maximal exercise was determined.

Methods.—Eight stable patients receiving hemodialysis (mean age, 37 years) and 8 healthy individuals (mean age, 44 years) were included in the study. All subjects exercised to exhaustion on a graded cycle ergometer test.

Findings.—The 2 groups did not differ significantly in exercise performance as assessed by peak work rate, maximal oxygen intake, or rate pressure product. Although baseline potassium levels were greater in the dialysis group than in the control group, the patterns of increase during exercise and return to baseline after exercise were similar in the 2 groups. However, the dialysis group had a greater response to exercise and higher

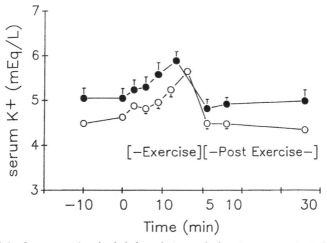

FIGURE 1.—Serum potassium levels before, during, and after vigorous exercise in hemodialysis patients (*solid circles*) and healthy volunteers (*open circles*). Baseline potassium level was higher in the dialysis patients, but both groups had a similar incremental rise in potassium level with exercise and a similar fall in potassium level during recovery. (Courtesy of Clark BA, Shannon C, Brown RS, et al: Extrarenal potassium homeostasis with maximal exercise in end-stage renal disease. *J Am Soc Nephrol* 7(8):1223–1227, 1996.)

basal norepinephrine levels, basal insulin levels, insulin postexercise levels, and basal aldosterone levels, with an increased response to exercise (Fig 1).

Conclusion.—Although patients receiving dialysis have higher basal potassium levels, their potassium responses to maximal exercise are normal. Extrarenal potassium homeostasis in ESRD may be maintained partly by more vigorous insulin, catecholamine, and aldosterone levels.

▶ α-Adrenergic stimulation, acidosis, and uremia all tend to diminish cellular potassium uptake, thus tending to cause high serum potassium levels in ESRD.[1] Although such patients benefit greatly from exercise programs (conveniently performed during the course of dialysis) there have been fears that the same factors that contribute to a high resting serum potassium value might lead to further dangerous increments in concentrations of this ion during exercise. However, these data from Clark et al. suggest that potassium remains well regulated and that the increments seen during exercise are no greater than would be anticipated in an individual with normal kidneys.

R.J. Shephard, M.D., Ph.D., D.P.E.

Reference

1. Brown RS: Extrarenal potassium homeostasis. *Kidney Int* 30:116–127, 1986.

Effects of Medium-chain Triglyceride Ingestion on Fuel Metabolism and Cycling Performance
van Zyl CG, Lambert EV, Hawley JA, et al (Univ of Cape Town, South Africa)
J Appl Physiol 80:2217–2225, 1996   7–25

Background.—Many athletes believe that a high-carbohydrate diet before an endurance event and carbohydrate (CHO) ingestion during the event is needed for optimal performance. The effects of ingesting medium-chain triglycerides (MCTs), which are rapidly absorbed into the hepatic portal system as glycerol and medium-chain free fatty acids, on the rate of CHO oxidation have attracted researchers' attention. The metabolic effects of ingesting a large amount of MCTs alone and combined with CHO during about 3 hours of cycling were documented.

Methods.—On 3 occasions 10 days apart, 6 endurance-trained cyclists rode for 2 hours at 60% of peak oxygen intake, then performed a simulated 40-km time trial. While riding, the cyclists ingested 2 L of a [U-^{14}/C] glucose-labeled beverage with 10% glucose, 4.3% MCTs, or 10% glucose plus 4.3% MCTs.

Findings.—Replacing CHO with MCTs slowed the time trials from 66.8 to 72.1 minutes. Adding MCTs to CHO improved the trials from 66.8 to 65.1 minutes. Faster time trials with CHO plus MCTs were associated with increased final circulating levels of free fatty acids and ketones and reduced final circulating levels of glucose and lactate. Adding MCTs to ingested CHO decreased total CHO oxidation rates from 14 to 10 mmol/

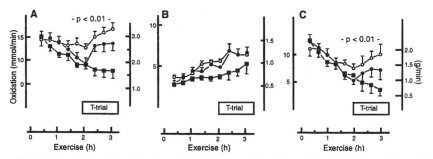

FIGURE 5.—Effects of carbohydrates (*CHO*) (*open circle*), medium-chain triglycerides (*MCT*) (*solid square*), and CHO + MCT (*solid circle*) ingestion on rates of CHO oxidation [total CHO (**A**), plasma glucose (**B**), and muscle glycogen (**C**)]. Values are means ± standard error. *P* values extending from 90 minutes of exercise to end of simulated 40-km cycling time trial (*T-trial*) in A and C are from comparisons between CHO and CHO + MCT trials. (Courtesy of van Zyl CG, Lambert EV, Hawley JA, et al: Effects of medium-chain triglyceride ingestion on fuel metabolism and cycling performance. *J Appl Physiol* 80:2217–2225, 1996.)

min at 2 hours and from 17 to 14 mmol/min in the time trial but had no effects on the corresponding 5- and 7-mmol/min rates of [^{14}/C]glucose oxidation (Fig 5).

Conclusion.—Medium-chain triglyceride oxidation appears to reduce the direct and/or indirect oxidation of muscle glycogen. Diminished reliance on CHO oxidation at a given oxygen uptake is comparable to an endurance-training effect, which may explain improved performance.

▶ A trip to Bordeaux at the time of the Tour de France bicycle races several years ago unearthed a rumor that one whole team of cyclists had become very ill from the IV infusion of fatty acids. Unfortunately, the trophy-winning infusion had turned rancid in the trunk of a coach's car! The possible role of MCTs in endurance performance, thus, has more than academic interest.

Traditional wisdom has been that the competitor in ultra-endurance events is best served by adopting a high CHO intake during the event. However, such an approach does not reduce the utilization of muscle glycogen reserves until these have fallen below 40 mmol/kg wet weight.[1] In contrast to long-chain fatty acids (which enter the body quite slowly through the lymphatic system), MCTs (C_8–C_{10}) are rapidly absorbed via the hepatic portal system and oxidized by the mitochondria.

The data presented here show that relative to 10% glucose, 4.3% MCTs yielded not only a reduction of glycogen usage but also an appreciable (2.5%) enhancement of performance in a simulated time trial.

R.J. Shepard, M.D., Ph.D., D.P.E.

Reference

1. Bosch AN, Dennis SC, Noakes TD: Influence of carbohydrate ingestion on fuel substrate turnover and oxidation during prolonged exercise. *J Appl Physiol* 76:2364–2372, 1994.

Combined Aerobic Training and Dichloroacetate Improve Exercise Capacity and Indices of Aerobic Metabolism in Muscle Cytochrome Oxidase Deficiency

Taivassalo T, Matthews PM, De Stefano N, et al (Montreal Neurological Inst; McGill Univ, Montreal)
Neurology 47:529–534, 1996   7–26

Background.—Mitochondrial myopathy can result in impaired oxidative phosphorylation and aerobic adenosine triphosphate production, exercise intolerance, and lactic acidosis. Treatments to date have not been effective. The protein kinase that inhibits pyruvate dehydrogenase by phosphorylation is inhibited by dichloroacetate. In patients with secondary lactic acidosis, dichloroacetate lowers systemic lactate in open clinical trials. In patients with mitochondrial disorders, short-term treatment with dichloroacetate reduces blood lactate at rest and during exercise, and improves indices of brain oxidative metabolism in a double-blind, placebo-controlled study. However, biochemical indices of muscle oxidative metabolism do not improve. The effects of aerobic training with and without treatment with dichloroacetate on exercise tolerance in a patient with mitochondrial myopathy were investigated.

Methods.—The subject was a 25-year-old woman with mitochondrial myopathy from cytochrome oxidase deficiency. The patient underwent aerobic training for 14 weeks. After 8 weeks of training, therapy with oral dichloroacetate, 25 mg/kg twice a day for 6 weeks, was begun. Aerobic power and oxidative metabolism were measured.

Results.—There were substantial improvements in aerobic power and oxidative metabolism. At rest and after a constant amount of work, venous lactate concentrations decreased by about 50% after 8 weeks of aerobic training alone (Fig 3). With aerobic training and treatment with dichloroacetate, lactate concentrations decreased by more than 70%. The heart rate decreased progressively at rest and after a constant amount of submaximal work. A graded submaximal exercise test was used to predict

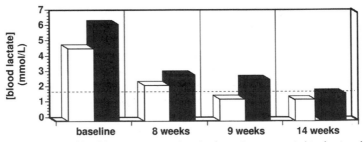

FIGURE 3.—Venous blood lactate concentrations in the patient at rest (*white bars*) and after a constant amount of work (*gray bars*). Measurements were performed at baseline, after aerobic training alone (8 weeks), and after combined dichloroacetate treatment and aerobic training (9 and 14 weeks). The *dotted line* indicates the upper limit (95%) of normal resting blood lactate. (Courtesy of Taivassalo T, Matthews PM, De Stefano N, et al: Combined aerobic training and dichloroacetate improve exercise capacity and indices of aerobic metabolism in muscle cytochrome oxidase deficiency. *Neurology* 47:529–534, 1996, by permission of Little, Brown and Company, Inc.)

aerobic power, which improved by 71% by the end of the study. After 8 weeks of training alone, there was a 1.7-fold increase in ^{31}P magnetic resonance spectroscopy measurements of rate constants for recovery of muscle phosphocreatine, and a 2.8-fold increase in metabolically active adenine diphosphate. After 14 weeks of training and therapy with dichloroacetate, there was a a 4.5-fold increase in ^{31}P magnetic resonance spectroscopy measurements of rate constants for recovery of muscle phosphocreatine, and a 23.0-fold increase in metabolically active adenine diphosphate. The patient indicated a significant reduction in handicap on a health survey questionnaire.

Conclusion.—These findings indicate that poor exercise performance in this patient resulted from chronic inactivity and a direct effect of mitochondrial dysfunction on muscle metabolism. It can be difficult to distinguish these 2 factors in patients with mitochondrial diseases. Aerobic training and treatment with dichloroacetate may improve exercise tolerance in these patients, but their independent effects cannot be determined from these data. Mitochondrial disorders are very heterogeneous, and results from this study of a single patient may not apply to other patients.

▶ Any possible new approach to the treatment of myopathy is welcome. This article is based on a single case, but nevertheless, a dramatic response to aerobic conditioning is reported. This response is apparently further enhanced by the administration of dichloroacetate (although the progressive benefit observed could also represent a continuing response to training). There are sound biochemical arguments for administering dichloroacetate (it inhibits a specific protein kinase, thus increasing the activity of pyruvate dehydrogenase). Nevertheless, it is a little puzzling as to why dichloroacetate alone has little effect on muscle function[1] if the postulated mechanism of benefit is correct.

R.J. Shephard, M.D., Ph.D., D.P.E.

Reference

1. De Stefano N, Matthews PM, Ford B, et al: Short-term dichloracetate treatment improves indices of aerobic metabolism in patients with mitochondrial disorders. *Neurology* 45:1193–1198, 1995.

Pivalic Acid–induced Carnitine Deficiency and Physical Exercise in Humans
Abrahamsson K, Eriksson BO, Holme E, et al (Gothenburg Univ, Sweden)
Metabolism 45:1501–1507, 1996   7–27

Introduction.—Antibiotics conjugated with pivalic acid can cause loss of carnitine from the body stores. Carnitine depletion can affect the liver, heart, and skeletal muscle. The effects of secondary carnitine deficiency on metabolic and physiologic variables during exercise testing were evaluated

TABLE 2.—Physiologic and Biochemical Variables During Maximal Exercise Test Before and After Treatment with Pivmecillinam

Variable	Group 1		Group 2		
	0 d	10 d	0 d	16 d	54 d
$\dot{V}o_2$max (L/min STPD)	3.20 ± 0.84	3.28 ± 0.73	2.57 ± 1.07	2.47 ± 0.93	2.26 ± 0.93*
Maximal heart rate (beats/min)	180 ± 11	181 ± 10	178 ± 18	175 ± 17	165 ± 15*
Maximal ventilation (L/min BTPS)	138 ± 30	150 ± 41	103 ± 46	99 ± 37	84 ± 36*
Respiratory quotient at $\dot{V}o_2$max	1.20 ± 0.06	1.16 ± 0.04	1.14 ± 0.06	1.08 ± 0.04	1.09 ± 0.08
Blood lactate at $\dot{V}o_2$max (mmol/L)	14.9 ± 2.9	12.2 ± 2.9*	10.1 ± 2.7	8.4 ± 2.6*	6.5 ± 2.1*†

Note: Values are means.
*$P < 0.05$ vs. day 0.
†$P < 0.05$ vs. day 16.
Abbreviations: $\dot{V}o_2$max, maximal oxygen uptake; *STPD*, standard temperature and pressure; *BTPS*, body temperature, ambient pressure, saturated.
(Courtesy of Abrahamsson K, Eriksson BO, Holme E, et al: Pivalic acid–induced carnitine deficiency and physical exercise in humans. *Metabolism* 45:1501–1507, 1996.)

in healthy adults after short- and long-term treatment with antibiotics containing pivalic acid.

Methods.—Thirteen volunteers were placed in 1 of 2 groups: group 1 subjects were treated with pivmecillinam for 10 days and group 2 subjects were treated for 54 days with pivmecillinam at the same dosage. Maximal working capacity, maximal oxygen intake ($\dot{V}O_2$max), and blood components were measured, and muscle biopsy samples were obtained at baseline, at a mean of 16 days in group 2, and at completion of pivmecillinam treatment (10 days for group 1 and 54 days for group 2).

Results.—There was a successive decrease in serum free carnitine during treatment. The carnitine in muscle did not decrease significantly in the first 2 weeks, but a significant reduction (by nearly half) was detected at 54 days. At 10 and 16 days of treatment with pivmecillinam, the $\dot{V}O_2$max heart rate and ventilation were unchanged; however, they had decreased by day 54 and were significantly correlated with the decrease in muscle carnitine concentration (Table 2). There was a significant decrease in blood lactate levels in relation to treatment time. A submaximal test was performed because of decreased $\dot{V}O_2$max at 54 days. A slight increase in the concentration of 3-hydroxybutyrate detected in serum may have been caused by decreased fatty acid oxidation in the liver. A decreased consumption of muscle glycogen was detected, indicating reduced glycolysis in the skeletal muscles. It is presumed that the muscles had enough energy available because there was no significant decrease in the concentration of adenosine triphosphate and creatine phosphate during exercise.

Conclusion.—A 54-day treatment regimen with drugs containing pivalic acid reduces carnitine concentrations to levels at which altered metabolism is observed in both cardiac and skeletal muscle and in the liver.

▶ Chronic medication often has more side effects than we realize. Here, chronic use of antibiotics for urinary infection apparently led to a 12% decrease in $\dot{V}O_2$max. Other studies by the same investigators have shown a 20% decrease in left ventricular mass[1] with a similar pattern of treatment. Both experimental subjects and controls were initially healthy, so that the deterioration in performance seems to be a real effect of using an antibiotic conjugated with pivalic acid and resulting severe carnitine depletion.

R.J. Shephard, M.D., Ph.D., D.P.E.

Reference

1. Abrahamsson K, Mellander M, Eriksson BO, et al: Transient reduction of human left ventricular muscle mass in carnitine depletion induced by antibiotics containing pivalic acid. *Br Heart J* 74:656–659, 1995.

Leptin Is Related to Body Fat Content in Male Distance Runners

Hickey MS, Considine RV, Israel RG, et al (East Carolina Univ, Greenville, NC; Thomas Jefferson Univ, Philadelphia; Colorado State Univ, Fort Collins)
Am J Physiol 271:E938–E940, 1996   7–28

Introduction.—There is poor understanding of the biological mechanisms that contribute to the chronic imbalance between energy intake and expenditure in obesity. In humans, it has been recently reported that circulating OB protein (leptin) is positively correlated with body fat. In obese persons, leptin concentrations are fourfold higher than in humans of normal body mass. Little is known about the association between physical activity and leptin turnover. The influence of chronic endurance training and the effect of acute exercise on serum leptin levels in humans were studied.

Methods.—Blood samples were obtained from 13 male distance runners after an overnight fast and after they had completed a 20-mile treadmill run at 70% of maximal oxygen intake under controlled environmental conditions. The men had a mean age of 32.2 ± 2.5 years, a mean height of 1.76 ± 0.02 m, a mean body mass of 71.9 ± 6.9 kg, a mean percentage fat of 9.7 ± 0.9%, and maximal oxygen intake of 62.9 ± 2.2 mL/kg per minute.

Results.—In the runners, serum leptin was closely related to fat mass. Serum leptin levels were not affected by acute exercise. Before exercise, the serum leptin levels were 2.19 ± 0.32 ng/mL, and after exercise they were 2.14 ± 0.36 ng/mL. The mean fasting plasma insulin value of 28.3 ± 3.9 pm/L was not related to leptin concentration.

Conclusion.—The circulating leptin concentration is closely related to fat content, even at a biological extreme of body fat. Acute exhaustive exercise has no immediate effect on the circulating leptin concentration in trained individuals with low leptin concentrations. Chronic changes in energy metabolism may be related to the dynamics of leptin production and/or clearance.

▶ There has been vigorous debate as to how far obesity can be blamed on a person's heredity. We have known for some time that it is possible to breed a form of mouse with a specific *ob* gene that makes it highly prone to obesity. Recently, Zhang et al.[1] have found a human homologue of the obese mouse gene. It has also been shown that the adipocytes produce a chemical that regulates the intake of food.[2] One component of such "satiety information" seems to be the chemical leptin. It is remarkable that even in such thin individuals as distance runners, there is a consistent ranking of plasma leptin levels with the percentage of body fat.

R.J. Shephard, M.D., Ph.D., D.P.E.

References

1. Zhang Y, Proenca R, Barone M, et al: Positional cloning of the mouse obese gene and its human homologue. *Nature* 372:425–432, 1994.

2. Flier JS: The adipocyte: Storage depot or node on the energy information super-highway? *Cell* 80:15–18, 1995.

The Association Between Secondary Amenorrhea and Common Eating Disordered Weight Control Practices in an Adolescent Population
Selzer R, Caust J, Hibbert M, et al (Royal Children's Hosp, Parkville, Australia; Univ of Melbourne, Australia)
J Adolesc Health 19:56–61, 1996   7–29

Introduction.—Only 1 epidemiologic trial has addressed the association between disordered eating and amenorrhea. All other trials used patients attending a gynecologic service or selected university students. The peak prevalences of eating pathology and secondary amenorrhea occur during adolescence. The association between eating disorder and secondary amenorrhea was analyzed using a cross-sectional survey of students attending 43 schools in Australia.

Methods.—The mean age of the 1,025 female students surveyed was 15 years. The Branched Eating Disorders Test was administered via notebook computer. This questionnaire was used to assess amenorrhea and symptoms of eating disorder.

Results.—The response rate was 86% (886 students). Two hundred five students (23%) reported either fasting or purging in the previous month. Thirty-five students (4.1%) reported secondary amenorrhea of at least 3 months' duration. Of the 35 students who reported secondary amenorrhea, 14 (40%) had fasted or purged in the previous month, compared with 191 (22%) in the eumenorrheic group. There was no significant correlation between amenorrhea and body mass index. The strongest association between amenorrhea and eating disorder was observed in the heaviest students.

Conclusion.—Adolescent girls of normal and above normal weight who engage in eating-disordered weight control practices may experience secondary amenorrhea. Disordered eating should be considered in adolescent females with amenorrhea. Preventive measures should be introduced before these unhealthy behaviors become entrenched.

▶ This large, cross-sectional survey of 15-year-old Australian schoolgirls finds that 23% had fasted or purged within the month and 4% had had secondary amenorrhea for at least 3 months. Amenorrhea did not corrrelate with body mass index but was twice as common (at about 7%) among girls who fasted or purged as among those who did not. In this community setting, then, amenorrhea was more strongly tied to behaviors (typical of eating disorders) than to weight. A limitation of the study is that exercise habits were not gauged; perhaps amenorrheic girls were so because they were athletes who consumed insufficient calories for their energy needs. How to recognize, treat, and prevent the "female athlete triad" (disordered eating, amenorrhea, and osteopenia) was covered in a recent 2-part roundtable.[1, 2]

E.R. Eichner, M.D.

References

1. Joy E, Clark N, Ireland ML, et al: Team management of the female athlete triad. Part 1: What to look for, what to ask. *Physician Sportsmed* 25:95–110, 1997.
2. Joy E, Clark N, Ireland ML, et al: Team management of the female athlete triad. Part 2: Optimal treatment and prevention tactics. *Physician Sportsmed* 25:55–69, 1997.

Menstrual Dysfunction in Swimmers: A Distinct Entity

Constantini NW, Warren MP (Wingate Inst, Netanya, Israel; St Luke's-Roosevelt Hosp, New York)
J Clin Endocrinol Metab 80:2740–2744, 1995   7–30

Introduction.—Reproductive system dysfunction is often seen in female ballet dancers, runners, gymnasts, and figure skaters. Swimming athletes start at a young age and perform strenuous endurance training throughout the year. It is not known whether the physical and mental demands of swimming are comparable to those of long-distance runners. Menstrual dysfunction in swimmers was evaluated to determine whether it is similar to or different from the typical hypogonadotropic hypogonadism observed in athletes with low body weight.

Methods.—Sixty-nine competitive swimmers and 279 age-matched controls older than 12 years of age completed questionnaires regarding exercise levels, height, weight, age at menarche, and menstrual history. A girl with 2 consecutive menstrual cycles shorter than 21 days or longer than 45 days was considered to have menstrual irregularity. Research subjects underwent physical examination, anthropometric measurements, determination of pubertal progression using Tanner's stages of breast and pubic hair development, and blood tests.

Results.—The mean age at menarche was significantly delayed in swimmers, compared with controls. Swimmers had a significantly higher prevalence of menstrual irregularities immediately post menarche compared with controls (82% vs. 40%) with significantly longer duration (16 months vs. 4 months). Swimmers had above average luteinizing hormone and follicle-stimulating hormone levels. The 17β-estradiol (E_2) levels were significantly higher in premenarche than in postmenarche swimmers (Table 2); they were within normal limits in all postmenarche swimmers. Both androstenedione (A) and dehydroepiandrosterone (DHEA-S) values were within normal range, but were markedly increased and above the average for sedentary girls matched for pubic hair development. All groups had normal thyroid function tests and prolactin levels.

Conclusion.—The most important finding was that swimmers did not have the low levels of gonadotropins and E_2 observed in long-distance

TABLE 2.—Hormone Concentrations in Swimmers According to Menstrual Status

Menstrual group	LH (IU/L)	FSH (IU/L)	LH/FSH ratio	E_2 (pmol/L)	Test (nmol/L)	A (nmol/L)	DHEA-S (μmol/L)
Pre-M (n = 9)	15.3 ± 1.7*	10.6 ± 0.9*	1.5 ± 0.2	383 ± 44*	1.8 ± 0.1†	6.3 ± 0.6	4.6 ± 0.6*
Nonathletes (n = 80)	1.6 ± 0.1	2.8 ± 0.1	0.6	126 ± 15	1.4 ± 0.1		2.7 ± 0.2
Post-M (n = 15)							
Regular (n = 6)	20.5 ± 2.9*	10.1 ± 1.2*	1.9 ± 0.4	247 ± 37	2.1 ± 0.2	7.0 ± 0.8	10.5 ± 1.6†
Irregular‡ (n = 9)	16.7 ± 1.7*	11.2 ± 1.3*	1.6 ± 0.2	296 ± 26	2.2 ± 0.2	7.2 ± 0.6	7.0 ± 0.9†
Nonathletes (n = 41)	2.8 ± 0.3	4.5 ± 0.3	0.6	313 ± 39	2.1 ± 0.2	4.2 (2.8–10.5)§	4.7 ± 0.3

Note: Data are summarized as the mean ± standard error with the range in parentheses. Normal levels for all hormones except androstenedione are taken from the report of Warren and Brooks-Gunn.
*$P < 0.0001$, swimmers vs. nonathletes.
†$P < 0.05$, swimmers vs. nonathletes.
‡Irregular indicates oligomenorrhea and amenorrhea.
§Normal levels of androstenedione are taken from the report of Winter et al., 1978.
Abbreviations: *LH*, luteinizing hormone; *FSH*, follicle-stimulating hormone; E_2, 17β-estradiol; *Test*, testosterone; *A*, androstenedione; *DHEA-S*, dehydroepiandrosterone; *M*, menarche.
(Courtesy of Constantini NW, Warren MP: Menstrual dysfunction in swimmers: A distinct entity. *J Clin Endocrinol Metab* 80(9):2740–2744, copyright 1995, The Endocrine Society.)

runners and ballet dancers. The androgen levels (A and DHEA-S) were significantly higher in swimmers than in controls. The reproductive profile in athletes who are required to maintain low body weight is different from that found in swimmers. Other mechanisms need to be considered in sports that require strength and not leanness.

▶ Concluding that the hormonal profiles of 9 swimmers with menstrual irregularities represent an entity distinct from that reported for amenorrheic runners and dancers should be no surprise. Blood samples taken from oligomenorrheic swimmers on a "random day" might well reflect normal levels of reproductive hormones as the swimmers were not amenorrheic. In this study, "irregular" was defined as a cycle less than 21 days or longer than 45 days, whereas most studies of amenorrheic athletes rely on determination of E_2 levels as part of their inclusion criteria. Only a comparison of swimmers and runners with similar menstrual patterns can determine whether different mechanisms are at work.

The hormone data for the control group apparently were taken from a study conducted several years before this one. This raises a number of questions regarding the validity of this comparison. Other investigators will have to replicate these results before I am convinced that 2 mechanisms are at work here.

B.L. Drinkwater, Ph.D.

Nutritional and Endocrine-Metabolic Aberrations in Amenorrheic Athletes
Laughlin GA, Yen SSC (Univ of California, San Diego)
J Clin Endocrinol Metab 81:4301–4309, 1996   7–31

Introduction.—Menstrual disorders in female athletes who do not have adequate compensatory increases in dietary intake may be caused by adaptive mechanisms working to conserve metabolic fuel. The interrelationship of energy balance and regulators of metabolic fuel and the link between the suppression of luteinizing hormone (LH) pulsatility and putative metabolic signals were evaluated in 24 women with exercise-induced menstrual disorders.

Methods.—Women were assigned to 1 of 3 groups based on menstrual status and exercise training level: normal menstrual cycles and little exercise activity (cyclic sedentary; CS), normal menstrual cycles and a regular, high level of exercise (cyclic athletes; CA), and amenorrhea for at least 6 months and high exercise levels equal to those in the cyclic athletes group (amenorrheic athletes; AA). There were 8 women in each group. Dual energy x-ray absorptiometry (DEXA) was used to determine body composition. Nutritional intake, insulin sensitivity (by rapid IV glucose tolerance test), and 24-hour dynamics of insulin/glucose, cortisol, somatropic growth hormone (GH)/GH-binding protein (GHBP)/insulin-like growth factor I (IGF-1)/IGF-binding proteins (IBFBPs), and LH axes were simultaneously characterized in the CS, CA, and AA groups. Seven-day diet records were kept by all women.

Results.—The CA group had significantly higher maximum oxygen consumption than the AA group. Basal body temperature was significantly lower in AA, compared with CA or CS (Table 1). All 3 groups were within the follicular phase range for levels of LH, follicle-stimulating hormone, androstenedione, and testosterone. The daily caloric intakes were similar in all 3 groups, despite an average of 900–1000 calories per day expended during exercise in CA and AA. The AA group consumed significantly less fat and more carbohydrate than did CA and CS. The average relative fat content of AA, CA, and CS diets was 13.2%, 24.4%, and 31.6%, respectively. Average percent of carbohydrate consumption was 70.2%, 53.8%, and 51.6%, respectively, for AA, CA, and CS, and average dietary protein consumption was 11.8%, 12.4%, and 17.5%, respectively. Compared with CS, insulin sensitivity was significantly increased in AA and CA. The plasma glucose levels were significantly lower and were accompanied by more pronounced hypoinsulinemia during feeding and fasting in AA than CA and CS. The greater degree of hypoinsulinemia in AA was correlated with a marked rise in IGFB-1 concentrations throughout the day. Compared with CS, the 24-hour mean levels of cortisol were significantly increased in CA and AA. Pulse amplitude was increased 60% in CA with no change in pulse number; in AA, the GH pulse frequency and interpulse GH levels were elevated. There were no between-group differences in 24-hour mean LH pulse amplitude and integrated levels. Compared with CS, the LH pulse frequency was decreased 30% and 50% in CA and AA, respectively, during waking hours but not during sleep. Cortisol and IGFBP-1 were significant independent negative factors and accounted for 65% of variance in LH pulse frequency.

TABLE 1.—Clinical Characteristics of CS, CA, and AA

	CS (n = 8)	CA (n = 8)	AA (n = 8)
Age (yr)	27.5 ± 1.8	30.7 ± 1.2	26.3 ± 1.5
H (cm)	168 ± 3	170 ± 1	169 ± 2
W (kg)	57.5 ± 3.1	58.1 ± 1.6	55.2 ± 2.2
BMI (kg/m²)	20.2 ± 0.6	19.6 ± 0.4	19.4 ± 0.6
% Body fat[a]	23.4 ± 0.9	15.9 ± 1.3[b]	16.0 ± 1.5[b]
% Lean body mass[a]	71.0 ± 0.7	78.7 ± 1.1[b]	78.3 ± 1.5[b]
Basal oral temperature (°F)	97.8 ± 0.1	97.5 ± 0.2	96.8 ± 0.3[b,c]
Age at menarche (yr)	12.9 ± 0.4	13.4 ± 0.4	14.3 ± 0.5
Gynecological age (yr)	14.7 ± 2.0	17.3 ± 1.4	11.9 ± 1.2
Duration of amenorrhea (yr)			4.1 ± 0.6
Resting heart rate (beats/min)	62.1 ± 2.3	46.6 ± 2.0[b]	48.1 ± 2.0[b]
Maximal aerobic capacity (ml/kg · min)[d]	39.0 ± 0.8	60.8 ± 3.0[b]	53.8 ± 1.0[b,c]
Duration of aerobic training (yr)		7.1 ± 1.7	6.6 ± 1.6
Exercise energy expenditure (Cal/day)	62 ± 19	906 ± 68[b]	1074 ± 106[b]

(Courtesy of Laughlin GA, Yen SSC: Nutritional and endocrine-metabolic aberrations in amenorrheic athletes. *J Clin Endocrinol Metab* 81:4301–4309, 1996.)

Values are the mean ± SE.
a Measured by DEXA.
b *P* <0.001 *vs.* CA.
c *P* <0.05 *vs.* CA.
d Measured by a running protocol.

Conclusion.—The lower levels of insulin and glucose in AA, along with manifestations of hypothyroidemia, decreased basal body temperature, and resting metabolic rate, suggest an overall negative energy balance in AA, compared with CA. The greater reduction in gonadtropin-releasing hormone/LH generator activity may be related to the dual impacts of a decreased stimulatory effect of IGF-1 consequent to increased IGFBP-1 and central inhibitory effects of corticotropin-releasing factor.

▶ Evidence is accumulating that the cause of the amenorrhea experienced by some athletes may be traced to an imbalance between the energy expended and that provided by dietary intake. Although the precise mechanism by which this imbalance interrupts the normal cycle is of interest to scientists, coaches and health professionals responsible for the welfare of the athlete should ensure that their athletes have access to nutritional counseling. Amenorrhea is not an indication of peak conditioning as some athletes believe but should be viewed as a "red flag"—a warning that they should seek the advice of their physician.

B.L. Drinkwater, Ph.D.

Hypoestrogenemia and Rhabdomyelysis (Myoglobinuria) in the Female Judoist: A New Worrying Phenomenon?

de Crée C, Lewin R, Barros A (Inst for Gyneco-Endocrinological Research, Leuven, Belgium; Univ of Copenhagen; Univ of Coimbra, Portugal)
J Clin Endocrinol Metab 80:3639–3646, 1995   7–32

Introduction.—To meet weight categories, many lightwight and middleweight judoists use diet and long-distance running to lose a lot of weight in a short period. Judo is an intense sport with complex demands on aerobic and anaerobic resistance and endurance, raising questions about its catabolic effect on muscle and bone. Menstruation and bone and muscle metabolism were assessed in female judoists.

Methods.—Three groups of nulliparous young women were studied: 17 competitive judoists, 12 top-class rowers, and 12 sedentary controls. Information on athletic history, menstrual and gynecologic history, injury history, and eating behavior was collected from all subjects. Physical examination and physiologic tests were performed to determine anthropometric values, body fat percentage, peak and submaximal oxygen consumption, functional aerobic power, blood pressure, heart rate, and ECG results. Pretraining maximal exercise tests were performed during the follicular phase and the luteal phase of the menstrual cycle. The same tests were repeated in the judoists after a 5-week, pre-Olympic program of aerobic, anaerobic, and weight training. Laboratory tests included blood hormone analyses, blood biochemical studies, and urine biochemical studies. From 2 days before to 2 days after the urine samples were collected, the women followed a recommended dietary allowance–sufficient lactovegetarian diet.

Results.—The 3 groups were similar in age, height, and at menarche. There were significant differences in percent body fat and percentage of ideal body weight, with percent body fat being lowest in the judoists. Aerobic capacity was higher in the judoists than in the sedentary controls but not as high as in the endurance-trained rowers. Five weeks of vigorous training produced significant reductions in body weight and percent body fat in the judoists. The percentage of judoists with oligomenorrhea in-

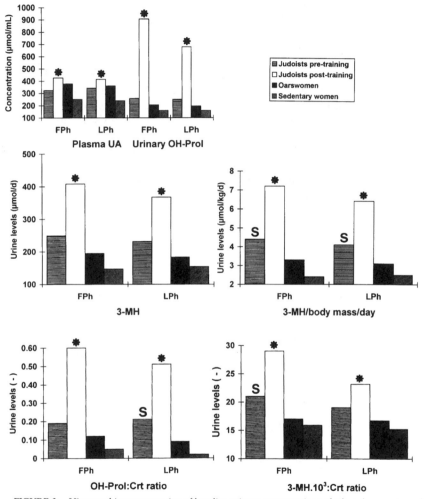

FIGURE 3.—Histographic representation of baseline urinary concentrations of selected parameters of bone and collagen turnover in judoists (before and after training) and in reference groups. *Asterisk* indicates significant difference ($P < 0.05$) compared with pretraining levels; *s* indicates significant difference ($P < 0.05$) between pretraining levels in judoists and those in a reference group of rowers. *Abbreviations:* *FPh,* follicular phase; *LPh,* luteal phase; *UA,* uric acid; *OH-Prol,* hydroxyproline; *Crt,* creatinine; *3-MH,* 3-methylhistidine. (Courtesy of de Crée C, Lewin R, Barros A: Hypoestrogenemia and rhabdomyelysis (myoglobinuria) in the female judoist: A new worrying phenomenon? *J Clin Endocrinol Metab* 80(12): 3639–3646, copyright 1995, The Endocrine Society.)

creased from 23.5% before training to 52% afterward. The 2 groups of athletes had significantly lower estrogen levels than the sedentary controls and in comparison with reference laboratory values. In the judoists, plasma myoglobin increased sharply after training, in association with muscle soreness, limited muscle recovery, and mild training injuries. The judoists also had high bone turnover, as evidenced by a rise in urinary hydroxyproline levels (Fig 3). Estrogen status was significantly and negatively correlated with rhabdomyelysis.

Conclusion.—This study of female judoists during rigorous training shows extremely high levels of blood diagnostic enzymes, together with low estrogen levels, high bone turnover, and muscle catabolism findings. The results imply a form of acute, possibly hypoestrogenic, rhabdomyelysis. High circulating levels of stress hormones could provoke hypothalamic hypoestrogenemia in athletes, thus playing a role in muscle catabolism and bone turnover. Data on endogenous excretion of 3-methylhistidine and its level in skeletal muscle during vigorous training suggest rapid wasting of muscle mass and thus a large increase in the risk of muscle injury.

▶ It is always disturbing to read articles that ascribe menstrual irregularities among some female athletes to "...strenuous engagement in aerobic endurance sports..." as these authors do in their abstract. To my knowledge, the cause of these irregularities is still undetermined. The most recent work in this area has focused on the interaction of caloric intake and energy expenditure. As the authors point out, judo has strict weight categories and many "...judoists have to engage in rigorous dieting and long distance running to lose much weight in a short period of time."

The decrease in body weight and percent body fat in these judoists indicates a caloric deficit and perhaps a nutritional deficit as well. Whether the caloric restriction in an attempt to meet weight played a part in the increase in muscle catabolism was not addressed. In addition, the biochemical marker for bone turnover is not specific to bone and does not provide any information about the balance between bone resorption and formation.

B.L. Drinkwater, Ph.D.

8 Medical Conditions

Cardiovascular Preparticipation Screening of Competitive Athletes
American Heart Association (Dallas)
Med Sci Sports Exerc 28:1445–1452, 1996   8–1

Background.—The sudden death of a competitive athlete is a shocking event that raises many ethical and practical issues. Recommendations for the preparticipation cardiovascular screening of competitive athletes were developed by a panel appointed by the American Heart Association.

Preparticipation Cardiovascular Screening.—Some form of preparticipation cardiovascular screening for high school and collegiate athletes is warranted. The best available and most practical approach to screening populations of competitive athletes of any age includes a complete and careful personal and physical examination to identify or raise suspicion of cardiovascular lesions known to cause sudden death or disease progression in young athletes. The physical examination must include precordial auscultation in the supine and standing positions to identify heart murmurs consistent with dynamic left ventricular outflow obstruction; femoral artery pulse assessment to exclude coarctation of the aorta; a check for the physical stigmata of Marfan syndrome; and brachial blood pressure measures obtained in the sitting position. Important information to note during history taking includes the previous occurrence of exertional chest pain or discomfort or syncope/near-syncope as well as excessive, unexpected, and unexplained shortness of breath or fatigue associated with exercise; previous detection of a heart murmur or increased systemic blood pressure; and family history of premature death, sudden or otherwise, and significant disability from cardiovascular disease in close relatives younger than 50 years of age or occurrence of certain conditions, such as hypertrophic cardiomyopathy, dilated cardiomyopathy, long QT syndrome, Marfan syndrome, or clinically important arrhythmias. Screening should be done before participation and every 2 years thereafter. An interim history should be obtained between these screening sessions. A national standard should be developed for preparticipation medical evaluations.

Conclusions.—Preparticipation cardiovascular screening of competitive athletes is advised. When cardiovascular abnormalities are suspected or identified, the patient should be referred to a cardiovascular specialist for further assessment.

▶ The issue of the sudden cardiovascular death of young athletes during competition is attracting growing attention. This paper from the American Heart Association also has the endorsement of the American Academy of Pediatrics, the American College of Cardiology, and the American College of Sports Medicine—a pretty impressive list of credentials, although many of the same people were probably expressing their opinions through each of these organizations.

The big question is whether vulnerable individuals can be detected by extensive preliminary screening. The development of echocardiography offered the hope that measurement of cardiac dimensions might identify many of those at risk. However, time has seen a progressive shift in the supposed upper limits of normal ventricular dimensions, and it is now recognized that even if extensive screening has been undertaken, hypertrophic cardiomyopathy is rarely detected before death. The potential value of genetic screening also attracted interest for a brief period, but it was soon recognized that a variety of genetic abnormalities can cause abnormalities in myocardial development and that people with such abnormalities live to a ripe old age. Probably the best warning of danger still comes from the premature death of other family members. A key sentence in the American Heart Association report should put to an end the time and money that has been wasted on ill-conceived screening in cardiac departments: "... it is not prudent to recommend routine use of such tests as 12-lead electrocardiography, echocardiography or graded exercise testing for detection of cardiovascular disease in large populations of young or older athletes."

R.J. Shephard, M.D., Ph.D., D.P.E.

Circulatory Responses to Weight Lifting, Walking, and Stair Climbing in Older Males
Benn SJ, McCartney N, McKelvie RS (McMaster Univ, Hamilton, Ont, Canada)
J Am Geriatr Soc 44:121–125, 1996   8–2

Introduction.—Although weight lifting and stair climbing are becoming more common in exercise training programs, little is known about the relative circulatory responses to these forms of exercise in older people. More detailed information regarding the circulatory responses was provided for horizontal treadmill walking with and without load carrying, walking uphill, stair climbing, and weight lifting. Continuous, intra-arterial measurements of blood pressure were compared among the exercises.

Methods.—Seventeen healthy males aged 64.4 ± 0.6 years had intrabrachial artery catheterization to compare arterial blood pressure and heart responses during various exercises: 10 repetitions of the single-arm curl and single-arm overhead military press; 12 repetitions of the single- and double-leg press weight-lifting exercises; 10 minutes of horizontal tread-mill walking at 4 km/h holding a 9 kg (20-lb) weight in minutes 4–6 and a 13.6 kg (30-lb weight) in minutes 8–10; 4 minutes of treadmill walking at 4.8 km/h up an 8% incline; and 12 flights of stair climbing at 60–65 steps/min. There were continuous intra-arterial measurements taken of systolic, diastolic, and mean arterial pressure, as well as heart rate and rate-pressure product.

Results.—Among the various activities, the peak values of heart rate, arterial blood pressure, and rate-pressure product were not systematically ordered. During the initial 4 minutes of horizontal treadmill walking, the lower peak values for all variables were recorded. Higher heart rates were found with stair climbing (151 ± 3.2 bpm) and treadmill walking up an 8% incline (121 ± 3.4 bpm) than for single-arm curls (100 ± 4.8 bpm), and single-arm overhead military presses (113 ± 3.8 bpm). Diastolic pressure, however, was higher for the weightlifting exercises with single-arm curls (128 ± 6.3 mm Hg) and single-arm overhead military presses (151 ± 4.8 mm Hg) than for treadmill walking (101 ± 2.5 mm Hg) and treadmill walking holding a 13.6 kg weight (118 ± 3.4 mm Hg). The mean arterial pressure was 145 ± 4.5 mm Hg for single-arm curls and 158 ± 4.8 mm Hg for single-arm military presses, whereas it was 129 ± 3.4 mm Hg for treadmill walking up an 8% incline, 148 ± 3.8 mm Hg for treadmill walking holding a 9 kg weight, and 157 ± 4.1 mm Hg for stair climbing. In the stair climbing, the peak systolic pressure was greatest with 271 ± 9.6 mm Hg. The peak rate-pressure product descended in sequence as follows: stair climbing, single-arm presses, treadmill walking at an 8% incline, double-leg press, treadmill walking holding a 13.6 kg weight, single-leg press, treadmill walking holding a 9 kg weight, and single-arm curl.

Conclusion.—Weight lifting with heavy submaximal loads will not cause more peak circulatory stress in older males than that created while walking on a treadmill at an incline. Peak circulatory demands caused by climbing 3–4 flights of stairs at a moderate pace are similar to the peak circulatory demands caused by 10 minutes of horizontal walking intermit-tently carrying a 13.6 kg weight or 4 minutes of walking up a moderately steep slope. Stair climbing, however, causes circulatory responses that are more pronounced than responses to the other forms of exercise. When older adults incorporate stair climbing, the circulatory responses should be monitored closely.

▶ A surprisingly large percentage of old people are unable to perform daily tasks such as grocery shopping alone because of a progressive deterioration in arm strength. There is, thus, growing interest in the potential for slowing, and even reversing, the loss of muscle function by participation in various forms of resistance exercise.[1] Occasionally, concerns are raised regarding the possible impact of such exercise on elderly individuals with an ischemic myocardium.

This study of 65-year-old individuals makes a useful comparison between moderate-paced walking while intermittently carrying a 20- or 30-lb load and another form of exercise commonly recommended for the elderly: climbing

3–4 flights of stairs at a moderate pace. The peak blood pressures reached under the 2 conditions are quite similar, but the stair climbing is probably more dangerous than load carrying, because the peak pressures are reached much more rapidly. The professor emeritus who walks briskly to work carrying a heavy briefcase in each hand may well be performing close to an optimum workout.

R.J. Shephard, M.D., Ph.D., D.P.E.

Reference

1. Fiatarone M, O'Neill EF, Doyle Ryan N, et al: Exercise training and nutritional supplementation for physical frailty in very elderly people. *N Engl J Med* 330:1769–1775, 1994.

Sedentary Lifestyle and Risk of Coronary Heart Disease in Women
Eaton CB, Lapane KL, Garber CA, et al (Brown Univ, Providence, RI; Mem Hosp of Rhode Island, Pawtucket)
Med Sci Sports Exerc 27:1535–1539, 1995   8–3

Introduction.—Reports vary regarding the relationship of sedentary lifestyle and coronary heart disease (CHD) in women. With the use of a nested case-control design, the effect of sedentary lifestyle on CHD in women was prospectively evaluated after adjusting for the potential confounders of hypertension, cigarette smoking, high-density lipoprotein (HDL) cholesterol, and diabetes mellitus.

Methods.—Data were collected from the Pawtucket Heart Health Program demonstration project that has conducted 6 biennial surveys of single, randomly selected adults aged 18–64 years living in randomly selected households. Fifty women with acute CHD and 150 age-matched controls (matched for gender, age, and city of intervention) without evidence of CHD were interviewed in their homes regarding activity level, blood pressure, total serum cholesterol, HDL cholesterol, body mass index (BMI), and cigarette smoking.

Results.—Women with CHD were more likely to have higher systolic blood pressure, higher total cholesterol, lower HDL cholesterol, higher BMI, history of diabetes mellitus, history of present and/or past smoking, and sedentary lifestyle, compared with controls. Women with sedentary lifestyle from both groups had risk factor profiles similar to those of women with CHD. Lower HDL cholesterol, slightly higher BMI, cigarette smoking, and diagnosis of diabetes were observed more frequently in sedentary than in active women. The adjusted odds ratio of CHD for sedentary lifestyle for women in this cohort was 2.3 (Table 3).

Conclusion.—These findings cannot be considered conclusive as the results are open to several contradictory interpretations. Further investigation is needed before a relationship between sedentary lifestyle and CHD in women can be established.

TABLE 3.—Adjusted Odds Ratio Relating Sedentary Lifestyle to Coronary Heart Disease in Women

	Adjusted OR*	95% Confidence Interval
Sedentary lifestyle	2.3	(1.0–5.7)
Low HDL (<35 mg · dl⁻¹)	6.5	(2.0–21.4)
Diabetes mellitus	4.0	(1.2–13.8)
Smoking	2.5	(1.1–5.8)
Hypertension	1.5	(0.6–3.4)
Born in U.S.	4.0	(0.6–25.4)

*Estimated using conditional maximum likelihood regression.
Abbreviations: OR, odds ratio; HDL, high-density lipoprotein.
(Courtesy of Eaton CB, Lapane KL, Garber CA, et al: Sedentary lifestyle and risk of coronary heart disease in women. *Med Sci Sports Exerc* 27(11):1535–1539, 1995.)

▶ Conclusions about the role of physical activity in decreasing the risk of CHD in women have been mixed in previous studies. Considering that CHD is a major cause of mortality in older women, there is a need for a definitive study on the question. Do we or do we not encourage women to become more physically active because it will decrease their risk of CHD? And how do we define "active"? In this study, active was defined as more than 1 hour of activity per week or an activity that resulted in sweating. To most of us, this definition falls short in discriminating an active woman from her sedentary peer. More thought needs to be given to not only the amount of activity but the quality of it as well.

B.L. Drinkwater, Ph.D.

Maximal Exercise Hemodynamics and Risk of Mortality in Apparently Healthy Men and Women

Kohl HW III, Nichaman MZ, Frankowski RF, et al (Childhood & Adolescent Health, Dallas; Univ of Texas-Houston Health Science Ctr)
Med Sci Sports Exerc 28:601–609, 1996   8–4

Background.—Risk factor screenings and resting ECG patterns appear to be of limited value in predicting death from cardiovascular disease (CVD) in otherwise healthy individuals. Exercise tests provide additional information, yet the positive predictive value of exercise ECG abnormalities relative to the development of either coronary heart disease (CHD) or CHD mortality in apparently healthy men and women has ranged from 5% to 46%. Participants in an ongoing prospective cohort study were followed to determine the association of maximal exercise hemodynamic responses with risk of mortality from all causes, CVD, and CHD.

Methods.—As part of a longitudinal study conducted at a preventive medicine clinic, 43,164 individuals were evaluated during 1971–1989. Participants underwent clinical examinations, laboratory tests, and maximal exercise treadmill tests and completed a medical history questionnaire. Those with a history of high blood pressure, stroke, diabetes,

TABLE 4.—Multivariate-adjusted Relative Risk Estimates for All-Cause, Cardiovascular Disease (CVD), and Coronary Heart Disease (CHD) Mortality for Specific Differences in Maximal Exercise Hemodynamic Responses in 20,387 and 6,234 Apparently Healthy Men and Women: ACLS, 1971–1989

Hemodynamic Factor	Difference*	Relative Risk	95% CI
All-cause mortality			
Men			
Maximal SBP (mm Hg)	55	1.30	0.97–1.72
Maximal HR (bpm)	35	0.51	0.37–0.71
Women			
Maximal SBP (mm Hg)	55	1.08	0.51–2.29†
Maximal HR (bpm)	35	1.22	0.57–2.60
CVD mortality			
Men			
Maximal SBP (mm Hg)	55	1.31	0.78–2.20
Maximal HR (bpm)	35	0.63	0.34–1.17
Women			
Maximal SBP (mm Hg)	55	3.46	0.71–16.9
Maximal HR (bpm)	35	0.92	0.18–4.63
CHD mortality (men)			
Maximal SBP (mm Hg)	55	1.54	0.80–2.98
Maximal HR (bpm)	35	0.57	0.26–1.27

Note: Each model for men and women was adjusted for age, body mass index, resting systolic blood pressure, treadmill time, fasting serum cholesterol and glucose, family history of CVD, abnormal exercise ECG, and smoking habit. Models included 20,371 men and 6,203 women.

*Difference calculated between mean of fourth and first quartiles of specific hemodynamic factor.

Abbreviations: SBP, systolic blood pressure; HR, heart rate; ACLS, Aerobics Center Longitudinal Study.

(Courtesy of Kohl HW III, Nichaman MZ, Frankowski RF, et al: Maximal exercise hemodynamics and risk of mortality in apparently healthy men and women. *Med Sci Sports Exerc* 28:601–609, 1996.)

myocardial infarction, or an abnormal resting or maximal exercise ECG at baseline were excluded. The final analysis cohort included 20,387 men and 6,234 women who were followed for an average of approximately 8 years.

Results.—There were 414 known deaths in the study cohort during follow-up (348 men and 66 women). Fifty-six men died of CHD and 92 died of CVD; among the women, CHD was the cause of 4 and CVD the cause of 13 deaths. Both maximal heart rate and maximal systolic blood pressure (SBP) measured during the maximal exercise test were related to risk of all-cause, CVD, and CHD mortality (Table 4). Men who died had an age-adjusted mean maximal SBP that averaged 2.4 mm Hg higher than that of surviving men; men who survived had a significantly higher maximal heart rate (4.3 beats per minute) than those who died. These measures did not differ significantly for surviving and nonsurviving women. After adjustment for confounding variables, men with a maximal SBP >200 mm Hg were at a 37% increased risk of death from all causes when compared with men whose pressures increased <171 mm Hg. A 35 beats per minute higher value of maximal heart rate was associated with a 36% decreased CVD mortality in men and an 8% lower risk in women.

Discussion.—In a large group of apparently healthy individuals followed for an average of 8 years, there was a direct association between maximal exercise SBP and mortality and an inverse association between maximal exercise heart rate and mortality. After adjustment for potential confounding variables, the association between maximal exercise SBP and mortality from all causes, CVD, and CHD was nonsignificant, whereas the inverse association between maximal exercise heart rate and all-cause mortality was significant in men. Findings among women were of limited value because of the small number of deaths in this cohort.

▶ Bruce has long argued that when the maximal oxygen intake is being measured, much can be learned not only from the peak oxygen transport itself, but also from other characteristics of the test performance.[1] The present data set provides a sustained (8-year) follow-up of a population that was initially apparently healthy. After careful statistical adjustment for other cardiac risk factors, prognosis was significantly influenced by the peak heart rate attained during treadmill exercise, and in the men (although not in the smaller sample of women) there was close to a significant relationship between prognosis and maximal SBP. The heart rate effect might be thought to indicate a "sick sinus syndrome" response or impaired left ventricular function secondary to silent myocardial ischemia. If so, it is important to emphasize that even the lowest heart rates exceeded the traditional threshold for the diagnosis of sick sinus syndrome (85% of the age-predicted maximal value). The apparent adverse influence of a high exercise blood pressure probably reflects the tendency for such individuals to have either hypertension[2, 3] or left ventricular hypertrophy,[3] both of which would increase the risk of subsequent death. Although the data seem to support the views of Bruce regarding the value of "ancillary information," it is important to note that the statistical significance of the findings depended in part on a huge sample size (20,387 men and 6,234 women). There was much interindividual variation, and it is less certain that we can advise the individual about prognosis on the basis that they have a low peak heart rate or a high exercise blood pressure during maximal testing.

R.J. Shephard, M.D., Ph.D., D.P.E.

References

1. Bruce RA, Derouen TA, Hossack KF: Value of maximal exercise tests in risk assessment of primary coronary heart disease events in healthy men. *Am J Cardiol* 46:371–378, 1980.
2. Amery A, Julius S, Whitlock LS, et al: Influence of hypertension on the hemodynamic response to exercise. *Circulation* 36:231–237, 1967.
3. Mahoney LT, Schieken RM, Clarke WR, et al: Left ventricular mass and exercise response predict future blood pressure. *Hypertension* 12:206–213, 1988.

Acute Aerobic Exercise Reduces Ambulatory Blood Pressure in Borderline Hypertensive Men and Women

Brownley KA, West SG, Hinderliter AL, et al (Univ of North Carolina, Chapel Hill)

Am J Hypertens 9:200–206, 1996   8–5

Background.—Postexercise hypotension (PEH)—a sustained blood pressure (BP) decrease to less than control levels after one bout of exercise—is a possible mechanism underlying the association of regular physical activity and reduced risk of hypertension, coronary heart disease, and mortality. The relationship of PEH with ambulatory BP in a sample of normotensive and borderline hypertensive men and women was investigated.

Methods.—Eleven subjects with increased resting and ambulatory BP and 20 normotensive subjects underwent ambulatory BP monitoring after 20 minutes of moderate aerobic cycle ergometry and after an equivalent rest period. For each individual, mean BP and heart rate (HR) levels were determined on an hourly basis and at work, at home, and during sleep.

Findings.—In patients with increased BP, a lower BP at work was documented on the exercise day compared with the control day. Hourly analyses demonstrated that the exercise-induced reduction in BP was significant for 5 hours, declining between 6 and 9 hours (Fig 3). These effects were not explained by marked mood differences, total daily stress, posture, or activities between test days. Exercise was uncorrelated with differences in sleep BP or in the 24-hour HR profile. In the normotensive group, exercise did not affect BP or HR. However, the exercise-induced decrease in mean arterial BP for 2–5 hours had a significant positive association with control day mean arterial BP levels at work in the entire sample.

Conclusions.—In individuals with borderline hypertension, ambulatory blood pressures are reduced for about 5 hours after 1 episode of moderate aerobic exercise. Such exercise appears to have no effect on ambulatory BP or HR in normotensive individuals.

► The "white-coat" effect and habituation to a doctor's office are important considerations when analyzing BPs. The authors of this report note that some earlier studies claiming a reduction of BP with exercise failed to use a balanced design, so that part of the apparent benefit of exercise could have arisen from habituation. Brownley et al. avoided this pitfall and demonstrated that the beneficial effect of exercise gradually waned during the first 5 hours after an exercise bout. Further, they argued that frequent repetition of a 5-hour reduction of pressures translates into improved cardiovascular health.

R.J. Shephard, M.D., Ph.D., D.P.E.

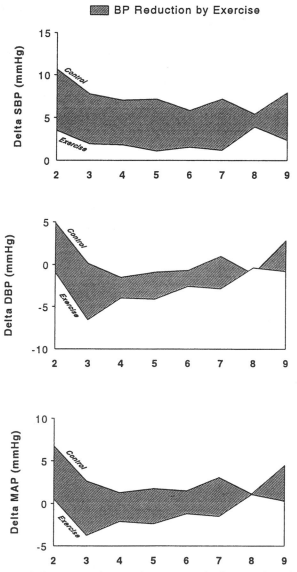

FIGURE 3.—Hour-by-hour contrast between change in control and exercise day ambulatory systolic, diastolic, and mean arterial blood pressures in the 11 subjects in the elevated blood pressure group. Exercise values are significantly less than control values for hours 2–5 for all 3 measurements ($P < 0.047$). *Abbreviations: BP,* blood pressure; *SBP,* systolic blood pressure; *DBP,* diastolic blood pressure; *MAP,* mean arterial pressure. (Reprinted by permission of Elsevier Science Inc. from Brownley KA, West SG, Hinderliter AL, et al: Acute aerobic exercise reduces ambulatory blood pressure in borderline hypertensive men and women. *Am J Hypertens* 9:200–206, Copyright 1996 by American Journal of Hypertension, Inc.)

Anticipatory Blood Pressure Response to Exercise Predicts Future High Blood Pressure in Middle-aged Men

Everson SA, Kaplan GA, Goldberg DE, et al (Western Consortium for Public Health, Berkeley, Calif; California Dept of Health, Berkeley; Univ of Kuopio, Finland)

Hypertension 27:1059–1064, 1996   8–6

Background.—Increased blood pressure in anticipation of exercise reflects cardiovascular adjustments to psychological and behavioral stress and is known as cardiovascular reactivity. Such increases in blood pressure have not been studied in relation to risk of hypertension. There is evidence that behavior-induced cardiovascular reactivity may be a risk marker for hypertension. Men at high risk for hypertension show the greatest blood pressure responses during casual stethoscopic readings and during standard laboratory challenges. There is little information on this reactivity hypothesis. The relationship between cardiovascular reactivity to psychological stimuli and future hypertension was investigated.

Methods.—In 508 randomly selected, population-based, middle-aged men, blood pressure data were obtained on 2 occasions. Blood pressure was first taken at seated rest and then 1 week later after subjects had been sitting on a cycle ergometer for 5 minutes but before exercise testing had begun. Blood pressure was again assessed in these subjects 4 years later.

Results.—Anticipatory systolic and diastolic blood pressure responses were calculated as the difference between mean blood pressure at seated rest and blood pressure while seated on the cycle ergometer. There was a graded association between quartiles of reactivity and risk of future hy-

TABLE 2.—Association Between Blood Pressure Change in Anticipation of Exercise and Incidence of High Blood Pressure 4 Years Later: Kuopio Ischemic Heart Disease Risk Factor Study

	OR	95% CI
SBP Δ		
<10 mm Hg	Referent	...
10–19 mm Hg	2.28	1.12–4.63
20–29 mm Hg	3.02	1.51–6.07
≥30 mm Hg	4.13	2.00–8.52
DBP Δ		
<5 mm Hg	Referent	...
5–9 mm Hg	1.52	0.79–2.94
10–15 mm Hg	2.14	1.05–4.39
>15 mm Hg	3.43	1.72–6.82

Note: SBP Δ indicates difference between seated SBP measurement before exercise and average seated resting SBP measured 1 week earlier; DBP Δ, difference between seated DBP measurement before exercise and average seated resting DBP measured 1 week earlier. The OR values are from logistic regression models with adjustment for age, baseline resting SBP (baseline resting DBP in DBP Δ model), smoking, physical activity, alcohol consumption, body mass index, and maternal and paternal histories of hypertension. For SBP Δ analyses, $n = 508$; DBP Δ, $n = 501$. Cases of high blood pressure, $n = 116$.

Abbreviations: OR, odds ratio; CI, confidence interval; SBP, systolic blood pressure; DBP, diastolic blood pressure.

(Courtesy of Everson SA, Kaplan GA, Goldberg DE, et al: Anticipatory blood pressure response to exercise predicts future high blood pressure in middle-aged men. *Hypertension* 27:1059–1064, 1996. Reproduced with permission [*Hypertension*]. Copyright 1996 American Heart Association.)

pertension. Men with systolic responses of 30 mm Hg or greater or diastolic responses greater than 15 mm Hg had almost 4 times the risk of having hypertension compared with subjects with the lowest reactions (Table 2). These associations did not change after adjustment for traditional risk factors for hypertension.

Conclusions.—These findings show an association between cardiovascular reactivity to psychological stimuli and future high blood pressure. Even in very healthy subjects, greater blood pressure responses during anticipation of exercise were related to greater risk of hypertension, which suggests that cardiovascular reactivity may have negative consequences even when there is no clinical disease.

▶ It is widely accepted that an excessive blood pressure response during exercise is a harbinger of future hypertension.[1] Everson and colleagues argue that the critical factor is the extent of psychological reactivity and that an abnormal response can be seen during the anticipatory phase, immediately before the onset of exercise. A decrease in autonomic reactivity may explain much of the benefit that is obtained from regular exercise.

Reference

1. Chaney RH, Eyman RK: Blood pressure at rest and during maximal exercise and isometric exercise as predictors of systemic hypertension. *Am J Cardiol* 62:1058–1061, 1988.

R.J. Shephard, M.D., Ph.D., D.P.E.

Exaggerated Blood Pressure Response to Maximal Exercise in Endurance-trained Individuals
Tanaka H, Bassett DR Jr, Turner MJ (Univ of Tennessee, Knoxville)
Am J Hypertens 9:1099–1103, 1996   8–7

Purpose.—There is evidence that people with an exaggerated blood pressure response to maximal exercise may be prone to later development of hypertension. Little is known about how the maximal blood pressure response to exercise differs in trained vs. untrained individuals. Physical training is known to reduce the risk of hypertension; if trained subjects have an exaggerated blood pressure response to exercise, such a response would not be a useful indicator of future hypertension risk. The blood pressure responses of trained and untrained subjects to maximal exercise were compared.

Methods.—The study included 26 trained endurance athletes of both sexes and 31 untrained subjects. All had normal blood pressure and no apparent cardiovascular disease. Participants in both groups performed a maximal, graded cycle ergometry test with continuous monitoring of oxygen intake. Blood pressure was measured every minute throughout the exercise test, and the blood pressure response to maximal exercise was analyzed.

Results.—The mean maximal oxygen intake was 59 mL/kg/min in the trained group vs. 45 mL/kg/min in the untrained group. The maximal work rates were 322 W 267 W, respectively. Resting blood pressure was similar in the 2 groups. However, the trained subjects had a maximal systolic blood pressure of 225 mm Hg during exercise, compared with 204 mm Hg in the untrained subjects. The difference in systolic pressure became significant beginning at work rates of 180 W.

Conclusion.—Trained subjects have a greater blood pressure response to maximal exercise. The maximal systolic blood pressure response to exercise in endurance athletes is usually in the range of 200 to 220 mm Hg, which would usually be classified as an exaggerated blood pressure response. Because these individuals are known to have a lower risk of future hypertension, the blood pressure response to maximal exercise appears not to be be a valid predictor of hypertension risk in this population.

▶ Maurice Jetté[1] has argued strongly that an excessive blood pressure response to exercise offers a warning of future hypertension. In population terms, he is correct: several different studies have shown that hyperresponders have a twofold to tenfold increase in the risk of hypertension. However, as is so frequently the case with statistical increases in risk, it is difficult to use an excessive test response to advise the individual; well-trained individuals not only have a reduced risk of future hypertension, they also have an above average increase in blood pressure during maximal exercise.

R.J. Shephard, M.D., Ph.D., D.P.E.

Reference

1. Jetté M, Landry F, Sidney KH, et al: Exaggerated blood pressure response to exercise in the detection of hypertension. *J Cardiopulmon Rehabil* 8:171–177, 1988.

Physical Activity and Stroke Incidence in Women and Men: The NHANES I Epidemiologic Follow-up Study
Gillum RF, Mussolino ME, Ingram DD (Ctrs for Disease Control and Prevention, Hyattsville, Md)
Am J Epidemiol 143:860–869, 1996   8–8

Introduction.—Although numerous studies confirm a protective effect of physical activity for coronary heart disease, the value of exercise in reducing the risk of stroke has not been demonstrated. Data from a longitudinal cohort study were analyzed to test the hypothesis that physical inactivity is associated with increased stroke risk.

Methods.—The source of data was the National Health and Nutrition Examination Survey I (NHANES I) Epidemiologic Follow-up Study. Analysis was based on 3 waves of follow-up data collected during 1982–1984, 1986, and 1987 for participants aged 45–74 years at the initial examina-

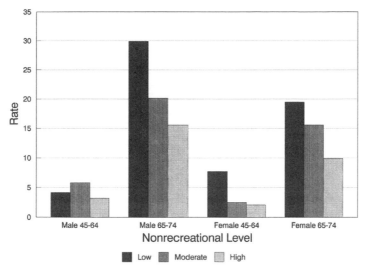

FIGURE 2.—Stroke incidence rate per 1,000 person-years by age, sex, and nonrecreational physical activity level in whites, National Health and Nutrition Examination Survey I Epidemiologic Follow-up Study, 1971–1987. (Courtesy of Gillum RF, Mussolino ME, Ingram DD: Physical activity and stroke incidence in women and men: The NHANES I Epidemiologic Follow-up Study. *Am J Epidemiol,* 143:860–869, 1996.)

tion (1971–1975). After excluding those with missing data and individuals with a positive history of stroke at baseline, 5,852 survey participants (5,081 whites and 771 blacks) remained for the analyses. Baseline medical surveys included questions on level of regular physical activity. Instances of fatal and nonfatal stroke were recorded during an average follow-up of 11.6 years and compared with the data on physical activity.

Results.—There were 623 incident cases of stroke during follow-up, 249 in white women, 270 in white men, and 104 in blacks. After adjustment for baseline factors, white women aged 65–74 years with a low level of nonrecreational activity had an increased risk of stroke (relative risk = 1.82). A similarly increased stroke incidence rate was observed in white men aged 65–74 years (Fig 2) but not in blacks. Low recreational activity was associated with increased stroke risk in men and women aged 65-74 years, but blacks exhibited no significant associations of recreational activity level with stroke risk. Among blacks, however, there was a significant association of pulse rate with the risk of stroke (comparing a pulse rate of >84 with a pulse rate of <74 beats per minute). Higher pulse rate was not associated with an increased risk of stroke in whites.

Conclusion.—Self-reported sedentary behavior was associated with an increased risk of stroke, particularly for white women. Increases in both recreational and nonrecreational activity may help to reduce the risk of stroke.

► Although the value of regular exercise in protecting against ischemic heart disease is now well accepted, there is much less evidence concerning the impact of physical activity on the incidence of stroke. [1, 2] The NHANES surveys unfortunately asked only one very simple question on each of recreational and nonrecreational activity. Nevertheless, the data show some significant associations between a sedentary lifestyle and the subsequent incidence of stroke. Possible factors contributing to the preventive value of physical activity include a reduction of systemic blood pressure, a raising of high-density lipoprotein cholesterol, a reduced probability of smoking, and an enhancement of cardiorespiratory fitness, with associated reductions in myocardial oxygen demand during daily life.

R.J. Shephard, M.D., Ph.D., D.P.E.

References

1. Shinton R, Sagar G: Lifelong exercise and stroke. *BMJ* 307: 231–234, 1993.
2. Wannamethee G, Shaper AG: Physical activity and stroke in British middle-aged men. *BMJ* 304: 597–601, 1992.

Impaired Heart Rate Response to Graded Exercise: Prognostic Implications of Chronotropic Incompetence in the Framingham Heart Study
Lauer MS, Okin PM, Larson MG, et al (Cleveland Clinic Found, Ohio; New York Hosp-Cornell Med Ctr; Boston Univ; et al)
Circulation 93:1520–1526, 1996   8–9

Introduction.—In heart disease, there has been increasing interest in the role of autonomic nervous system regulation. An important marker of risk among survivors of myocardial infarction has been heart rate variability, a marker of autonomic activity. An investigation was made to find the heart rate response to a standard, graded exercise test and to test the hypothesis that a reduced heart rate variability is associated with an adverse outcome. The relationship between exercise heart rate response and prognosis in asymptomatic patients was determined.

Methods.—Patients had participated in the Framingham Heart Study, which is an epidemiologic study of cardiovascular disease precursors. There were 1,575 male participants (mean age, 43 years) who were free of coronary heart disease in this prospective cohort investigation. All had submaximal treadmill exercise testing, and none were taking β-blockers. Their heart rate response was assessed by the actual increase in heart rate from rest to peak exercise; the ratio of heart rate to metabolic reserve, called the chronotropic response index; and failure to achieve 85% of the age-predicted maximum heart rate, considered to be the traditional definition of chronotropic incompetence. During the 7.7 years of follow-up, proportional hazard analyses were used to evaluate the associations of heart responses with coronary heart disease incidence and all-cause mortality.

Results.—There were 95 incidents of coronary heart disease and 55 deaths, 14 of which were caused by coronary heart disease. Total mortality and incident coronary heart disease were significantly predicted by failure

TABLE 6.—Late (After 2 Years of Follow-up or More) Coronary Heart Disease Incidence: Results of Multivariable Cox Proportional Hazards Regression Analyses

End Point/Heart Rate Variable	Hazard Ratio*	95% CI	P
Coronary heart disease (82 events)			
(a) Failure to achieve target HR†	1.59	0.98–2.56	.06
(b) Heart rate increase to peak†	1.24	1.05–1.46	.01
(c) Chronotropic response index			
at stage 2†	1.30	1.07–1.57	.008

*Hazard ratio to compare (1) failure vs. ability to achieve target heart rate, (2) 1 SD decrease in heart rate change from rest to peak exercise (12 bpm) or (3) 1 SD decrease in the ratio of heart rate to metabolic reserve used by stage 2 of exercise (0.20).

†Adjusted for age, ST-segment response, body mass index, smoking status, hypertension, hypertension treatment, diabetes, physical activity index, and total cholesterol/high-density lipoprotein cholesterol ratio.

Abbreviations: HR, heart rate; *CI*, confidence interval.

(Courtesy of Lauer MS, Okin PM, Larson MG, et al: Impaired heart rate response to graded exercise: Prognostic implications of chronotropic incompetence in the Framingham Heart Study. Circulation 93:1520–1526. Reproduced with permission of *Circulation*, copyright 1996, American Heart Association.)

to achieve target heart rate, a smaller increase in heart rate with exercise, and the chronotropic response index (Table 6). Incident coronary heart disease was predicted by failure to achieve the target heart rate, even after adjustments were made for age, physical activity, and traditional coronary disease risk factors. Total mortality and coronary heart disease were inversely predicted by an increase in exercise heart rate. Total mortality and coronary heart disease were also predicted by the chronotropic response index.

Conclusion.—Increased mortality and coronary heart disease incidence are predicted by an attenuated heart rate response to exercise, a manifestation of chronotropic incompetence.

▶ The sick sinus syndrome has traditionally been diagnosed when patients fail to reach 85% of the predicted maximal heart rate for their age. Unfortunately, the apparent prevalence of the disorder thus depends very much on the assumptions that the investigator makes regarding the aging of maximal heart rate.[1] However, both the causes and the prevalence of the condition merit further study, given the present analysis, which shows that chronotropic incompetence is a substantial predictor of both all-cause mortality and ischemic heart disease death after control of the data for other major risk factors.

R.J. Shephard, M.D., Ph.D., D.P.E.

Reference

1. Shephard RJ: The sick sinus syndrome (letter). *Med Sci Sports* 3:iii–iv, 1980.

Antiarrhythmic Mechanisms During Exercise

Paterson DJ (Univ Lab of Physiology, Oxford, England)
J Appl Physiol 80:1853–1862, 1996   8–10

Background.—Exercise constitutes a major disturbance of homeostasis, disturbing both cardiac sympathovagal and ionic balance. During vigorous exercise, the plasma potassium level in arterial blood is doubled, pH is reduced by 0.4, and catecholamines are elevated 15-fold. At rest, these same changes would pose an increased risk of arrhythmia and cardiac arrest. The mechanism by which the heart is protected against the chemical stress of exercise is unknown. Current knowledge of the body's protective mechanisms against the chemical stress of exercise was reviewed.

Findings.—It may be that the chemical changes mentioned above have a mutual antiarrhythmic effect. In vitro and in vivo studies have shown that catecholamines can counterbalance the harmful effects of hyperkalemia and acidosis on the heart. In potassium-depolarized ventricular myocytes, catecholamines can produce improvement in action potential characteristics. In these situations, adrenergic and noradrenergic hormones modulate an increase in the inward Ca^{2+} current. On the other hand, an elevated potassium level has protective effects against arrhythmias induced by norepinephrine. The mutual antagonism of this antiarrhythmic mechanism is lessened in the presence of acidosis, hyperkalemia, and high norepinephrine levels in a heart with regional ischemia or a small area of infarction. The period after exercise—with its low plasma potassium level and high adrenergic tone—may be the time of greatest risk. Abnormalities in the regulation of electrolytes and cardiac sympathovagal balance after exercise may lead to a higher incidence of arrhythmia, particularly in hearts with underlying ischemia. These observations may be relevant to the occurrence of exercise-related myocardial infarction and sudden death, particularly in sedentary individuals with coronary artery disease. These subjects may have disruption of the heart's normal mechanisms to protect against exercise.

Summary.—The chemical changes occurring in the body during exercise are normally well tolerated by the heart, as the potentially harmful effects of each chemical are offset by the others. There is evidence of synergy between hyperkalemia and hypercalcemia and mutual antagonism between the sympathetic nervous system and the by-products of muscle contraction. Dysrhythmias may develop in the face of abnormal cardiac sympathovagal regulation during and after exercise, particularly in a heart with regional ischemia or an old infarct. Episodes of sudden cardiac death occurring after vigorous exercise may be related to disruption of the heart's normal mechanism for coping with the chemical stress induced by exercise.

▶ Paterson discusses an interesting paradox: the manner in which the various ionic and hormonal changes associated with vigorous exercise offset one another so that a heart attack is avoided. A study of these checks and balances and the manner in which they are disturbed by myocardial ischemia may give new insights into the factors provoking heart attacks.

R.J. Shephard, M.D., Ph.D., D.P.E.

Improvement in Ischemic Parameters During Repeated Exercise Testing: A Possible Model for Myocardial Preconditioning
Maybaum S, Ilan M, Mogilevsky J, et al (Shaare Zedek Med Ctr, Jerusalem)
Am J Cardiol 78:1087–1091, 1996   8–11

Background.—Myocardial preconditioning, or protection against further ischemic damage, occurs in animals exposed to repeated, brief episodes of coronary occlusion. It also occurs in humans undergoing balloon angioplasty. This may be related to the phenomenon of "warmup" angina, in which the subject stops exercise because of angina but is later able to resume exercise without pain. Patients with coronary artery disease were studied to see whether the myocardial ischemia produced by repeated exercise testing can reduce the ischemia produced by subsequent tests.

Methods.—The study included 26 patients with coronary artery disease, as confirmed by a positive stress test. Each patient performed 5 treadmill exercise tests over 3 consecutive days. The first 2 tests were performed on consecutive days to eliminate or reduce the "training effect." The last 3 tests were performed on a single day at intervals of 30 minutes apart. The 3 tests on the study day were all at a similar workrate. The extent of improvement in ischemic parameters between these tests was analyzed.

Results.—Total ischemic time decreased from 633 to 399 seconds from the first to the second test, and recovery time decreased from 259 to 126 seconds. Neither parameter changed significantly from the second to the third test. The ischemic threshold appeared to be higher for the second test, as evidenced by a longer time to 1mm ST-segment depression (487 vs. 593 seconds) and a greater double product at 1 mm ST-segment depression (20,322 vs. 22,325 mm Hg/second). Ninety-six percent of patients had at least 10% improvement in at least 1 ischemic parameter, and 76% had improvement in at least 2 parameters. Total ischemic burden, the most sensitive parameter, improved in 85% of patients.

Conclusion.—In patients with coronary artery disease, repeated exercise tests performed after brief intervals are associated with improvement in ischemic parameters. The mechanism of protection against ischemia is unclear. However, any repeated ischemic challenge—whether the result of reduced coronary flow or increased demand—appears to lead to myocardial preconditioning.

▶ Cardiologists have long argued that a warmup exercise reduces the risk and/or the severity of myocardial ischemia. This is one important reason why a warmup is recommended as part of a well-conceived exercise prescription. Much of the explanation of the protective effect of a warmup lies in peripheral vasodilation and reduced cardiac after-loading, and because the warmup itself does not usually cause myocardial ischemia, coronary vasodilation is unlikely to be a major factor. In my view, it is incorrect to describe an initial maximal test that has been pursued to ischemia as a "warmup", even though there is an analogous reduction of myocardial ischemia in subsequent bouts of exercise.

R.J. Shephard, M.D., Ph.D., D.P.E.

Accurate Detection of Coronary Artery Disease by Integrated Analysis of the ST-segment Depression/Heart Rate Patterns During the Exercise and Recovery Phases of the Exercise Electrocardiography Test

Lehtinen R, Sievänen H, Viik J, et al (Tampere Univ of Technology, Finland; UKK Inst for Health Promotion Research, Tampere, Finland; Univ of Tampere, Finland)
Am J Cardiol 78:1002–1006, 1996   8–12

Background.—The diagnostic accuracy of the standard end-exercise ST-segment criterion of the exercise ECG in detecting coronary artery disease (CAD) in clinical populations is limited. The diagnostic accuracy of a novel computerized diagnostic variable—ST-segment depression/heart rate (ST/HR) hysteresis—which integrates the efficient ST/HR analysis during the exercise and postexercise recovery phases of the ECG, was compared with that of methods using exercise or recovery phase alone.

Methods.—Three hundred forty-seven patients referred for a routine cycle exercise ECG were studied. One hundred twenty-seven had angiographically proved CAD, 13 did not, and 18 had no perfusion defect on technetium-99m sestamibi single-photon emission CT. One hundred eighty-nine had clinically normal hearts.

Findings.—The area under the receiver-operating characteristic curve of the ST/HR hysteresis was 89%. This was significantly greater than that of the end-exercise ST depression, recovery ST depression, and ST/HR index, indicating the superior diagnostic ability of the ST/HR hysteresis independent of the partition value selection (Fig 2).

Conclusion.—The diagnostic performance and clinical usefulness of the exercise ECG for detecting CAD can be significantly improved by computerized analysis of the HR-adjusted ST-segment depression pattern during the exercise phase, integrated with the HR-adjusted ST-segment depression pattern during the recovery phase after exercise. The ST/HR hysteresis tries to account for the complex pattern of the ST/HR diagram by allocating the ST-segment depression pattern in the first 3 minutes of the recovery phase after exercise to the ST-segment depression pattern of the exercise phase in a heart rate–adjusted manner.

▶ If information is indeed to be gained from ST-segment depression, it seems logical that this will be maximized by integrating changes over the exercise and recovery cycle, rather than by making measurements at a fixed time. Modern computers now enable this to be done, and as Lehtinen and

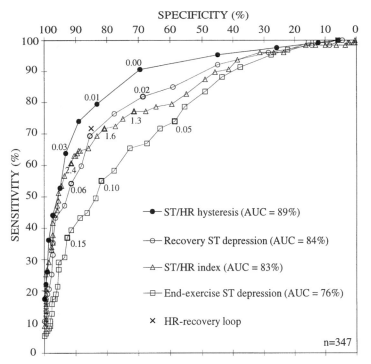

FIGURE 2.—Receiver-operating characteristic curves for the continuous diagnostic variables and the operating point for the dichotomous heart rate (*HR*) recovery loop. The *curve symbols* refer to the partition values of the variables. Some of these values are specified, expressed in millivolts for the ST segment depression/heart rate (*ST/HR*) hysteresis and ST depressions, and in millivolts per beats/per minute for the ST/HR index. *Abbreviation: AUC*, area under the receiver-operating characteristic curve. (Reprinted by permission of the publisher, courtesy of Lehtinen R, Sievänen H, Viik J, et al: Accurate detection of coronary artery disease by integrated analysis of the ST-segment depression/heart rate patterns during the exercise and recovery phases of the exercise electrocardiography test. *American Journal of Cardiology* 78:1002–1006, copyright 1996 by Excerpta Medica, Inc.)

associates demonstrate, there is an appeciable improvement in the specificity and sensitivity of the test.

R.J. Shephard, M.D., Ph.D., D.P.E.

Acute Effects of β Blockade and Exercise on Mood and Anxiety

Head A, Kendall MJ, Ferner R, et al (Univ of Birmingham, England)
Br J Sports Med 30:238–242, 1996   8–13

Background.—Exercise is increasingly recommended as a way to improve health, including psychological well-being. Previous studies have shown that β-blockers induce adverse changes in mood state and anxiety measures. Whether prolonged aerobic exercise can attenuate such mood modifications was investigated.

Methods.—Twenty healthy volunteers were included in the study. Treatment with comparable doses of propranolol, metoprolol, or placebo was given for 4 days, after which the subjects walked on a treadmill for 1 hour at 50% maximum oxygen uptake. Mood and anxiety states were determined before and after exercise.

Findings.—Compared with placebo, propranolol was associated with significantly higher resting tension, depression, and total mood disturbance. However, all were reduced with exercise. Propranolol was also associated with fatigue and confusion, which were not alleviated by exercise. More fatigue was also associated with metoprolol after exercise, compared with placebo. Anxiety was not affected by drugs or exercise.

Conclusion.—Exercise significantly reduces the tension and depression associated with propranolol treatment. Thus, exercise may be a highly desirable adjuvant therapy.

▶ Many years ago, we noted that a major depression affected many patients after myocardial infarction,[1] and a reviewer at that time questioned how much the depression might be a secondary consequence of medication. The use of β-blocking agents was much less common when our study was done, and we were convinced that in most of the patients, the cause of the depression was the clinical incident rather than subsequent medication. Nevertheless, as in the study of Head and associates, we found that exercise played an important role in bringing those who were depressed back to normal mental health.

R.J. Shephard M.D., Ph.D., D.P.E.

Reference

1. Kavanagh T, Shephard RJ, Tuck JA: Depression after myocardial infarction. *Can Med Assoc J* 113:23–27, 1975.

Effects of Exercise Training on Left Ventricular Filling at Rest and During Exercise in Patients With Ischemic Cardiomyopathy and Severe Left Ventricular Systolic Dysfunction
Belardinelli R, Georgiou D, Cianci G, et al (Ospedale Cardiologico "GM Lancisi," Ancona, Italy; South Valley Cardiovascular Group, Gilroy, Calif)
Am Heart J 132:61–70, 1996   8–14

Introduction.—Patients with ischemic cardiomyopathy can achieve improved exercise tolerance with exercise training. This probably happens mostly through peripheral adaptations, but changes in left ventricular (LV) systolic or diastolic function or both should not be excluded. The effects of exercise training on 43 consecutive patients with ischemic cardiomyopathy and severely depressed LV was evaluated prospectively to determine whether exercise training can induce changes in LV diastolic filling at rest and during exercise that can account for improved exercise capacity.

Methods.—Patients were randomly divided into training (T) and sedentary control (C) groups. Group T patients participated in a supervised exercise group that met 3 times weekly for 8 weeks. Patients exercised at 60% of peak oxygen intake. Group C patients did not exercise. Patients in both groups underwent an upright exercise test with gas-exchange analysis and a radionuclide ventriculography at baseline and at 8 weeks.

Results.—Group T patients had significant increases in peak oxygen intake and peak exercise work rate, compared to controls. Patients in group T had a slightly reduced heart rate at rest and during submaximal exercise. The heart rate did not change significantly in either group during peak exercise. There were no significant between-group differences in systolic blood pressure, diastolic blood pressure, or LV ejection fraction. At peak exercise, there was a slight increase in cardiac index in group T only. Group T but not group C patients had slightly reduced end-diastolic and end-systolic volume indexed at peak exercise and a mild increase in submaximal and peak exercise ejection fraction. Significant increases in resting peak early filling rate and peak filling rate were observed in group T, but not group C patients (Table 3). The observed single peak filling rate in group T patients was significantly correlated to the increase in cardiac index, changes in end-systolic volume index, and LV ejection fraction. The predictors of pretraining peak oxygen intake were resting heart rate and peak atrial filling rate. The best predictors of change in peak oxygen intake were changes in peak power output and peak early filling rate.

Conclusions.—Exercise training was shown to increase exercise tolerance in patients with ischemic cardiomyopathy and severely depressed LV systolic function. There was a high correlation between the training-induced increases in peak oxygen intake and LV diastolic filling at rest and during exercise. Peripheral adaptations were also important contributors

TABLE 3.—Radionuclide Left Ventricular Diastolic Filling Variables Before and After Exercise Testing

Variable	T		C	
	Before	*After*	*Before*	*After*
PEFR (EDV/sec)	1.50 ± 0.4	1.64 ± 0.4*	1.54 ± 0.3	1.58 ± 0.4
PEFR (ml/sec/m²)	141 ± 23	157 ± 20*	149 ± 29	154 ± 30
PAFR (EDV/sec)	0.61 ± 0.3	0.56 ± 0.2	0.60 ± 0.3	0.60 ± 0.3
PAFR (ml/sec/m²)	58 ± 19	54 ± 18	55 ± 16	54 ± 15
TPEFR (msec)	156 ± 14	155 ± 12	159 ± 24	152 ± 25
TPAFR (msec)	177 ± 63	236 ± 86*	165 ± 73	188 ± 80†
TPFR (msec)	129 ± 27	128 ± 26	138 ± 52	136 ± 19
DFP (msec)	389 ± 108	441 ± 129*	323 ± 114	311 ± 108†
RFF (%)	58.6 ± 13	64.5 ± 8*	59.0 ± 9	58.0 ± 8†
AFF (%)	33.0 ± 12	28.0 ± 11*	34.1 ± 14	33.2 ± 13†

*$P < 0.05$ vs. that before training.

†$P < 0.05$ vs. the same variable of group T. The exact P values are given in the text. Data are expressed as mean ± SD.

Abbreviations: PEFR, peak early filling rate; PAFR, peak atrial filling rate; PFR, peak filling rate; TPEFR, time to PEFR; TPAFR, time to PAFR; TPFR, time to PFR; DFP, diastolic filling time; RFF, rapid filling fraction; AFF, atrial filling fraction; EDV/sec, end-diastolic volume per second.

(Courtesy of Belardinelli R, Georgiou D, Cianci G, et al: Effects of exercise training on left ventricular filling at rest and during exercise in patients with ischemic cardiomyopathy and severe left ventricular systolic dysfunction. *Am Heart J* 132:61–70, 1996.)

to improved aerobic power. It is possible that the increases in early diastolic filling at rest and during exercise contribute to the improvement in peak oxygen intake.

▶ In the past few years, there has been increasing evidence of the value of exercise programs in patients with congestive failure resulting from ischemic cardiomyopathy.[1] A variety of mechanisms have been suggested,[2, 3] ranging from the peripheral (a correction of abnormalities of muscle metabolism or muscle weakness) to the central (a strengthening of residual myocardial function or an effect upon ventilatory abnormalities). A further factor is a slowing of diastolic relaxation, and Belardinelli, et al. provide good evidence that training can (through some mechanism yet to be elucidated) restore a more normal rate of ventricular filling.

R.J. Shephard, M.D., Ph.D., D.P.E.

References

1. Shephard RJ: Value of exercise training in congestive heart failure. *Sports Med* 1996, in press.
2. Massie B, Conway M, Yonge R, et al: Skeletal muscle metabolism in patients with congestive heart failure: Relation to clinical severity and blood flow. *Circulation* 76:1009–1019, 1987.
3. Wilson JR, Ferraro N: Exercise intolerance in patients with chronic left heart failure: Relationship to oxygen transport and ventilatory abnormalities. *Am J Cardiol* 51:1358–1363, 1983.

Prolonged Impairment of Regional Contractile Function After Resolution of Exercise-induced Angina: Evidence of Myocardial Stunning in Patients With Coronary Artery Disease
Ambrosio G, Betocchi S, Pace L, et al (Johns Hopkins School of Medicine, Baltimore, Md; Federico II School of Medicine, Naples, Italy)
Circulation 94:2455–2464, 1996   8–15

Introduction.—Myocardial stunning refers to delayed recovery of contractile function in the face of a return of normal perfusion. This phenomenon has been observed in animal models of exercise-induced myocardial ischemia. It is unknown whether stunning can occur after episodes of exercise-induced angina in patients with coronary artery disease. Contractile recovery and regional myocardial perfusion were monitored after exercise-related angina.

Methods.—The study included 31 patients with coronary artery disease. All underwent an exercise test to produce the typical symptoms of angina. Contractile function was then monitored for up to 4 hours in 1 of 2 ways: technetium-99m radionuclide angiography to measure regional ejection fraction (17 patients, group A) or computer-assisted echocardiographic measurement of systolic wall thickening (14 patients, group B). The patients in group B also underwent ^{99m}Tc-sestamibi single-photon emission CT to assess myocardial perfusion.

Results.—Substantial contractile dysfunction occurred with the onset of angina. The ischemic changes in hemodynamic and ECG parameters promptly returned to normal. By 30 minutes after cessation of exercise, the patients in group B had no detectable perfusion defects. However, their contractile dysfunction continued to be impaired. In group A, regional ejection fraction in the areas that had been ischemic during angina was 83% of baseline at 30 minutes after cessation of exercise. In group B, systolic thickening of the previously ischemic areas averaged 34% 1 hour after the end of exercise, compared with 41% at baseline. By the end of the second hour after cessation of exercise, the contractile impairment had resolved completely.

Conclusion.—In patients with coronary artery disease, myocardial stunning can occur after an episode of exercise-related angina. These patients have impaired regional myocardial function even though the ischemic episode has ended and perfusion is normal. The contractile abnormalities last for an hour or 2, but ultimately resolve. This finding may have important clinical implications; even if the contractile dysfunction is relatively modest, repeated episodes could have a cumulative effect.

▶ Parker et al.[1] demonstrated some 30 years ago that myocardial ischemia could precipitate cardiac failure. However, this paper provides a nice demonstration of the time course of ischemic dysfunction. It also shows rather beautifully that the problem of myocardial contractility after ischemia is limited to the ischemic segment of the myocardium—indeed, there seems to be some attempt at compensation by other segments of the myocardium.

R.J. Shephard, M.D., Ph.D., D.P.E.

Reference

1. Parker JO, DiGiorgi S, West RO. A hemodynamic study of acute coronary insufficiency precipitated by exercise: With observations on the effects of nitroglycerin. *Am J Cardiol* 17:470–483, 1966.

Kinetics of Oxygen Consumption During and After Exercise in Patients With Dilated Cardiomyopathy: New Markers of Exercise Intolerance With Clinical Implications
de Groote P, Millaire A, DeCoulx E, et al (Centre Hospitalier Régional et Universitaire, Lille, France)
J Am Coll Cardiol 28:168–175, 1996   8–16

Introduction.—The kinetics of oxygen consumption during a short recovery period have been evaluated in a small series of patients with dilated cardiomyopathy. The clinical relevance of indices of recovery has never been investigated. The kinetics of oxygen consumption during a prolonged recovery period were evaluated in 153 patients with stable dilated cardiomyopathy and 53 normal controls. Prognostic information on indices of recovery was evaluated in ambulatory patients with stable dilated cardiomyopathy.

Methods.—Patients were placed in subgroups according to peak oxygen consumption: group 1—15 or more mL/min/kg; group 2—less than 15 and more than 10 mL/min/kg; and group 3—10 or less than 10 mL/min/kg. Thirty healthy controls were aged 18–35 years and 25 were aged 36–71 years. An upright electromagnetically braked cycle ergometer was used to calculate the ratio between total oxygen consumption during exercise and recovery (RVO_2), the half-recovery time of peak oxygen consumption ($\frac{1}{2}$ pVO_2), the time constant of recovery, the recovery time (RT), and the ratio between duration of exercise and RT.

Results.—All indices of recovery differed significantly between subgroups. Compared to those of controls, the RVO_2 and all indices related to

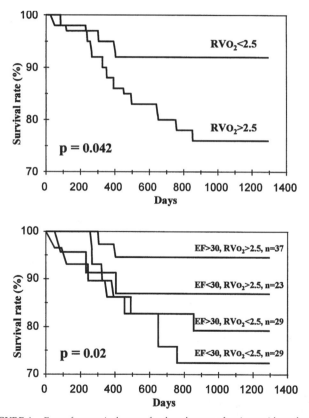

FIGURE 4.—Event-free survival curves for the subgroup of patients with moderate exercise intolerance (percent maximal predicted oxygen consumption [VO_2] >40%). **Top,** patients stratified by the median value of the ratio between total oxygen consumption during exercise and during recovery (RVO_2 <2.5 or >2.5). **Bottom,** patients stratified by the median values for both left ventricular ejection fraction (EF <30% or >30%) and RVO_2 <2.5 or >2.5. (From de Groote P, Millaire A, DeCoulx E, et al: Kinetics of oxygen consumption during and after exercise in patients with dilated cardiomyopathy: New markers of exercise intolerance with clinical implications. *J Am Coll Cardiol* 28:168–175, 1996. Reprinted with permission from the American College of Cardiology.)

recovery were significantly reduced in the patient group. Mean age and peak oxygen consumption were the only significant differences between the younger and older control subgroups. Compared to controls, patients in groups 2 and 3 (peak oxygen consumption less than 15 ml/[kg·min] had significantly lower oxygen consumption at rest and at the end of recovery. The RVO_2 was the most closely correlated index of recovery with peak oxygen consumption, followed by RT, age, and ½ pVO_2. In the patient groups, there were 24 cardiovascular deaths and 16 heart transplants during a median follow-up of 439 days. Survival rates at 6, 12, and 18 months were 97.4%, 90.2%, and 87.6%, respectively. With inclusion of heart transplants, the event-free survival rates were 91.5%, 83%, and 77.8%, respectively. Independent predictors of survival were percent maximal predicted peak oxygen consumption and ejection fraction. Independent predictors of survival were RVO_2 and the ejection fraction in a subgroup of 35 patients with a maximal peak oxygen consumption of less than 40%. Patient subgroups were stratified by RVO_2 and ejection fraction (Fig 4). Median RVO_2 was 2.5. In a subgroup of 14 patients (74%) with a major event, the median RVO_2 value was less than 2.5. Regardless of the value of the ejection fraction, survival was better when RVO_2 was greater than 2.5.

Conclusion.—Compared to normal controls, patients with stable dilated cardiomyopathy had delayed kinetics of oxygen consumption during recovery. Independent predictors of survival in the patient group were percent maximal predicted value of oxygen consumption and left ventricular ejection fraction. The RVO_2 and ejection fraction were independent predictors of survival in a subgroup of patients with a peak oxygen consumption of less than 40%.

▶ In recent years, attention has focused on the exercise response rather than the subsequent recovery process, but this study by de Groote and associates suggests that it may sometimes be useful to look at both variables. In a subgroup of their patients with dilated cardiomyopathy (those with moderate exercise intolerance), a poor prognosis was associated with a slow recovery from exercise, independently of such traditional markers of poor prognosis as a low ejection fraction. The authors suggest that the recovery process may be serving as a marker of peripheral functional limitations such as impaired muscle metabolism or muscle atrophy.

R.J. Shephard, M.D., Ph.D., D.P.E.

Does Appropriate Endurance Exercise Training Improve Cardiac Function in Patients With Prior Myocardial Infarction?
Adachi H, Koike A, Obayashi T, et al (Musashino Red Cross Hosp, Tokyo; Tokyo Med and Dental Univ; Yokosuka Kyosai Hosp, Kanagawa-ken, Japan)
Eur Heart J 17:1511–1521, 1996   8–17

Background.—Home-based physical training is becoming very popular among patients who have had myocardial infarction. In such patients,

TABLE 3.—Measures of Exercise Capacity Obtained During the Incremental Exercise Test

	Control group (Group 1)			Low intensity training group (Group 2)			High intensity training group (Group 3)		
	Before	After	P value	Before	After	P value	Before	After	P value
Heart rate at peak exercise (beats . min^{-1})	149 ± 23	142 ± 24	0·185	145 ± 23	145 ± 22	0·976	157 ± 14	152 ± 13	0·166
Blood pressure at peak exercise									
Systolic (mmHg)	192 ± 21	195 ± 20	0·528	191 ± 25	188 ± 25	0·509	169 ± 28	182 ± 39	0·154
Diastolic (mmHg)	101 ± 11	104 ± 10	0·533	103 ± 20	91 ± 27	0·103	99 ± 16	107 ± 29	0·180
Peak oxygen uptake (ml . min^{-1})	1196 ± 241	1333 ± 328	0·093	1106 ± 248	1211 ± 388	0·201	1335 ± 437	1560 ± 424	0·030*
Maximal work rate (watts)	98·4 ± 19·9	106·4 ± 22·5	0·065	93·1 ± 16·0	105·3 ± 22·9	0·025*	109·5 ± 21·6	125·0 ± 29·8	0·024*
Exercise time (s)	470·1 ± 120·3	518·1 ± 135·5	0·061	439·0 ± 96·3	511·5 ± 137·1	0·025*	536·3 ± 129·2	628·9 ± 178·5	0·023*

Note: Values are expressed as the mean ± SD. P value was determined by the paired t-test.
*Significant difference between before and after training.
(Courtesy of Adachi H, Koike A, Obayashi T, et al: Does appropriate endurance training improve cardiac function in patients with prior myocardial infarction? Eur Heart J 17:1511–1521, 1996. Reprinted by permission of the publisher, WB Saunders Company Limited, London.)

exercise capacity is known to improve with training. However, the most appropriate intensity of training for improving exercise capacity in this population has not been established.

Methods.—Twenty-nine patients who had had myocardial infarction were assigned to a control group (group 1), low-intensity training (group 2), or high-intensity training (group 3). Groups 2 and 3 did 15 minutes of home-based physical training twice daily 5 days a week for 2 months. Before and after training, the patients performed 2 constant work rate tests and a symptom-limited incremental exercise test.

Findings.—In all 3 groups, heart rates at rest and during exercise declined significantly after 2 months. Stroke volume at rest increased significantly only in group 3. Group 2 and 3 patients also had significant increases in stroke volume after 6 minutes of heavy-intensity exercise. However, the ejection fraction at 6 minutes of heavy-intensity exercise increased significantly in group 3 only. Groups 2 and 3 had significant increases in the maximal work rate attained during incremental exercise testing (Table 3).

Conclusions.—Both exercise groups showed the benefits of physical training on maximal exercise capacity. However, improved cardiac function at rest and during exercise was noted only in the high-intensity training group. Thus, relatively high-intensity training may improve exercise capacity and cardiac function in patients who have had myocardial infarction.

▶ It is a useful corrective to the current enthusiasm for low-intensity aerobic exercise to recall that most studies, beginning with that of Paterson and colleagues,[1] have found that high-intensity programs are more effective than low-intensity in the area of cardiac rehabilitation. This paper, although confirming such a view, is particularly interesting in that central cardiac benefit was seen after as little as 8 weeks of rehabilitation. The time of entry to the trial after infarction is not clearly indicated, but it seems to have been much later than in many previous studies.

R.J. Shephard, M.D., Ph.D., D.P.E.

Reference

1. Paterson D, Shephard RJ, Cunningham D, et al: Effects of physical training upon cardiovascular function following myocardial infarction. *J Appl Physiol* 47:482-489, 1979.

Exercise Training in Patients With Heart Failure
Keteyian SJ, Levine AB, Brawner CA, et al (Henry Ford Heart and Vascular Inst, Detroit)
Ann Intern Med 124:1051–1057, 1996   8–18

Introduction.—Reports vary regarding exercise benefit in patients with symptomatic heart failure. Functional capacity and cardiorespiratory fitness were measured before and after exercise training in patients with compensated heart failure in order to determine exercise benefit and to describe physiologic changes associated with exercise training.

Methods.—Forty men with compensated heart failure and left ventricular dysfunction were randomly assigned to an exercise group or a control group. Nineteen men participated in a supervised exercise program that met 3 times weekly for 24 weeks. The 19 men in the control group did not exercise. Before randomization and at weeks 12 and 24, patients underwent symptom-limited maximal exercise testing, using an upright cycle ergometer, and gas exchange analysis.

Results.—Fifteen of 21 patients in the exercise group and 14 of 19 patients in the control group completed the trial. There were no significant between-group changes over time in resting heart rate, heart rate during exercise at 50 W, ventilation at 50 W, or resting systolic or diastolic blood pressures. Men in the exercise group experienced a significant decrease in heart rate during exercise at a standardized submaximal power output of 50 W. This significant decrease was not observed in the control group. Compared to controls, absolute peak oxygen consumption ($\dot{V}O_2$), relative peak $\dot{V}O_2$, exercise duration, and peak power output were significantly increased over time in the exercise group (Table 2). There were no significant between-group differences in ventilatory derived anaerobic threshold over time. Peak heart rate over time was significantly decreased in the exercise group, compared to controls. Much of the increase (46%) in peak $\dot{V}O_2$ could be attributed to the increase in peak heart rate.

Conclusion.—There seem to be no cardiac-related contraindications to exercise training in patients with compensated heart failure. Peak $\dot{V}O_2$, peak heart rate, peak ventilation, peak power output, and exercise duration were significantly improved in patients who participated in exercise training. The improved exercise tolerance was partly the result of an increase in peak heart rate.

▶ We have recently demonstrated that the majority of patients with stable congestive heart failure can participate in an exercise program successfully for as long as a year.[1] Moreover, such rehabilitation not only yields gains of physiologic performance, but also enhances various measures of the quality of life. In our study, we demonstrated in matched but not randomly assigned controls that there were no significant changes over 3 months of normal treatment. The study of Keteyian and associates is useful because of its substantial sample size (40 patients), randomization, and a substantial period of observation (24 weeks). The ejection fraction (an average of 22%) was the same as in our study, and the proportion who completed the exercise trial (15 of 21) also coincides with our experience.

R.J. Shephard, M.D., Ph.D., D.P.E.

TABLE 2.—Changes in Cardiorespiratory Responses During Peak Exercise in Patients in the Exercise Group and Patients in the Control Group

Variable	Control Group (n = 14)			Exercise Group (n = 15)			Difference between Groups (Exercise - Control) For Change from Baseline to Week 24 (95% CI)
	Baseline	Change from Baseline		Baseline	Change from Baseline		
		Week 12	Week 24		Week 12	Week 24	
Exercise duration, *min*	10.3 ± 1.0	0.2 ± 0.4	0.5 ± 0.5	10.6 ± 0.8	1.9 ± 0.4	2.8 ± 0.6*	2.3 (0.7 to 3.9)
Power output, W	89 ± 8	0 ± 5	2 ± 5	92 ± 7	10 ± 5	20 ± 6†	18 (3 to 33)
Oxygen consumption; *mL/min*	1224 ± 112	86 ± 27	58 ± 38	1412 ± 74	197 ± 37	231 ± 54†	173 (37 to 309)
Oxygen consumption, *mL/kg of body weight per min*	14.7 ± 1.1	1.0 ± 0.4	0.5 ± 0.5	16.0 ± 0.9	2.2 ± 0.5	2.5 ± 0.6†	2.0 (0.4 to 3.6)
Ventilation, *L/min*	61 ± 5	-4 ± 2	-4 ± 3	58 ± 4	8 ± 2	12 ± 3*	16 (8 to 24)
Ventilatory derived anaerobic threshold, *mL/min*	930 ± 74	105 ± 43	94 ± 37	1048 ± 74	100 ± 38	65 ± 65	-29 (-184 to 126)
Oxygen pulse, *mL/beat*	9.3 ± 1.0	0.3 ± 0.2	0.5 ± 0.3	10.7 ± 0.7	0.7 ± 0.4	0.8 ± 0.3	0.3 (-0.5 to 1.1)
Respiratory exchange ratio	1.24 ± 0.04	-0.10 ± 0.03	-0.07 ± 0.04	1.13 ± 0.02	0.04 ± 0.02	0.04 ± 0.02	0.11 (-0.02 to 0.24)
Blood pressure, *mm Hg*							
Systolic	147 ± 9	3 ± 4	5 ± 4	160 ± 8	-3 ± 5	4 ± 3	-1 (-11 to 9)
Diastolic	76 ± 3	3 ± 2	2 ± 3	78 ± 5	1 ± 4	-2 ± 3	-4 (-14 to 6)
Rate pressure product, *mm Hg/min* ($\times 10^2$)‡	203 ± 17	9 ± 9	11 ± 8	208 ± 15	33 ± 18	25 ± 8	14 (-9 to 37)
Rating of perceived exertion	17.4 ± 0.5	-1.5 ± 0.8	-0.2 ± 0.6	17.5 ± 0.4	-1.8 ± 0.5	-1.0 ± 0.7	-0.8 (-2.5 to 0.9)

Note: Values are expressed as the mean ±SE.
*$P < 0.01$ for significant differences in overall change across time for control group compared with exercise group.
†$P > 0.01$ but < 0.05 for significant differences in overall change across time for control group compared with exercise group.
‡Rate pressure product = heart rate × systolic blood pressure.
(Courtesy of Keteyian SJ, Levine AB, Brawner CA, et al: Exercise training in patients with heart failure. *Ann Intern Med* 124:1051–1057, 1996.)

Reference

1. Kavanagh T, Myers MG, Baigrie RS et al: Quality of life and cardiorespiratory function in congestive heart failure: Effects of 12 months' aerobic training. *Heart* 76:42–49, 1996.

High Intensity Knee Extensor Training, in Patients With Chronic Heart Failure: Major Skeletal Muscle Improvement

Magnusson G, Gordon A, Kaijser L, et al (Karolinska Inst, Stockholm; Deaconess Inst, Oulu, Finland)

Eur Heart J 17:1048–1055, 1996   8–19

Background.—Designing an effective rehabilitation program for patients with chronic heart failure (CHF) requires a determination of the appropriate type, intensity, and duration of local muscle exercise. The efficacy of a period of high-intensity training involving 1 muscle group in inducing significant muscular adaptations and improving exercise capacity in patients with CHF was investigated.

Methods and Findings.—Eleven patients with CHF were randomly assigned to either a strength or an endurance training group. The quadriceps femoris muscles were exercised 3 days a week for 8 weeks. In all 11 patients, maximal exercise intensity tolerated on the cycle ergometer was increased after training, from an average of 99 to 114 W. The peak dynamic knee extensor work rate showed the largest increase, at 40%, after endurance training. After strength training, maximal dynamic and isometric strength were increased by 40% to 45%. The cross-sectional area of the quadriceps femoris muscle was increased by 9% in the legs undergoing strength training. The capillary-per-fiber ratio of the vastus lateralis muscle was increased by averages of 47% and 58% in the legs undergoing endurance training. The oxidative enzyme activity in the vas-

TABLE 1.—Physical Characteristics, Ejection Fraction, and Maximal Oxygen Uptake Before and After 2 Months of Knee Extensor Training

Variable	S group (n=5)	E group (n=6)	All patients (n=11)
Age (years)	57 (11)	55 (8)	56 (9)
Height (cm)	176 (5)	178 (8)	177 (7)
Weight (kg) B	88·8 (22·7)	86·8 (14·3)	87·7 (17·6)
Weight (kg) A	88·0 (21·8)	87·1 (13·9)	87·6 (17·3)
EF (%) B	11·4 (5·4)	28·2 (9·1)*	19·8 (11·3)
EF (%) A	13·6 (8·5)	29·6 (5·6)*	21·6 (10·8)
$\dot{V}O_2$ (ml . kg^{-1} . min^{-1}) B	13·8 (3·3)	16·2 (2·3)	15·1 (2·9)
$\dot{V}O_2$ (ml . kg^{-1} . min^{-1}) A	14·4 (3·8)	17·3 (3·6)	15·9 (3·8)

Note: Values are given as the mean with standard deviation in parentheses.
$P < 0.05$ for the difference between the strength and endurance groups.
Abbreviations: S, strength; E, endurance; B, before; A, after; EF, ejection fraction; $\dot{V}O_2$, systemic oxygen uptake.
(Courtesy of Magnusson G, Gordon A, Kaijser L, et al: High intensity knee extensor training in patients with chronic heart failure. *Eur Heart J* 17:1048–1055, 1996.)

tus lateralis muscle was increased significantly to more than 50% after endurance training. Glycolytic enzyme activity was not affected (Table 1).

Conclusion.—In patients with CHF, the peripheral skeletal musculature adapts fairly quickly to high-intensity knee extensor training, resulting in a marked increase in local work capacity and a small increase in total work capacity. This indicates the maintenance of skeletal muscle plasticity in patients with CHF.

▶ Peripheral muscle weakness is an important factor contributing to the poor exercise performance of patients with CHF. Moreover, the skeletal muscles are much more receptive to training than is the weakened myocardium. The gains of extensor strength are large (40% to 45% over 8 weeks), reflecting mainly an enhanced coordination of muscle contraction, but there are also objective increases in muscle cross-sectional area. Particularly with local endurance training, an increased capillary-per-fiber ratio and an augmentation of oxidative enzyme activity have also been observed. Plainly, local muscle training should be an important component of rehabilitation for the patient with stable congestive heart failure.

R.J. Shephard, M.D., Ph.D., D.P.E.

Influence of the Exercise Protocol on Hemodynamic, Gas Exchange, and Neurohumoral Responses to Exercise in Heart Transplant Recipients
Gullestad L, Myers J, Noddeland H, et al (Univ Hosp, Oslo, Norway; Stanford Univ, Calif)
J Heart Lung Transplant 15:304–313, 1996   8–20

Introduction.—Maximum oxygen uptake ($\dot{V}O_{2max}$) is used to define the limits of the cardiopulmonary system. Results vary according to the method used. Patients with severe heart failure who have undergone heart transplantation have delayed oxygen kinetics that must be considered when choosing protocol for determining $\dot{V}O_{2max}$. Two different protocols (one with rapid and one with modest increments in work rate) were used to determine how each would affect gas exchange, hemodynamic, and neurohumoral responses to exercise after heart transplantation.

Methods.—Nine patients performed the 2 incremental maximal cycle ergometry tests 3 hours apart. Exercise duration was 5 minutes with the shorter protocol and 15 minutes with the longer protocol. The absolute work rates were equivalent for both protocols, but stage duration was 1 minute in 1 test and 3 minutes in the other. Matched work rate increments ranged from 30 to 40 W. Arterial blood was drawn periodically and 30 to 40 W. Arterial blood was drawn periodically and oxygen uptake was measured continuously.

Results.—Exercise time for the 1-minute stage test was 6.4 minutes and 15.3 minutes for the 3-minute stage test. The maximal workrate achieved was significantly higher for the 1-minute protocol than for the 3-minute protocol. There were no significantly between-group differences in $\dot{V}O_{2max}$.

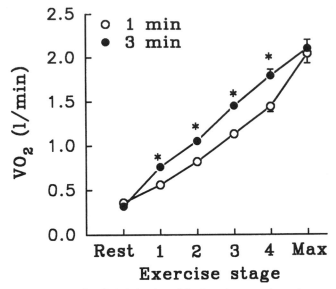

FIGURE 7.—Oxygen uptake ($\dot{V}O_2$) during 1- and 3-minute incremental exercise protocols at rest, during submaximal and maximal (Max) exercise. Results are given as mean ± SE. *Error bars* not shown when smaller than symbol size. *$P < 0.001$. (Courtesy of Gullestad L, Myers J, Noddeland H, et al: Influence of the exercise protocol on hemodynamic, gas exchange, and neurohumoral responses to exercise in heart transplant recipients. *J Heart Lung Transplant* 15:304–313, 1996.)

Strong correlations were observed between $\dot{V}O_2$ and heart rate and $\dot{V}O_2$ and norepinephrine. Patients had higher $\dot{V}O_2$ and ventilation, but did not differ at exhaustion or recovery, when performing the 3-minute protocol during submaximal exercise (Fig 7) compared with performing the 1-minute protocol. Maximum heart rate did not differ between protocols, but heart rates were higher than during the latter stages of the 3-minute protocol. Diastolic blood pressure remained about the same during all stages of both protocols. Systolic pressure increased in a parallel fashion for the 1- and 3-minute protocols. During the 3-minute protocol, patients had significantly higher natriuretic factor and growth factor, but not epinephine, norepinephrine, and insulin responses, compared to the 1-minute protocol.

Conclusion.—The maximal oxygen intake was independent of the exercise protocol. Metabolic and hormonal responses were significantly affected by the protocol. Delayed oxygen intake and hormonal responses suggest a significant physiologic lag time during the more rapidly incremental protocol. Work rate and stage duration should be carefully considered in patients who have undergone heart transplantation.

▶ It is now well recognized that in the transplanted heart, heart rate and oxygen consumption increase only slowly during exercise, and this has important implications for the choice of test protocol.[1] A progressive test with rapid increments of work rate leads to unacceptably large errors in predictions of maximal oxygen intake. The solution to this problem, as shown in the present paper, is to measure the symptom-limited maximal oxygen intake. Scores for this measurement remain relatively independent of protocol, even if there is a slow acceleration of heart rate.

R.J. Shephard, M.D., Ph.D., D.P.E.

Reference

1. Shephard RJ, Kavanagh T, Mertens D, et al: Kinetics of the transplanted heart. Implications for the choice of field-test exercise protocol. *J Cardiopulm Rehabil* 15:288–296, 1995.

Persistent Exercise Intolerance Following Cardiac Transplantation Despite Normal Oxygen Transport
Mettauer B, Lampert E, Petitjean P, et al (Univ Hosp, Strasbourg, France)
Int J Sports Med 17:277–286, 1996   8–21

Background.—Although heart transplantation can transform the quality of life of patients severely disabled with heart failure, the exercise capacity of transplant recipients is still limited. Questions remain regarding the cardiac output, oxygen extraction, and anaerobic contribution during exercise after heart transplantation. The respective roles of the periphery and central oxygen transport in the exercise limitation of heart transplant recipients were defined.

Methods and Findings.—Eleven transplant recipients were compared with 6 age- and weight-matched healthy subjects during an incremental exercise test up to peak exercise level. The control subjects stopped at between 120 and 240 W, compared with 90 W in the patient group. Patients had significantly lower peak oxygen intake, cardiac index, and arteriovenous oxygen difference values than controls. Lactate values in the 2 groups were similar. At the 90-W step, the control subjects were close to their anaerobic threshold, having similar parameters of oxygen transport but lower lactate levels than the transplant group. At the same intermediate exercise levels, oxygen intake, cardiac index, and arteriovenous oxygen difference were similar in the 2 groups, whereas the closely matched lactate values and ventilation increased faster in the patients, reaching significantly greater levels as soon as the 30-W step (Fig 4).

Conclusion.—Despite the denervation of the transplanted heart, recipients' central oxygen transport remains sufficient during exercise at submaximal work rates and adequately related to the power produced. The peripheral metabolic energy production relies more on anaerobic processes, as suggested by a faster blood lactate accumulation than that seen in healthy subjects. Thus peripheral factors appear to make a large contribution to exercise limitation in heart transplant recipients. Further research is needed to investigate the reversibility of the muscular changes

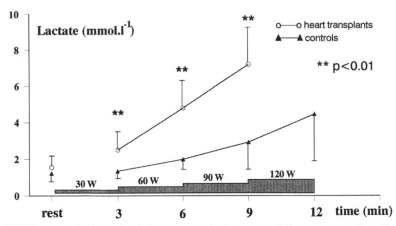

FIGURE 4.—Arterial lactate in relation to exercise time/power. Arterial lactate, expressed in millimoles per liter, increases faster in heart transplant patients (*HTR; open circles*) than in normal sedentary controls (*C; solid triangles*), with an almost linear pattern above 30 W in HTR. In C, its increase becomes curvilinear and significant only at and above 90 W. As before, the HTR values are presented up to the peak W level they all reached. The C values are presented only up to the 120 W level they also all reached but do not represent peak exercise values because of the variable maximal tolerated power in this group. Values are expressed as means ± standard deviation; *double asterisks* indicate $P < 0.01$ HTR vs. C at the same exercise time. (Courtesy of Mettauer B, Lampert E, Petitjean P, et al: Persistent exercise intolerance following cardiac transplantation despite normal oxygen transport. *Int J Sports Med* 17:277–286, 1996.)

induced by heart failure and the muscular impact of the immunosuppressive drugs.

▶ This paper shows clearly that during a progressive exercise test, the patient who has undergone cardiac transplantation accumulates unusually large amounts of lactate, even at very light workloads. Detraining effects—such as muscle weakness, impaired muscle perfusion, and loss of tissue enzyme activity—may arise from prior congestive heart failure or limitation of activity associated with major surgery, but such factors are unlikely to be operative at loads as low as 30.

Here, the abnormal lactate buildup is probably related mainly to a slow increase of cardiac output at the onset of exercise.[1] There are possibly also some contributions from an enhanced secretion of catecholamines and, thus, a greater reliance on glycolytic metabolism,[2] together with effects of immunosuppressant drugs upon mitochondrial proton transport.[3] Irrespective of mechanisms, there is evidence that the limitation of aerobic power after cardiac transplantation can be substantially alleviated by an endurance training program,[4] possibly with a speeding of oxygen on-transients.[2]

R.J. Shephard, M.D., Ph.D., D.P.E.

References

1. Shephard RJ, Kavanagh T, Mertens DJ: et al: Kinetics of the transplanted heart. Implications for the choice of field test protocol. *J Cardiopulmon Rehabil* 15:288–296, 1995.

2. Brooks GA: Current concepts in lactate exchange. *Med Sci Sports Exerc* 23:895–906, 1991.
3. Mercier J, Hokanson JF, Brooks GA: Effects of cyclosporine on skeletal muscle mitochondrial respiration and endurance time in rats. *Am J Respir Crit Care Med*, in press.
4. Kavanagh T, Yacoub M, Mertens DJ, et al: Cardiorespiratory responses of exercise training after orthotopic cardiac transplantation. *Circulation* 77:162–171, 1988.

Influence of Post-surgery Time After Cardiac Transplantation on Exercise Responses

Mercier J, Ville N, Wintrebert P, et al (Hôpital Arnaud de Villeneuve, Montpellier, France; Univ of Montpellier I, France)
Med Sci Sports Exerc 28:171–175, 1996   8–22

Introduction.—The influence of time postsurgery on the exercise responses of patients with orthotopic heart transplantation (OHT) is under-investigated. It is possible that cardiorespiratory and metabolic responses to exercise in patients with OHT may change with time postsurgery independently of training or transplant rejection. The exercise responses of patients with OHT who did not participate in formal exercise training and were free of rejection in the year after transplantation were evaluated. The transplanted heart rate and oxygen intake were observed during submaximal and peak exercise in the period postsurgery.

Methods.—Nine patients with OHT received appropriate donor-recipient matches. All patients were given standard triple-drug therapy for immunosuppression, and none were treated with β-blockers. All patients were functional class I (according to the New York Heart Association criteria) after transplantation and were free of acute rejection and systemic infection. Patients did not participate in an exercise program. Graded exercise tests were conducted at 1, 3, 6, 9, and 12 months after surgery, using cycle ergometry and an automated exercise metabolic system.

Results.—No patients had a decrease in oxygen saturation of more than 4% and none developed adverse cardiac rhythm changes during exercise testing. Patients experienced a persistent mean tachycardia of 90 beats per minute at rest in the first month after surgery. This increased significantly, to a mean of 104 beats per minute, by 12 months after transplantation. During peak exercise, oxygen intake ($\dot{V}O_2$, mL/kg^{-1} min) normalized minute ventilation ($\dot{V}E$) and O_2 did not change significantly between months 1 and 12 after surgery. The transplanted heart rate (HR_t) and delta heart rate (the peak exercise heart rate − resting heart rate) increased significantly between months 1 and 12, particularly between months 1 and 3 (Fig 1). A significant negative correlation was observed between O_2 and HR_t at peak exercise. There was no correlation between delta heart rate and delta $\dot{V}O_2$ (peak exercise $\dot{V}O_2$ − resting $\dot{V}O_2$, 1/min^{-1}). From rest to peak exercise, $\dot{V}E$, $\dot{V}O_2$, HR_t, and O_2 pulse increased significantly. In relation to postsurgery time, only HR_t increased significantly. The $\dot{V}O_2$-HR_t relationship shifted toward higher values of HR_t in relation to postsurgery time.

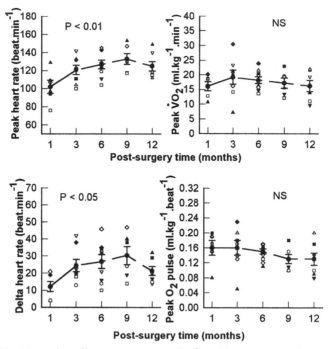

FIGURE 1.—Mean values of heart rate, oxygen uptake (V̇O₂), delta heart rate (peak exercise − resting heart rate), and oxygen pulse measured at peak exercise in relation to postsurgery time. Individual data are represented by different symbols; *dashed lines* represent the mean. (Courtesy of Mercier J, Ville N, Wintrebert P, et al: Influence of post-surgery time after cardiac transplantation on exercise responses. *Med Sci Sports Exerc* 28:171–175, 1996.)

Conclusion.—During graded exercise the denervated heart rate of patients with OHT not participating in a rehabilitation program increased greatly in relation to time postsurgery in the first year after transplantation. This increase was not correlated with changes in submaximal or peak oxygen intake.

▶ A number of authors, most notably Kavanagh and associates,[1] have demonstrated a substantial enhancement of aerobic power in patients who have been enrolled in a progressive exercise program subsequent to OHT. However, the authors of these studies have believed sufficiently strongly in the virtues of exercise that they have not generally included control groups. This has left the nasty lingering suspicion that some, if not all, of the reported benefits might reflect the natural history of the recovery process after transplantation. It is thus very valuable to have careful documentation of time-related changes in the exercise performance of cardiac transplant patients who did not receive formal exercise rehabilitation. During the first 12 months, such patients show a dramatic increase of peak heart rate, but there is no significant change in peak oxygen intake. The reason for the increase in peak heart rate remains unclear; there is little evidence of anatomical reinnervation in the first 12 months after surgery.[2, 3] and the explanation may lie in an altered sensitivity of myocardial receptors to circulating catecholamines.[4, 5] Irrespective of mechanisms, we can now accept with greater confidence the earlier reports showing that functional gains can be realized through an exercise-centered rehabilitation program.

R.J. Shephard, M.D., Ph.D., D.P.E.

References

1. Kavanagh T, Yacoub M, Mertens D, et al: Cardiorespiratory responses to exercise training after orthotopic cardiac transplantation. *Circulation* 77:162–171, 1988.
2. Fallen E, Kamath M, Ghista D, et al: Spectral analysis of heart rate variability following human heart transplantation: Evidence for functional reinnervation. *J Auton Nerv Syst* 23:199–206, 1988.
3. Wilson R, Christensen B, Olivbari M, et al: Evidence for structural sympathetic reinnervation after orthotopic cardiac transplantation in humans. *Circulation* 83:1210–1220, 1991.
4. Borow K, Neuman A, Arensman F, et al: Clinical evidence of differential sensitivity of alpha and beta adrenergic receptors after cardiac transplantation. *Circulation* 72: S111–S129, 1985.
5. Zerkowski H, Kahamssi, M, Brodde O: Development of beta adrenoceptor number and subtype distribution in the transplanted human heart. *Eur Heart J* 12:S124–S126, 1991.

Iron Deficiency in Distance Runners: A Reinvestigation Using[59] Fe-Labelling and Non-invasive Liver Iron Quantification
Nachtigall D, Nielsen P, Fischer R, et al (Universitätskrankenhaus Eppendorf, Hamburg, Germany)
Int J Sports Med 17:473–479, 1996
8–23

Background.—The term "sports anemia" describes hemoglobin levels that are low-normal or below normal in endurance athletes, although the cause of this condition is unknown. It does not appear that iron deficiency plays a major part in sports anemia, but various studies have reported low iron stores in endurance runners and other athletes. This negative iron balance in runners may be caused by decreased food iron absorption resulting from malnutrition or malabsorption of iron and by increased loss of iron in sweat, urine, and feces. Whether deficiency in these individuals is a real or apparent event is unclear, because low serum ferritin does not necessarily indicate low iron stores under conditions of intense exercise. Iron metabolism in male endurance runners was reinvestigated using liver iron quantification.

Methods.—The subjects were 45 male middle-or long-distance runners of regional or national class. Blood parameters of iron metabolism were determined. A radioimmunoassay was used to measure ferritin in serum and lysates from purified erythrocytes. Intestinal iron absorption was measured in 8 of the 45 subjects. Liver iron concentrations were measured with a SQUID biomagnetometer. Age-matched control subjects were also studied.

Results.—Serum ferritin values were less than 20 µg/L in 7 athletes and less than 12 µg/L in 1 athlete. Only 1 of 112 controls had serum ferritin less than 20 µg/L. In a test of intestinal iron absorption, 5 of 8 athletes absorbed and retained more than 50% of the test dose. This was the typical upregulation of iron absorption in iron deficiency. In athletes, mean liver iron concentration was significantly lower than in controls. To obtain individual ^{59}Fe elimination rates during periods of endurance training, ^{59}Fe whole-body retention was measured periodically in the 3–4 months after the absorption test. In the majority of athletes, ^{59}Fe elimination rates were somewhat higher. After 164 stool samples were collected under various training conditions, small but significant increases in ^{59}Fe activity were noted in each of the athletes. During periods when the subject did not run, a fecal excretion of ^{59}Fe equivalent to 1.5 mL blood loss/day was noted; this represents normal iron excretion. During periods of intensive racing, a significant increase up to 4.9 to 6.6 mL blood loss/day occurred (Fig 2), but excretion of ^{59}Fe in urine and sweat was insignificant. Gastrointestinal blood loss was primarily responsible for the slightly negative iron balance in athletes. Gastrointestinal bleeding was associated more with intensity than with distance. Mean blood volume was 6,190 mL in the athletes, which was about 25% greater than normal. The difference represents an additional iron mass of 590 mg, which is captured in the hemoglobin pool while endurance activity is maintained.

Discussion.—The reduced liver iron concentration seen in these athletes does not support the Magnusson hypothesis that increased red blood cell catabolism in endurance athletes may result in a shift from iron of reticuloendothelial cells to parenchymal cells in the liver. The amount of iron excreted through sweat glands and kidneys is small and has a negligible

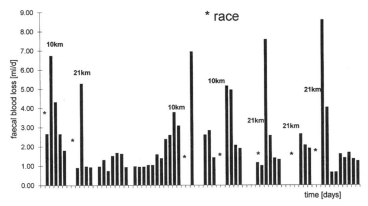

FIGURE 2.—Gastrointestinal blood loss after different competition races (5–21 km) in a top long-distance runner. Collected 24-hour stool samples were analyzed for ^{59}Fe activity. The maximum fecal ^{59}Fe activity was 1–3 after the race. Breaks of the X-axis indicate time intervals (5 days to 4 wks) during normal training (data not shown). (Courtesy of Nachtigall D, Nielsen P, Fischer R, et al: Iron deficiency in distance runners: A reinvestigation using ^{59}Fe-labelling and non-invasive liver iron quantification. *Int J Sports Med* 17:473–479, 1996.)

effect on total iron loss in runners. This is consistent with the low value of sweat iron observed by Brune et al. In the present study, no relevant amounts of [^{59}Fe]hemoglobin (greater than 0.3 mL blood loss per day) were found in urine samples, even though each athlete had signs of hemolysis after a test race. It is unknown whether iron medication benefits runners without anemia. Given that the normal excretion of iron almost doubles because of the significant fecal excretion of iron during intensive training, oral iron therapy is recommended for all male runners that have low serum ferritin. The situation in female runners may be more serious. Self-medication with iron without blood tests can be dangerous because of the prevalence of homozygous or heterozygous hemochromatosis.

▶ This research emphasizes gastrointestinal blood loss as the main cause of the slightly negative iron balance in distance runners compared with controls. Granted, 7 of the 45 male distance runners—vs. only 1 of 112 controls—had a serum ferritin level less than 20 µg/L, but the expansion of blood (and muscle) volume in such athletes "locks up" iron in hemoglobin (and myoglobin), and thus lowers serum ferritin. And the increase in plasma volume in athletes dilutes down serum ferritin, so athletes should have lower ferritin levels than nonathletes. This study does show, however, that intense training or racing increases the amount of occult blood lost in the stool (from about 1–2 mL/day to about 5–6 mL/day), and speculates that intestinal ischemia (or stress gastritis) plays a role. Finding liver iron stores low in runners with low ferritins refutes the hypothesis that low serum ferritin levels in endurance athletes result from a shift of iron (via intravascular hemolysis) from macrophages to hepatocytes.

E.R. Eichner, M.D.

Awareness and Identification of Athletes With Sickle Cell Disorders at Historically Black Colleges and Universities
Jones JD, Kleiner DM (LaGrange, Ga; Univ of North Florida, Jacksonville)
J Athletic Train 31:220–222, 1996   8–24

Background.—The incidence and complications of sickle cell disorders in athletes have not been well reported in the literature. The exposure that athletic trainers at historically black colleges and universities have to these individuals was evaluated, and the precautions, screening techniques, and therapies used in management of this disorder were described.

Definitions.—Sickle cell trait is a benign disorder associated with the heterozygous condition; sickle cell anemia is associated with the homozygous condition. Sickle cell disorder is the collective term. Individuals with sickle cell trait may have a greater amount of sickling with intense physical activity—thus initiating a "crisis" in which complications of sickling (including muscle cramps, tissue ischemia, and musculoskeletal pain) occur.

Methods.—Ninety-four 12-question surveys were mailed to the head athletic trainers of 94 historically black colleges and universities; 34 were returned.

Results.—Screening for sickle cell abnormalities was required by only 12% of the schools during their athletic preparticipation examinations. Respondents reported that 4.9% of athletes had the genetic trait. Three of the 4 schools requiring screening reported a total of 10 incidents of sickle cell crises among their athletes.

Conclusions.—Athletic trainers are likely to encounter athletes with sickle cell disorders, and further education regarding these disorders may be indicated. Athletes at risk should be identified and educated about their condition. Screening should be provided to student athletes during preparticipation examinations.

▶ Studies have suggested that athletes with sickle cell disorder may be susceptible to a crisis and because of this should not participate in intense activities.[1, 2] The authors state this practice is no longer accepted; however, they do stress the importance of black athletes being aware of their sickle cell status. The medical team caring for these athletes should certainly be aware of both sickle cell trait and sickle cell anemia and the complications associated with sickling.

Black athletes should be made aware of sickle cell disorders and be offered testing for these disorders if they so desire. The authors recommend that questions designed to identify sickle cell trait be included in the medical history and that screening be provided to athletes during their preparticipation examinations.

F.J. George, A.T.C., P.T.

References

1. Karh JA: Sickle-cell trait as a risk factor for sudden death in physical training. *N Engl J Med* 317:781–787, 1987.
2. Sears DA: The morbidity of sickle cell trait. A review of the literature. *Am J Med* 64:1021–1036, 1978.

Sport, Exercise, and the Common Cold
Weidner TG, Sevier TL (Ball State Univ, Muncie, Ind; Central Indiana Sports Medicine, Muncie)
J Athl Train 31:154–159, 1996   8–25

Objective.—Upper respiratory diseases may be the most common illnesses affecting athletes. Because of health consequences to athletes, health providers must be aware of the epidemiology, risks of infection, and transmission features of upper respiratory illnesses.

Epidemiology.—Studies have demonstrated that regular vigorous exercise increases the incidence and severity of upper respiratory illness with distance runners having the highest risk.

Risks of Upper Respiratory Infection.—Intense exertion may dampen immune system response, whereas moderate exercise and long-term conditioning may enhance the response of the immune system. Psychological and emotional stress coupled with overexertion may increase the risk of infection. Compromised acute phase response may also lower resistance to infection.

Communicability and Transmission of Upper Respiratory Illness.— Communicability of viruses is controversial although transmission is expected to be spurious among athletes, and the rate is anticipated to be low as a result of other studies.

Sport/Exercise Participation and Upper Respiratory Illness.—The effect of upper respiratory illness on pulmonary function during exercise has not been studied, although respiratory muscle strength and functional capacity of skeletal and cardiac muscles have been found to be reduced during infection. Isometric and dynamic strength and endurance also decrease during infection. Protracted infections, death, malaise, fatigue, lassitude, and aching muscles may occur. Symptoms may persist for months or years if the infecting agent is Coxsackie virus, which can also lead to arrhythmias or death. The potential impact of upper respiratory infection on sports performance should be determined.

Participation and Clinical Management Guidelines.—Resumption of training after symptoms subside is recommended whereas training during the incubation period is not. Supportive treatment in the form of rest, fluids, analgesics, and over-the-counter cold remedies for fever, headache, and muscle pain is appropriate.

Conclusion.—Although the risk of upper respiratory illness transmission among athletes is possibly high, the incidence is unknown. Athletic performance can be affected during illness, although the extent of decline is unknown and needs to be studied.

▶ An athletic trainer often has to decide whether an athlete with an upper respiratory illness should be allowed to practice or compete. The authors report on Eichner's recommended "neck check—" If the symptoms are located 'above the neck,' such as a stuffy or runny nose, sneezing, or scratchy throat with no constitutional symptoms, then the athlete should be allowed to proceed cautiously through the scheduled workout at half speed. After a few minutes, if the congestion clears and the athlete feels better, then intensity can be gradually increased. If the athlete feels worse, rest is recommended. The athlete with 'below the neck' symptoms, such as a fever, aching muscles, hacking or a productive cough, vomiting, or diarrhea, should not train.[1]

F.J. George, A.T.C., P.T.

Reference

1. Eichner ER: Neck check. *Runner's World* 27:16, 1992.

Plasma Glutamine and Upper Respiratory Tract Infection During Intensified Training in Swimmers

MacKinnon LT, Hooper SL (Univ of Queensland, Brisbane, Australia)
Med Sci Sports Exerc 28:285–290, 1996   8–26

Introduction.—Overtraining can lead to a generalized stress response in athletes, with poor performance, fatigue, and mood changes. Frequent illnesses, particularly upper respiratory tract infections (URTIs), can occur as well. Intense training can also affect various biochemical and immune variables, including plasma levels of the amino acid glutamine, which is required as a substrate for energy production and as a nitrogen source for nucleotide synthesis by lymphocytes. It has been suggested that low plasma glutamine levels associated with intensive training can compromise lymphocyte function and lead to an increase in infectious illnesses. The effects of intensive training on plasma glutamine concentrations and the link between plasma glutamine and URTIs were studied in swimmers.

Methods.—The subjects were 24 elite swimmers—16 females and 8 males—participating in a 4-week program of intensified training. During this period, the swimmers' already high level of training was increased in volume by about 10% per week. Plasma glutamine concentrations at rest were measured by high-performance liquid chromatography. The athletes were observed for signs of overtraining syndrome and URTIs.

Results.—Symptoms of overtraining syndrome (OT), such as decreased performance and persistent fatigue, developed in 8 subjects. Symptoms of URTI developed in 42% of the swimmers, including 1 in the OT group and 9 in the non-OT group. Although plasma glutamine concentration increased during the 4-week period, the increase was significant only in the OT group. The only time the plasma glutamine level was significantly lower in the OT group was at the midway time point. Glutamine levels were no different for athletes with or without URTI.

Conclusion.—Plasma glutamine levels do not necessarily decrease during periods of intensified training in athletes. Also, the occurrence of URTI in overtrained athletes is unrelated to their plasma glutamine concentration.

▶ The "glutamine hypothesis" has been advocated vigorously by Newsholme and his colleagues.[1] They argue that adequate plasma levels of glutamine are essential to lymphocyte proliferation. Moreover, they have accumulated evidence that both single bouts of prolonged exercise and periods of heavy training induce significant reductions in plasma glutamine levels, and they have hypothesized that these changes are of sufficient magnitude to increase the vulnerability of the athlete to viral infections.

The above paper found the expected vulnerability to URTIs during a period of intensive training (10 of 24 elite swimmers were affected). However, plasma glutamine levels showed very little decrease during the period of OT, and there was no evidence that glutamine concentrations were lower in those in whom infections developed compared with those in whom they did not. It is important to follow these observations with some further studies of immune function in relation to training-induced changes in plasma glutamine.

R.J. Shephard, M.D., Ph.D., D.P.E.

Reference

1. Parry-Billings M, Budgett R, Koutedakis Y, et al: Plasma amino acid concentrations in the overtraining syndrome: Possible effects on the immune system. *Med Sci Sports Exerc* 24:1353–1358, 1992.

Effects of a Single Bout of Ultraendurance Exercise on Lipid Levels and Susceptibility of Lipids to Peroxidation in Triathletes
Ginsburg GS, Agil A, O'Toole M, et al (Children's Hosp, Boston; Univ of Granada, Spain; Univ of Tennessee, Memphis; et al)
JAMA 276:221–225, 1996   8–27

Introduction.—Free radicals produced by vigorous exercise may promote tissue and vascular injury. If this is true, physical activity may actually be harmful. The effects of participation in the 1994 Hawaii Ironman World Championship Triathlon on lipid and lipoprotein levels and oxidative susceptibility of lipids were evaluated in 39 highly trained athletes.

Methods.—Blood samples were collected 2 days before the triathlon and within 15 minutes of triathlon completion in 26 male and 13 female volunteers. Participants answered questionnaires regarding demographic, training, dietary, and risk factor data. The triathlon consisted of a 3.9-km (2.4-mile) swim, 180.2-km (112-mile) bicycle race, and a 42.2-km (26.2-mile) marathon.

Results.—Compared to baseline, participants had significant decreases in triglycerides (39%), total cholesterol (9%), low-density lipoprotein cholesterol (11%), and apolipoprotein B (10%). The levels of peroxidation were similar prerace and postrace. At exercise completion, the susceptibility of plasma lipids to peroxidation was decreased by 47%, suggesting that exercise acutely produced a favorable balance of antioxidants and pro-oxidants. There were no pre- and postrace differences between athletes who reported use or nonuse of vitamins A or C. There was a tendency toward decreased pre-exercise susceptibility to peroxidation among vitamin E users. The susceptibility of lipids to peroxidation was reduced by exercise in both users and nonusers of vitamin E. Nonusers of vitamin E had a larger decrease in susceptibility of lipids to peroxidation with exercise, compared to users of vitamin E. Serum iron, a potential pro-oxidant, was decreased 45% with exercise. There was a weak association between the susceptibility to peroxidation after exercise and postrace iron levels.

Conclusion.—In both men and women, vigorous exercise improves lipid and lipoprotein risk factors for development of coronary artery disease.

Susceptibility to lipid peroxidation is significantly decreased with exercise. Antioxidant supplements may decrease the degree of acute skeletal muscle injury caused by exercise, but have no additional benefits in reducing the susceptibility of lipids to peroxidation beyond exercise itself.

▶ Debate continues as to whether exercise increases or decreases oxygen free radical stress. Often, it has been argued that the critical factor is the amount of exercise undertaken. However, in this study, even participation in the grueling Hawaiian "Ironman Triathlon" was associated with a substantial decrease of lipid peroxidation. The change was observed within 15 minutes of ceasing the race. It could not be explained by race-induced alterations in antioxidants such as vitamin C or vitamin E, but there was a weak statistically significant correlation with changes in serum iron levels. Possibly, the iron is a modulator of peroxidation. Strenuous exercise leads to losses of iron in sweat, and also increases binding in the reticuloendothelial system.[1]

R.J. Shephard, M.D., Ph.D., D.P.E.

Reference

1. Taylor C, Rogers G, Goodman C, et al: Hematologic, iron-related and acute-phase protein responses to sustained strenuous exercise. *J Appl Physiol* 62:464–469, 1987.

Extreme Exercise and Oxidative DNA Modification
Poulsen HE, Loft S, Vistisen K (Copenhagen Univ)
J Sports Sci 14:343–346, 1996   8–28

Background.—Species with high specific oxygen consumption rates live a shorter time and age earlier than those with a low oxygen consumption. Oxygen consumption and oxidative modification of proteins increase with exercise, so exercise might affect the rate of oxidative DNA damage. It is unknown whether long-term exercise has any such effect in humans. The effects of a period of extreme exercise on oxidative DNA modification were thus studied.

Methods.—Observations were made on 23 healthy men (average age, 22 years) who participated in a 30-day military physical training program. The men trained vigorously for 8–11 hr/day, 6 days/week. Before and after training, urinary excretion of the DNA repair product 8-oxo-7,8-dihydro-2'-deoxyguanosine (8-oxodG) was measured as an indicator of the rate of oxidative DNA modification.

Results.—There was an average 33% increase in creatinine-standardized 8-oxodG excretion from before to after the training period. Men who did not smoke had a significant 50% increase in 8-oxodG excretion, compared with a nonsignificant 25% increase in smokers (Fig 1).

Conclusion.—Extreme exercise appears to increase the rate of oxidative DNA modification in men. The health effects of this increase are unknown.

Non-smokers   Smokers

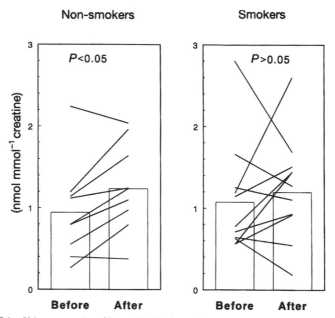

FIGURE 1.—Urinary excretion of 8-oxo-7,8-dihydro-2'-deoxyguanosine (*8-oxodG*) in nanomoles per millimole of creatine, in 9 nonsmokers and 11 smokers before and after a 30-day program of 8–11 hours of vigorous exercise 6 days/wk. In the group as a whole ($n = 20$), the excretion of 8-oxodG increased 33% (95% confidence limits, 3% to 67%) after the exercise program ($P < 0.02$). The lines represent pre-exercise and postexercise values in each individual. The histograms show the mean values. The P values for the smoking and the nonsmoking groups are also given. (Courtesy of Poulsen HE, Loft S, Vistisen K: Extreme exercise and oxidative DNA modification. *J Sports Sci* 14:343-346, 1996.)

However, the findings suggest that extreme exercise could potentially lead to cancer or premature aging.

▶ A number of European authors have recently commented on the development of DNA damage in response to bouts of very heavy exercise. The regimen adopted here—30 days of vigorous exercise, pursued for 8–11 hours per day—exceeds even the demands made on most international competitors. Nevertheless, the body appears to have responded positively to this strain, and indeed the DNA damage was only detected because of its stimulation of repair mechanisms.

One interesting point of reference is that the 33% increase in excretion of repair products was less than that seen normally in smokers (50%). Smokers also showed less increase in DNA repair after the period of exercise, suggesting that their repair mechanisms may already have been fully taxed in correcting the DNA damage inflicted by smoking.

R.J. Shephard, M.D., Ph.D., D.P.E.

DNA Damage After Exhaustive Treadmill Running in Trained and Untrained Men

Niess AM, Hartmann A, Grünert-Fuchs M, et al (Universität Ulm, Germany)
Int J Sports Med 17:397–403, 1996   8–29

Introduction.—Exercise increases the production of oxygen-derived free radicals, some of which may react with lipids, proteins, or nucleic acids. Thus, exercise may cause oxidative DNA damage. Regular training improves exercise tolerance and may shorten the recovery period. The effects of training on oxidative DNA damage after exhaustive exercise were assessed.

Methods.—Six trained distance runners and 5 untrained men participated in the study. Both groups completed an incremental exercise test to exhaustion. Before and after exercise, DNA damage in peripheral white blood cells was measured by single-cell gel electrophoresis. The maximal lactate levels were similar in the trained and untrained men: 12.9 and 12.2 mmol/L, respectively.

Results.—Exercise was associated with a significant increase in DNA migration, from 2.31 at rest to 2.65 tail moment 24 hours after exercise in the trained group and from 2.22 to 3.00 tail moment in the untrained group (Table 6). The percentage increase was 19% in the trained men vs. 36% in the untrained men. Neither group had a significant increase in the plasma malondialdehyde (MDA) level from before to after exercise. However, at rest and 15 minutes after exercise, MDA values were significantly lower in the trained group.

Conclusion.—Exhaustive exercise is associated with DNA damage in white blood cells, perhaps as a result of oxidative stress. This effect is shown in both trained athletes and sedentary men. Physical training may reduce the damaging effects of free radicals on DNA. However, causes and biological relevance of exercise-related DNA damage remain to be demonstrated.

▶ In contrast to the 30 days of sustained endurance exercise evaluated by Poulsen et al. (abstract 8–28), Niess and associates present evidence of

TABLE 6.—DNA Migration Before and After Treadmill Running

	n	Pre-exercise	15 min after exercise	24 h after exercise
DNA-migration (tail moment)				
Pooled	11	2.23 ± 0.19	2.22 ± 0.24	2.82 ± 0.38*
Untrained (UT)	5	2.22 ± 0.16	2.27 ± 0.23	3.00 ± 0.41*
Trained (TR)	6	2.31 ± 0.20	2.18 ± 0.25	2.65 ± 0.30*

Note: The results are shown as mean ± standard deviation.
*$P < 0.05$ postexercise vs. pre-exercise.
†$P < 0.05$ untrained vs. trained subjects.
(Courtesy of Niess AM, Hartmann A, Grünert-Fuchs M, et al: DNA damage after exhaustive treadmill running in trained and untrained men. *Int J Sports Med* 17:397–403, 1996.)

DNA damage in white blood cells after a single session of progressive exercise to exhaustion. Nevertheless, the adaptability of the body is again evidenced in that DNA damage seems greater in untrained than in trained subjects.

R.J. Shephard, M.D., Ph.D., D.P.E.

Effects of a Long-Term Training Program of Increasing Intensity on the Immune Function of Indoor Olympic Cyclists
Ferrández MD, Maynar M, De la Fuente M (Universidad Complutense, Madrid)
Int J Sports Med 17:592–596, 1996   8–30

Introduction.—Unlike overtraining, with its resultant immunodeficiency and increased susceptibility to infections, moderate and regular exercise can stimulate immune response and improve resistance to infections. The immunologic and hormonal status of elite cyclists was evaluated at 2 different time intervals, during a long-term training program, to determine the influence of intense exercise on immune response.

Methods.—Research subjects were 10 men from the Spanish Olympic Team of indoor cyclists who participated in the 1992 Olympic Games in Barcelona. Serum blood was collected in the third year of the program and 25 days before the Games (February 1991 and June 1992, respectively) to measure the concentration of immune cells, phagocytic response of lymphocytes to mitogens, ascorbic acid content of immunocompetent cells, and stress hormone status (cortisol, adrenocorticotropic hormone [ACTH], and β-endorphin). The steps of the phagocytic process of neutrophils were studied: adherence to endothelium, directed mobility or chemotaxis, ingestion of latex beads, and superoxide anion production measured by the nitroblue tetrazolium (NBT) reduction test.

Results.—There was a significant increase in chemotaxis and NBT reduction activity just before the games, compared with the first time point. There was a nonsignificant increase in the values of the proliferative capacity of lymphocytes in June 1992, compared with February 1991. Immediately before the games, there was a striking decrease in ascorbic acid content, particularly in lymphocytes. Compared with February 1991, there was an increase in serum ACTH and β-endorphin levels in June 1992.

Conclusion.—Findings suggest that no immunosuppression occurs at the end of a long-term training program. An important increase in the ACTH and β-endorphin levels was observed; this may be explained by the psychological stress associated with participation in an important event.

▶ Conventional wisdom has it that heavy acute or chronic exercise is associated with an increased risk of upper respiratory infections. Among runners, for example, one expert argues that the risk for such infections is elevated for the highest distance runners, especially during the first week or so after a marathon.[1] This study, however, finds that among men on the Spanish Olympic Indoor Cycling Team, long-term training did not cause immunosuppression clinically or by the immune markers gauged. Indeed, neutrophil and lymphocyte function tended to be improved, not compromised, by training for the Olympics, despite an increase in "stress hormones" as the games drew nigh. Other recent studies explore the role of cortisol in postexercise changes in lymphocyte subsets.[2] They find that both exercise itself and the associated rise in core temperature contribute to changes in leukocytes and subsets during and after moderate exercise,[3] and show that exercise causes similar immune changes in children as in adults.[4]

E.R. Eichner, M.D.

References

1. Nieman DC: The immune response to prolonged cardiorespiratory exercise. *Am J Sports Med* 24:S98–S103, 1996.
2. Shinkai S, Watanabe S, Asai H, et al: Cortisol response to exercise and post-exercise suppression of blood lymphocyte subset counts. *Int J Sports Med* 17:597–603, 1996.
3. Cross MC, Radomski MW, Vanhelder WP, et al: Endurance exercise with and without a thermal clamp: Effects on leukocytes and leukocyte subsets. *J Appl Physiol* 81:822–829, 1996.
4. Boas SR, Joswiak ML, Nixon PA, et al: Effects of anaerobic exercise on the immune system in eight- to seventeen-year-old trained and untrained boys. *J Pediatr* 129:846–855, 1996.

Blood Sampling in Doping Control: First Experiences From Regular Testing in Athletes

Birkeland KI, Donike M, Ljungqvist A, et al (Aker Hosp, Oslo, Norway; Deutsche Sporthochschule, Cologne, Germany; Internatl Amateur Athletic Foundation; et al)
Int J Sports Med 18:7–12, 1997   8–31

Background.—As controls on the use of traditional doping agents have become stricter, athletes are finding other ways to dope to improve performance, including blood doping and the misuse of commercially available recombinant peptide hormones. Thus, new methods for doping control are needed. The results of blood sampling for this purpose were reported.

Methods and Findings.—Samples were obtained from 99 athletes for doping control immediately after a sports event. Three control groups were studied for comparison. Blood doping was not detected with allogenic blood. The athletes' distribution of hemoglobin levels did not differ substantially from that in control subjects. Compared with control subjects, athletes had markedly lower erythropoietin (EPO) values. Fifty-eight percent had EPO values lower than the detection limit for the assay, which may be attributable to high-altitude residence before testing. Measurements of growth hormone (GH) and insulin-like growth factor–1 suggested no misuse of GH in the athletes assessed. One third of the male athletes had subnormal testosterone levels, possibly in part because sampling was done at night and after strenuous activity. Testosterone levels were grossly increased in 1 female athlete.

Conclusion.—The circumstances of sampling must be considered when interpreting the results of blood testing in athletes. More research is needed to develop more sensitive and specific tests for detecting doping with endogenous substances such as GH and EPO.

▶ This study of blood tests taken (after their events) from 99 "athletes" (probably mainly runners, as these tests were from 8 meets sanctioned by the International Amateur Athletic Federation) suggests that abuse of testosterone, GH, or EPO by such athletes may not be widespread. In sharp contrast, detailed investigative reports in the lay press (*Velonews,* February 1997; *Sports Illustrated,* April 14, 1997) charge that drug abuse (including EPO) is common yet largely undetected at the elite level in sports such as track and field, cycling, and swimming. What price glory?[1]

E.R. Eichner, M.D.

Reference

1. Eichner ER: Ergogenic aids: What athletes are using—and why. *Physician Sportsmed* 25:70–83, 1997.

Metabolic and Cardiovascular Effects of a Progressive Exercise Test in Patients With Chronic Fatigue Syndrome
Sisto SA, LaManca J, Cordero DL, et al (Univ of Medicine and Dentistry of New Jersey–New Jersey Med School, Newark; Graduate School of Biomedical Sciences Newark, NJ; VA Med Ctr, East Orange, NJ; et al)
Am J Med 100:634–640, 1996   8–32

Purpose.—Chronic fatigue syndrome (CFS) is defined as serious fatigue that lasts more than 6 months and is not attributable to any medical disease. The symptoms are worsened by even mild exertion, suggesting a possible abnormality of exercise tolerance or of the cardiovascular response to exercise. Previous studies of the response to exercise in patients with CFS have yielded conflicting results. Exercise tests were used to evaluate aerobic power in women with CFS vs. controls.

Methods.—The study included 21 women (mean age, 34 years) meeting the working case definition for CFS. A group of 22 sedentary healthy controls was studied as well. The women performed an incremental treadmill walking test to exhaustion. Expired gases were analyzed, continuous recordings of heart rate were made, and ratings of perceived exhaustion were recorded at each workload. The patient and control groups were further classified into women who did and did not achieve maximal oxygen intake ($\dot{V}O_2$ max)

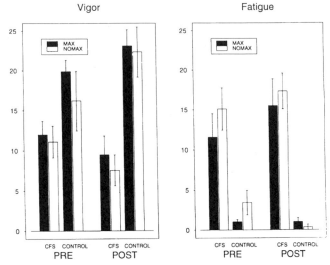

FIGURE.—The means and standard deviations of the Profile of Mood States (*POMS*) scores for vigor and fatigue just before and 4 days after the maximal treadmill test. Vigor increased for the control subjects ($P = 0.03$) and decreased for patients with chronic fatigue syndrome (*CFS*) ($P = 0.01$) when contrasting pre-POMS with post-POMS. No significant change was seen in the fatigue scores of either group, although the magnitude of decrease of fatigue for the CFS group was similar to that of the increase in vigor. (Reprinted by permission of the publisher, courtesy of Sisto SA, LaManca J, Cordero DL, et al: Metabolic and cardiovascular effects of a progressive exercise test in patients with chronic fatigue syndrome. *Am J Med* 100:634–640, copyright 1996 by Excerpta Medica, Inc.)

Results.—Ten women in the CFS group and 17 in the control group achieved $\dot{V}O_2$ max, with a mean value of 28 mL/kg per minute in the CFS group vs. 32 mL/kg per minute in the control group. Women who achieved $\dot{V}O_2$ max in the CFS group achieved values of 98% predicted. At identical absolute workrates, the women in the CFS group had a higher rating of perceived exhaustion than the women in the control group; however, this was not the case at the same relative workrates.

Conclusion.—Testing of aerobic power in women with CFS shows a fitness level in the low-normal range, with no evidence of any cardiopulmonary abnormality. At least in the group of women studied, patients with CSF could perform a maximal treadmill exercise test with no major worsening of their symptoms (figure). There appears to be little or no risk associated with maximal exertion in CFS, and, thus, the type of test used in this study can be included in the overall fitness evaluation of patients with CFS.

▶ Chronic fatigue syndrome is extremely debilitating and notoriously difficult to treat. It is common wisdom that even mild exercise worsens symptoms, and this belief tends to initiate a vicious cycle of decreasing daily activity, deterioration of physical condition, increased fatigue, and a further worsening of symptoms. This careful controlled study shows that well-defined patients with CFS are able to undertake a progressive treadmill measurement of maximal oxygen intake; the results of Profile of Mood

States testing suggest that 4 days after the test, there was some decrease of vigor and an increase in fatigue that was not seen in the control subjects, but the overall health impact of all-out exercise was minor.

Plainly, the implication is that the average patient with CFS could undertake more exercise than that patient does at present without prejudice to the overall condition. The $\dot{V}o_2$ max scores were lower than in the controls, as might be anticipated from the patients' restricted daily physical activity. However, no evidence was found for the early acidosis of exercising muscle that has previously been described in patients with chronic postviral fatigue.[1]

R.J. Shephard, M.D., Ph.D., D.P.E.

Reference

1. Taylor DJ, Arnold DL, Radda GK, et al: Excessive intracellular acidosis of skeletal muscle on exercise in a patient with a post-viral exhaustion/fatigue syndrome. *Lancet* ii:1367–1369, 1984.

Infectious Mononucleosis: Recognizing the Condition, 'Reactivating' the Patient
Eichner ER (Univ of Oklahoma, Oklahoma City)
Physician Sportsmed 24:49–54, 1996   8-33

Introduction.—Infectious mononucleosis (IM) can be a difficult condition to manage in athletes. In addition to the diagnostic difficulties, there are questions about when it is safe to return to competition, given concerns about the risk of splenic rupture. Current knowledge about infectious mononucleosis was reviewed, emphasizing its management in athletes.

Pathogenesis.—The cause of IM is the Epstein-Barr virus, and the disease has a two-stage pathogenesis. After the virus infects and propagates in epithelial cells, the progeny invade a secondary cell type, where they remain latent and establish a persistent infection. Infection of oropharyngeal epithelial cells causes pharyngitis and releases infectious viruses that invade B lymphocytes. Full-blown IM—with the classical triad of clinical, laboratory, and serologic features—is seen most often in adolescents. It is spread by intimate contact such as kissing, so no quarantine is necessary.

Diagnosis and Management.—The classic presentation of IM is a 3- to 5-day prodrome followed by a 1- to 2-week syndrome of fever, sore throat, and lymphadenopathy. Up to 75% of patients will have palpable splenomegaly by the second week of illness. There are new serologic tests for viral antigens, but the diagnosis is usually confirmed with a rapid kit test for heterophil antibody. Other conditions that may mimic IM include cytomegalovirus infection and severe pharyngitis from group A, beta-hemolytic streptococci. There is no specific treatment of IM. Supportive treatments may be helpful, including rest and fluids, aspirin or acetaminophen, and sore throat treatments. Most patients with IM feel better after a week and are well in 4–6 weeks.

Infectious Mononucleosis in Athletes.—There is some evidence that athletes may recover from IM faster than other patients; in mild cases, loss of stamina may be the predominant feature of IM in athletes. Still, it may take 3–6 months for an elite athlete to recover completely from IM. There is controversy as to when an athlete with IM should be allowed to return to competition, with recommendations for contact sports ranging from 3 weeks to 3 months. A reasonable approach to this problem is to wait until the spleen has returned to its usual size and location. Ultrasound is commonly used to assess the size of the spleen. As long as the spleen is normal-sized, the athlete should be able to resume contact sports 5–6 weeks after the onset of the illness.

Summary.—Infectious mononucleosis commonly occurs in athletes. Splenic rupture is a feared but rare complication. Athletes with IM should make a gradual return to activity, and should not resume participation in contact sports until splenomegaly has resolved.

▶ Frequently team physicians have to struggle with the vexing question of when to let an athlete with IM return to play. Controversy abounds here, and patients must be considered individually, but this article offers general guidelines. Most experts agree that it is reasonable to exclude vigorous sports until the spleen has returned to normal size and location (behind the rib cage, where it is protected against rupture). In many cases, physical examination can suffice to gauge the spleen, but more and more in these litigious times, ultrasonography is used as the "gold standard." As a rule of thumb, if the athlete feels well, and results of complete blood count and liver chemistries are again normal, he or she can resume easy training 3–4 weeks after the onset of illness. If the training goes well and the spleen returns to normal size, the athlete can resume contact sports (perhaps wearing a flak jacket at first) in 5–6 weeks after onset of illness

E.R. Eichner, M.D.

Obstructive Sleep Apnea Syndrome and Circadian Rhythms of Hormones and Cytokines

Entzian P, Linnemann K, Schlaak M, et al (Forschungsinstitut Borstel, Germany)
Am J Respir Crit Care Med 153:1080–1086, 1996   8–34

Introduction.—One of the most ancient circadian rhythms is the sleep-wake cycle, and understanding is growing regarding mechanisms by which sleep is disturbed. Several cytokines have been shown to enhance sleep, including interleukin-1 and endotoxin-induced tumor necrosis factor-α. The question of whether comparative cytokine measurements in patients with obstructive sleep apnea syndrome and healthy controls can add to the knowledge of sleep regulation was addressed. Nasal continuous positive airway pressure ventilation has been shown to treat patients with obstructive sleep apnea effectively.

Methods.—Ten patients with obstructive sleep apnea were studied to determine whether circadian rhythms of cytokine release were altered. They were compared with 10 healthy volunteers. After 3 months of therapy with nasal continuous positive airway pressure, the patients with obstructive sleep apnea were reexamined. Short-term cultures of blood samples were taken to investigate circadian cytokine release ex vivo. The cytokines investigated were interleukin-1, interleukin-6, γ-interferon, and tumor necrosis factor-α.

Results.—In patients with obstructive sleep apnea syndrome, the circadian rhythm of tumor necrosis factor-α was significantly disturbed (Fig 4). There was almost a complete disappearance of the nocturnal physiologic peaks in tumor necrosis factor-α and an additional daytime peak had developed. No differences compared with controls were found in the other cytokines.

Conclusion.—Tumor necrosis factor-α could well play a pathophysiologic role in patients with obstructive sleep apnea syndrome, particularly because this cytokine is a known modulator of sleep and because nasal continuous positive airway pressure mask ventilation did not normalize tumor necrosis factor rhythms. More studies should be conducted to

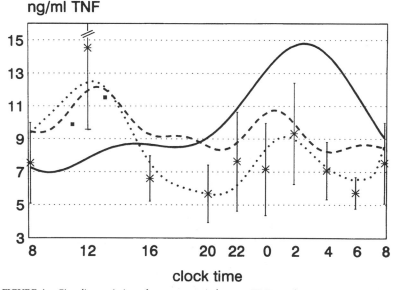

ng/ml TNF

clock time

FIGURE 4.—Circadian variation of tumor necrosis factor-α (*TNF-α*) release in normal volunteers (*n* = 10, *solid line*) and patients with obstructive sleep apnea syndrome (*OSAS*) before (*n* = 10, *broken line*) and during effective nasal continuous positive airway pressure ventilator (*nCPAP*) (*n* = 7, *dotted line*). Tumor necrosis factor concentrations were determined by bioassay. Data are provided in means ± standard error of the plus a fitted curve (OSAS patients undergoing nCPAP therapy), or in fitted curves only (normals and OSAS patients); the curves were calculated by complex overlapping cosine functions adapted with the nonlinear program Pharmfit. No significant circadian rhythm was found in untreated OSAS patients. The patients' maximum concentrations of TNF-α occurred at noon, whereas the normal nocturnal peak had almost disappeared. Effective nCPAP treatment did not restore the normal TNF rhythm. (Courtesy of Entzian P, Linnemann K, Schlaak M, et al: Obstructive sleep apnea syndrome and circadian rhythms of hormones and cytokines. *Am J Respir Crit Care Med* 153:1080–1086, 1996.)

determine whether there is a link between obstructive sleep apnea syndrome and tumor necrosis factor-α.

▶ It has long been argued that regular exercise promotes deep, slow-wave sleep. Recently, a physiologic explanation has begun to emerge in that several of the cytokines modulated by vigorous exercise (for example, interleukin-1 and tumor necrosis factor-α) have sleep-inducing properties.[1, 2] Thus, it is fascinating to find a disturbance in the normal circadian rhythm of tumor necrosis factor-α levels in patients with obstructive sleep apnea.

It is well recognized that such patients are obese; the average body mass in this series by Entzian and associates was 94.9 kg. It may, thus, be that a lack of adequate physical activity is producing both the obesity and a disturbance of normal sleep-wakefulness cycles. There would seem to be scope to examine whether regular exercise could normalize circadian rhythms of cytokine release and whether this, in turn, would help to normalize sleep patterns.

R.J. Shephard, M.D., Ph.D., D.P.E.

References

1. Krueger JM, Walter J, Dinarello CA, et al: Sleep-promoting effects of endogenous pyrogen (interleukin-1). *Am J Physiol* 246:R994–R999, 1984.
2. Pollmächer T, Schreiber W, Gudewill S, et al: Influence of endotoxin on nocturnal sleep in humans. *Am J Physiol* 264:R1077–R1083, 1993.

Exercise-induced Bronchodilatation in Asthmatic Athletes
Todaro A (Inst of Sport Science, Rome)
J Sports Med Phys Fitness 36:60–66, 1996   8–35

Background.—Muscular effort leads to bronchial spasms in most patients with asthma, yet many people with asthma can still participate in high-level athletics. Part of the reason is that training can modify the bronchial response, inducing bronchodilation and reducing the seriousness of bronchospasm. Changes in bronchial status were monitored in asthmatic athletes with chronic airways obstruction.

Methods.—Fourteen high-level athletes with chronic but clinically silent bronchial obstruction were studied. During the 4-day study period, the athletes underwent measurement of forced vital capacity, forced expiratory volume in 1 second, and other ventilatory and metabolic values before and after salbutamol inhalation and before and after maximal exercise tests.

Results.—The athletes had very high values for peak ventilation and peak oxygen intake during the maximal exercise test. Bronchodilation occurred at the end of the exercise test in all patients, with a slow return of bronchial patency values toward baseline during the recovery period. The effort did not worsen bronchial obstruction in any of the patients.

When inhaled salbutamol was given before the exercise test, an even greater degree of bronchodilation was achieved.

Conclusion.—Highly trained athletes with asthma have a persistent bronchodilatory response to exercise, which allows them to achieve high ventilation levels and perform in their sports without any respiratory limitations. Athletes with asthma may have an increased number or density of β-adrenergic receptors, thus enhancing the activity of catecholamines. The effort-related increase in bronchial caliber is great enough that pre-activity administration of bronchodilators is not likely to be useful under favorable climatic conditions.

▶ One of the paradoxes of Olympic competition is that a number of athletes with asthma have been gold medal winners. A possible clue lies in the effect of all-out exercise on bronchial dimensions. We described, many years ago, an increase in maximal voluntary ventilation after a bout of heavy endurance exercise,[1] and we suggested that ventilation had been facilitated by the liberation of catecholamines. Other possible explanations include mechanical effects of the hyperpnea and the release of prostaglandins.[2] Our subjects were ordinary laboratory volunteers, but it is conceivable that the rigorous training of the endurance competitor increases the density or the sensitivity of the β-adrenoreceptors and, thus, the bronchodilation induced by vigorous exercise. Certainly, salbutamol further enhances the ventilation of an athlete with asthma during the recovery period, but it adds little to the normal bronchodilator effect of vigorous exercise while the activity is under way.

R.J. Shephard, M.D., Ph.D., D.P.E.

References

1. Shephard RJ: The maximum sustained voluntary ventilation in exercise. *Clin Sci* 32:167–176, 1967.
2. Gelb AF, Tashkin DP, Epstein JD, et al: Exercise-induced bronchodilation in asthma. *Chest* 87:196–201, 1985.

Exercise-induced Asthma and Cardiovascular Fitness in Asthmatic Children

Thio BJ, Nagelkerke AF, Ketel AG, et al (Academisch Ziekenhuis Vrije Universiteit, Amsterdam, The Netherlands; Spaarneziekenhuis, Haarlem, The Netherlands; Free Univ, Amsterdam, The Netherlands)
Thorax 51:207–209, 1996   8–36

Purpose.—It has been suggested that normalizing cardiovascular fitness in asthmatic children could have important effects in preventing exercise-induced asthma. If this is so, there may be a significant association between an asthmatic child's level of cardiovascular fitness and the occurrence of exercise-induced asthma. Exercise tests were performed in asthmatic children to examine this association.

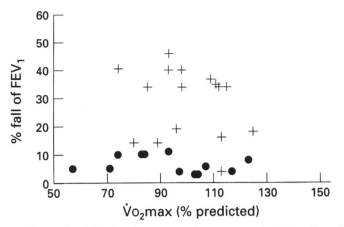

FIGURE.—Relation of % fall in forced expiratory volume in 1 second (FEV$_1$) to % predicted peak oxygen consumption rate (V̇O$_{2max}$) in asthmatic children taking steroids (*filled circles*) (*r*=−0.54) and in children not taking steroids (+) (*r*=0.44). (Courtesy of Thio BJ, Nagelkerke AF, Ketal AG, et al: Exercise-induced asthma and cardiovascular fitness in asthmatic children. *Thorax* 51:207–209, 1996.)

Methods.—The study included 31 children with mild to moderate asthma. Age range was 6 to 13 years; all of the children had dyspnea that limited their ability to play sports. The children performed an exercise test in which the heart rate was increased to 180 beats per minute and maintained at that level for 5 minutes. Forced expiratory volume in 1 second (FEV$_1$) was measured at intervals from 1 to 30 minutes after the exercise had stopped. Another exercise test was performed to assess peak oxygen consumption rate (V̇O$_{2max}$). Three children were excluded because they could not complete the exercise test.

Results.—The children's percent predicted V̇O$_{2max}$ was not significantly related to the percent decrease in FEV$_1$ (Figure). This was so for the 12 patients who were receiving maintenance therapy with inhaled corticosteroids as well as the 16 patients who were not receiving steroid treatment. The fall in FEV$_1$ was significantly greater for children who were not receiving steroids.

Conclusions.—Children with severe exercise-induced asthma can achieve normal cardiovascular fitness, and this level of fitness does not prevent severe exercise asthma. The findings confirm the importance of inhaled corticosteroid therapy in preventing exercise-induced asthma. For children who are taking steroids, the level of exercise used in this study does not produce substantial exercise-induced asthma. In these children, the symptoms of exercise-related dyspnea are probably related to their low level of cardiovascular fitness, which means that they must put forth a greater effort to keep up with other children.

▶ In this cross-sectional study of 28 children who completed both a maximal exercise test (after bronchodilator) and an asthma-provoking test (7-minute run with last 5 minutes at a heart rate of 180 beats per minute), there was no correlation between fitness and the occurrence of exercise-induced asthma. This study also shows that some children with exercise-induced asthma can achieve top fitness and suggests that inhaled steroids are a good "first-line therapy" for severe exercise-induced asthma. Even though fitness may not necessarily protect against exercise-induced asthma, other studies have shown that exercise training can benefit athletes with asthma by making their given event less of an effort.

Other recent studies show that inhaled salmeterol taken the evening before can improve lung function and protect against exercise-induced asthma the next morning[1]; exercise-induced asthma may correlate with increases in both seasonal and perennial allergies as gauged by specific immunoglobulin E levels[2]; a 10-week, high-intensity, swim-training program can benefit patients with asthma and possibly decrease their difficulties with exercise-induced asthma[3]; and in mild asthma, inhaled albuterol should be used not on a regular schedule, but only as needed.[4]

E.R. Eichner, M.D.

References

1. Carlsen KH, Roksund O, Olsholt K, et al: Overnight protection by inhaled salmeterol on exercise-induced asthma in children. *Eur Resp J* 8:1852–1855, 1995.
2. Brutsche M, Britschgi D, Dayer E, et al: Exercise-induced bronchospasm (EIB) in relation to seasonal and perennial specific IgE in young adults. *Allergy* 50:905–909, 1995.
3. Emtner M, Herala M, Stalenheim G: High-intensity physical training in adults with asthma. A 10-week rehabilitation program. *Chest* 109:323–330, 1996.
4. Drazen JM, Israel E, Boushey HA, et al: Comparison of regularly scheduled with as-needed use of albuterol in mild asthma. *N Engl J Med* 335:841–847, 1996.

Time Course of the Protective Effect of Inhaled Heparin on Exercise-induced Asthma

Garrigo J, Danta I, Ahmed T (Univ of Miami, Fla; Mount Sinai Med Ctr, Miami Beach, Fla)
Am J Respir Crit Care Med 153:1702–1707, 1996   8–37

Introduction.—Exercise-induced asthma has been prevented by inhaled heparin without influencing histamine-induced bronchoconstriction. It is not known whether inhaled heparin has the same time-dependent inhibitory effects on antigen-induced bronchoconstriction in humans as it has in sheep. The pharmacokinetics of the inhibitory action of inhaled heparin was investigated in patients with exercise-induced asthma. The antiasthmatic activity of inhaled heparin was also compared with that of cromolyn sodium.

Methods.—On 10 different experiment days, 9 patients with a history of exercise-induced asthma were studied. To document the presence of exercise-induced asthma, on day 1 the patients performed a standardized exercise challenge after their baseline pulmonary functions were obtained. Exercise challenge was performed on a treadmill with increasing workrate until 85% of predicted maximum heart rate was achieved. Exercise was

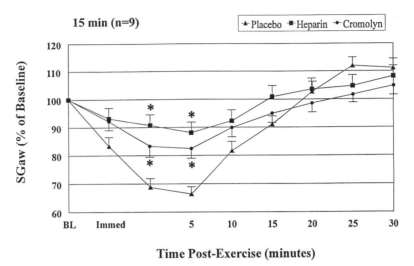

15 min (n=9)

Placebo ■ Heparin ● Cromolyn

Time Post-Exercise (minutes)

FIGURE 2.—Effect of pretreatment with aerosolized heparin (80,000 units) or cromolyn (20 mg) on exercise-induced changes in specific airway conductance (*SGaw*) in subjects with exercise-induced asthma. On different experiment days, heparin or cromolyn was administered 15 minutes before exercise challenge (*n* = 9). Data are shown as a mean ± standard error percent change from baseline (100%) for up to 30 minutes after exercise. No significant difference between cromolyn and heparin was observed. *Asterisk* indicates significant difference from placebo (*P* < 0.05). *Abbreviations: BL*, baseline; *Immed*, immediate. (Courtesy of Garrigo J, Danta I, Ahmed T: Time course of the protective effect of inhaled heparin on exercise-induced asthma. *Am J Respir Crit Care Med* 153:1702–1707, 1996.)

continued for 10 minutes. Before and after exercise, exercise-induced asthma was assessed by measurements of specific airway conductance. In a single-blind, randomized fashion, the patients inhaled 4 mL of heparin (20,000 units/mL), cromolyn (20 mg), or placebo solutions on experiment days 2–10. The drugs were given at increasing pretreatment intervals of 15 minutes, 1 hour, 3 hours, and 6 hours.

Results.—At 3 to 5 minutes after exercise, maximum decreases in specific airway conductance were reproducible on days of control (39 ± 2.1%) and of placebo (37 ± 2.6%). Baseline specific airway conductance was not affected by heparin or cromolyn (Fig 2); however, exercise-induced asthma was attenuated in a time-dependent fashion. When nebulized at 15 minutes before exercise, heparin inhibited the bronchoconstrictor responses to exercise by 58%. When nebulized at 1 hour before exercise, heparin inhibited the bronchoconstrictor responses to exercise by 78%. At 3 hours before exercise, the response to exercise was 67%. Cromolyn attenuated the response by 38% at 15 minutes, 46% at 1 hour, and 41% at 3 hours. When administered 6 hours before exercise, both agents were ineffective. At 1–3 hours, heparin offered greater protection than cromolyn.

Conclusion.—Inhaled heparin is more effective than cromolyn and prevents exercise-induced asthma for as long as 3 hours.

▶ The anti-inflammatory properties of heparin were discovered many years ago,[1] but they have recently been attracting renewed attention.[2] Among possible applications, heparin has been proposed as a treatment for exercise-induced asthma.[3] The demonstration in this study of a greater effectiveness than cromolyn strongly supports this suggestion.

R.J. Shephard, M.D., Ph.D., D.P.E.

References

1. Dolowitz DA, Dougherty TF: The use of heparin as an anti-inflammatory agent. *Laryngoscope* 70:873–884, 1960.
2. Nelson RM, Cecconi O, Roberts G, et al: Heparin oligosaccharides bind L- and P-selectin and inhibit acute inflammation. *Blood* 82:3253–3258, 1993.
3. Ahmed T, Garrigo J, Danta I: Preventing bronchoconstriction in exercise-induced asthma with inhaled heparin. *N Engl J Med* 329:90–95, 1993.

Dyspnea Ratings for Prescribing Exercise Intensity in Patients With COPD
Horowitz MB, Littenberg B, Mahler DA (Dartmouth Med School, Lebanon, NH; Washington School of Medicine, St Louis)
Chest 109:1169–1175, 1996   8–38

Objective.—Symptomatic patients with stable chronic obstructive pulmonary disease (COPD) were recruited for a trial designed to test the hypothesis that such patients can reproduce reliably an exercise intensity, as measured by oxygen consumption, using dyspnea ratings obtained from a previous graded exercise test. The ability to use dyspnea targets was examined over both short-term and long-term periods.

Methods.—Eligible patients were clinically stable, had no other significant illnesses, and were not taking β-adrenergic antagonists, calcium channel agents, oral corticosteroids, or supplemental oxygen. On the first visit the 15 participants (5 women and 10 men with a mean age of 68 years) were familiarized with the testing procedure. At 3 additional visits during a 7-week period patients estimated the heaviness of weights to evaluate their estimation of a nonrespiratory task and underwent spirometry to determine lung function. At the first and second visit (estimation trials 1 and 2), patients rated the intensity of dyspnea during an incremental symptom-limited exercise test. At visits 3 and 4 (production trials 1 and 2) they were asked to produce specific intensities of dyspnea (dyspnea targets) during submaximal exercise. Visit 2 took place on study days 5–7, visit 3 on days 10–14, and visit 4 on days 40–44.

Results.—All patients completed the study protocol and lung function was stable at all visits. At estimation trial 2, mean dyspnea ratings were 1.8 at 50% of peak oxygen consumption and 5.5 at anaerobic threshold (AT)/80% of peak oxygen consumption. (On the scale used, 0 represented no breathlessness and 10 represented the greatest breathlessness ever experienced.) Twelve of the 15 patients were able to exercise at an intensity within 15% of the 50% peak oxygen consumption target at visit 3; 9 patients achieved this accuracy at visit 4. And at the AT/80% peak oxygen consumption target, 13 patients at visit 3 and 12 at visit 4 exercised within 15% of the targets. Patients were more accurate when a higher dyspnea target was used, but maintained their ability to reproduce exercise intensities during a 1-month period. Two patients appeared to be unreliable raters, showing excessive variability in estimation of the heaviness of weights.

Conclusion.—Dyspnea ratings obtained during a graded exercise test may be used by patients with COPD as a target for regulation of steady-state exercise intensity. This technique offers a simple and inexpensive method for patients to monitor their exercise training intensity.

▶ Investigators continue to argue that ratings of perceived exertion or dyspnea provide a useful basis for the regulation of exercise prescription.[1] In the study of Horowitz, et al, such ratings brought only 12 of 15 patients to within 15% of the intended oxygen consumption at a high intensity of effort (80% of peak oxygen intake); at 50% of peak oxygen intake, a level more likely in the early stages of rehabilitation, only 9 of 15 participants attained the 15% level of accuracy. Some people may regard this as a useful check on exercise intensity, but in my view greater precision could be obtained by asking a person to walk a specific distance in a set time.

R.J. Shephard, M.D.

Reference

1. Shephard RJ, Kavanagh T, Mertens DJ, et al: The place of perceived exertion ratings in exercise prescription for cardiac transplant patients before and after training. *Br J Sports Med* 30:116–121, 1996.

Exostoses of the External Auditory Canal in Oregon Surfers
Deleyiannis FW-B, Cockcroft BD, Pinczower EF (Univ of Washington, Seattle; Providence Seaside Hosp, Seaside Ore)
Am J Otolaryngol 17:303–307, 1996   8–39

Background.—Exostoses of the external auditory canal can occur with exposure to cold water. The amount of cold water exposure necessary to produce this biological response was investigated in surfers along the Oregon and northern California coast.

Methods.—Free ear evaluations were offered at 2 surf shops in northern Oregon. Data on 21 surfers were analyzed. All underwent ear canal examination with an otoscope and received a summary score indicating the percentage of canal obstruction by exostoses.

Findings.—The extent of ear canal obstruction increased significantly with increasing number of years surfing and number of surfing sessions annually. The median summary score was 7.5 for those surfing 1–5 years, 63 for those surfing 6–15 years, and 93 for those surfing more than 15 years. Individuals surfing 50 sessions or less annually had a median summary score of 10, compared with 87.5 for those surfing more than 50

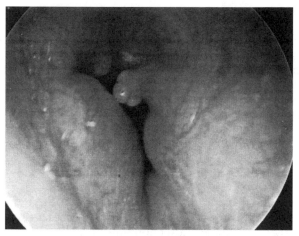

FIGURE 2.—Near total occlusion (90%) of the left external auditory canal by multiple exostoses. (Courtesy of Deleyiannis FW-B, Cockcroft BD, Pinczower EF: Exostoses of the external auditory canal in Oregon surfers. *Am J Otolaryngol* 17:303–307, 1996.)

sessions annually. Problems were minimal in most surfers with exostoses. Only 1 subject had had surgery for related complaints (Fig 2).

Conclusion.—Exostoses will probably not develop in surfers who have surfed for 5 years or less and for fewer than 50 sessions annually. In general, exostoses are a benign condition needing no surgical intervention.

► This novel report suggests that, over the years, cold water surfers can go deaf! Exostoses of the external auditory canal, it seems, are a normal biological response to cold water exposure. Rarely, such exostoses need to be removed surgically because they cause recurrent otitis externa or chronic hearing impairment. Indeed, 1 surfer here had near total occlusion of the left external auditory canal by multiple exostoses. Only 21 surfers were studied, but there was a rough correlation of degree of canal obstruction with years spent surfing. Other than occasional "ear plugging," however, this malady— "surfer's ear"—seems typically benign. The wearing of earplugs and hoods may prevent exostoses by preventing cold water from entering the external ear canal.

E.R. Eichner, M.D.

Cutaneous Manifestations of Sports Participation
Pharis DB, Teller C, Wolf JE Jr (Baylor College of Medicine, Houston)
J Am Acad Dermatol 36:448–459, 1997   8–40

Background.—Diagnosing skin problems associated with sports participation can be difficult without knowledge of these associations. Effective treatment often relies on an understanding of the unique factors that contributed to such dermatologic problems. The cutaneous manifestations of sports participation were reviewed and suggestions made for diagnosis, prevention, and treatment.

Traumatic Injuries.—Injury to the skin during sports participation is common, especially the skin of the feet. The main cause of traumatic skin lesions in athletes is the equipment used. Such injuries include friction blisters, calluses, corns, ingrown toenails, and black heels and palms. Piezogenic papules and multiple, skin-colored, painful papules, 2 to 5 mm, on the lateral or medial surfaces of the heel occur most often in long distance runners. Tennis toe is a painful, subungal bleeding that usually occurs in the first and second toes. The term is misleading because it is also caused by jogging, skiing, hiking, climbing, or any other sport that causes repetitive slippage of the foot anteriorly against the shoe or frequent dorsiflexion of the toes in a shoe with a limited toe box. Turf toe, seen in athletes who play on artificial turf, presents as a painful, red, swollen first toe. Jogger's nipples are painful, fissured, eroded nipples that occasionally bleed, occurring immediately after long-distance running in women not wearing a bra and in men wearing hard-fiber shirts. Striae develop in up to 90% of adolescent girls and 40% of adolescent boys, especially those who lift weights. Striae distansae is the most common type, caused by rupture of elastic fibers into the reticular dermis, probably resulting from a corticosteroid effect on elastic tissue. Striae are arranged perpendicular to lines of skin tension and usually occur over the anterior shoulders, lower back, and thighs. The finding of atrophic striae, especially combined with severe acne, a receding hairline, or hypertrichosis, suggests the use of anabolic steroids. Other manifestations are green hair in swimmers, athlete's nodules, golfer's nails, mogul skier's palm, pulling-boat hands, hooking thumb, swimmer's shoulder, runner's and rower's rump, jazz ballet bottom, and ping pong patches.

Environmental Injuries.—Extremes of temperature, wind, and sun exposure may also damage the skin. Such damage includes frostnip, frostbite, phototoxicity, and sunburn. Long-term sun exposure can result in photoaging, actinic keratosis, basal cell carcinoma, squamous cell carcinoma, and malignant melanoma. Allergic contact dermatitis and xerosis are also seen in athletes.

Infections.—Athletes are exposed to many common and uncommon infectious agents. Skin infections associated with sports participation include pitted keratolysis, swimmer's ear, herpes gladiatorum, impetigo, tinea corporis gladiatorum, tinea pedis, seabather's eruption, and swimmer's itch.

▶ This article is one of the few comprehensive reviews dealing with dermatologic problems confronting the sports medicine practitioner. Most noteworthy is the extensive and complete bibliography with 110 citations.

J.S. Torg, M.D.

Cutaneous Disease in Wrestlers and Other Athletes: Part II. Viral Infections

Bikowski J (Univ of Pittsburgh, Pa)
Athletic Ther Today 1:30–35, 1996   8–41

Introduction.—Some of the common viruses affecting athletes were reviewed. Contact-sport athletes, especially wrestlers, have greater risk of acquiring these infections because of increased skin-to-skin contact with less protective clothing.

Herpes simplex.—The herpes simplex viruses (HSV) may cause lesions above the waist (usually HSV-1) or below (usually HSV-2). Herpes simplex virus-1 generally appears as an isolated group of erythematous-based papules, vesicles, and pustules, and may occur anywhere on the body. Systemic antiviral therapy is most effective; the severity and duration of the attack may be decreased.

Varicella/Zoster.—Wrestlers with chickenpox should be withheld from practice and competition until all lesions are crusted over. Most cases resolve in 7–14 days with no specific therapy, but symptomatic therapy can alleviate itch and decrease the risk of secondary infection. Shingles is a return to activity of the virus in an individual who has already had chickenpox. The lesions of shingles are grouped together in "clumps" on only one side of the body. The rash usually resolves in 3–6 weeks. Individuals with an outbreak of shingles may transmit the virus to those who have never had it—resulting in chickenpox. Symptomatic treatment and systemic antiviral therapy may be helpful for shingles.

Molluscum Contagiosum.—This viral disease occurs most often in children, adolescents, and young adults and has a predilection for males. Discrete round papules that are flesh, pink, or white in color are characteristic. Lesions usually resolve spontaneously in 3–12 months; the incubation period is 2–8 weeks. Treatment is not always necessary, but centers around removal or destruction of the central curdlike core of the lesions. Second infections are rare.

Warts.—Warts are also caused by a viral infection of the skin and can be contagious. Warts need to be treated only when they are tender or painful.

Conclusions.—The athletic therapist should recognize contagious processes, restrict participation, recommend initial treatment, and ensure referral to a physician.

▶ Diseases of the skin can be a major problem for wrestlers because these lesions may eliminate them from practice or competition. The author recommends treating recurrent HSV infections with valacyclovir, 500 mg, 1 tablet twice a day for 5 days or famciclovir, 125 mg, 1 tablet twice a day for 5 days, in place of the previously used acyclovir. The newer drugs are better absorbed from the gastrointestinal tract and therefore only a twice a day dosing is required.

F.J. George, A.T.C., P.T.

Meningococcemia: Heading Off a Killer

Howe WB (Western Washington Univ, Bellingham)
Physician Sportsmed 24:57–60, 1996
8–42

Background.—Meningococcemia is a potentially lethal disease that requires early, aggressive treatment. It is frequently seen among closed groups, such as sports teams. The epidemiology, signs and symptoms, and proper treatment of meningococcemia were reviewed.

Managing Meningococcemia.—*Neisseria meningitidis*, the underlying organism, can be cultured in 5% to 15% of healthy individuals. Nasopharyngeal infection is associated with few, if any, symptoms. Typically, early disease manifests as acute febrile illness with malaise, nausea, aches, and chills. Patients usually get noticeably sicker, with toxemia and prostration. A high index of suspicion in the early stage of disease is key to effective treatment. In children, the preferred initial treatment is ceftriaxone, as septicemia with *Haemophilus influenzae* results in signs and symptoms similar to those of meningococcemia. After diagnosis, the public should be alerted, with wide publicity of the early symptoms of meningococcemia. Individuals in the potentially exposed population should be urged to seek immediate medical care if febrile illness develops. Affected patients should be isolated during the first 24–36 hours of antibacterial treatment. Individuals who have been in close contact with patients require chemoprophylaxis to eradicate meningococci from the nasopharynx. Rifampin is the drug of choice for this purpose. Patients with meningococcemia should also receive this prophylaxis before hospital discharge, as organisms are often recovered from the nasopharynx after treatment. A meningococcal vaccine is available and should be offered to patients with impaired resistance, such as those with no spleen or with a deficiency in terminal-component complement. Although universal immunization is not practiced, some authorities recommend immunization as a supplement to chemoprophylaxis to control outbreaks.

Conclusion.—Clinicians must maintain a high index of suspicion for meningococcemia when examining patients with acute febrile illness, especially those younger than 20 years of age. Antibiotics and intensive supportive care are required. To limit an outbreak of this potentially fatal disease, prophylaxis is indicated in individuals who have had close contact with the patient. Widely publicizing the early signs and symptoms of the disease is also necessary.

▶ This report—a different tack from the usual "infections in athletes" theme—reminds us of the potential for outbreaks of meningococcemia in relatively closed groups, such as sports camps and athletic teams. The clinical hallmarks of this grave illness are covered. For treating children, ceftriaxone is preferred. Once one case is diagnosed, the early symptoms of meningococcemia should be widely publicized and the public urged to rush to the doctor if a febrile illness develops. Those in close contact with the patient should be given chemoprophylaxis (first choice, rifampin) to eradicate meningococci from the nasopharynx. Patients should also receive chemoprophylaxis before hospital discharge. People with impaired resistance—such as those lacking a spleen or deficient in terminal-component complement—should be given the meningococcal vaccine. The vaccine can also serve as an adjunct to help curb some outbreaks. On the usual theme of "infections in athletes," a review of the immune response to exercise offers a timely, balanced update, including practical clinical implications.[1]

E.R. Eichner, M.D.

Reference

1. Nieman DC: The immune response to prolonged cardiorespiratory exercise. *Am J Sports Med* 24:S98–S103, 1996.

Pressor Response to Isometric Exercise in Patients With Multiple Sclerosis
Pepin EB, Hicks RW, Spencer MK, et al (Northeastern Univ, Boston)
Med Sci Sports Exerc 28:656–660, 1996   8–43

Introduction.—Neurocardiovascular involvement in multiple sclerosis (MS) is probable. About 50% of patients with MS who have participated in trials that tested autonomic cardiovascular reflexes have shown abnormal responses. Heart rate and arterial pressure responses were measured during sustained submaximal isometric handgrip exercise in patients with MS and normal controls to determine whether patients with MS have attenuated heart rate and/or pressor responses.

Methods.—One hundred and four patients with MS (mean age 41.6 years) and 25 healthy controls (mean age 34.3 years) underwent handgrip exercise testing, using a dynamometer connected to a load cell that was interfaced with a physiograph recorder. The best 2 of 3 maximal voluntary contractions (MVC) with the dominant hand were averaged. After a 5-minute recovery period, research subjects performed a handgrip contraction at a force output equal to 30% of MVC. This force was maintained until fatigue. Heart rate, systolic and diastolic blood pressure, rate of perceived exertion (RPE), and mean arterial pressure (MAP) were calculated at rest and at 20%, 40%, 60%, 80%, and 100% of time to fatigue. All participants underwent a neurologic examination. Patients with MS were also evaluated for disability.

Results.—Patients with MS were significantly older than controls. At baseline, MVC was significantly greater and the time to fatigue was about 50 seconds longer for controls, compared to patients with MS. The RPE at each percentage of exercise duration was about equal for patients and controls. There was a linear increase in systolic blood pressure, diastolic blood pressure, and MAP from rest to fatigue in both groups. For patients with MS, each of these responses were significantly attenuated at each percentage of exercise duration. The mean changes in MAP at fatigue were +47.9 mm Hg for controls and +28.2 mm Hg for patients with MS (Fig

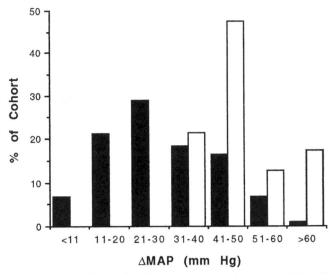

FIGURE 2.—Frequency distribution for change in mean arterial pressure (MAP) at fatigue during isometric handgrip exercise at 30% maximal voluntary contraction in patients with multiple sclerosis and controls. *Open bars*, % control; *filled bars*, % MS. (Courtesy of Pepin EB, Hicks RW, Spencer MK, et al: Pressor response to isometric exercise in patients with multiple sclerosis. *Med Sci Sports Exerc* 28:656–660, 1996.)

2). The distribution around the mean for the patient group was considerably wider than that of controls. The arterial pressure in 58% of patients with MS was below the lowest value recorded for a control research subject. Eighteen patients with MS had increases in MAP at the point of fatigue that ranged from −6 mm Hg to 15 mm Hg. At 20% of exercise duration, the heart rate for controls was significantly higher than in patients with MS. In patients with MS, the Incapacity Status Scale and age combined to account for 26% of the variability in change in MAP at the point of fatigue. No other variables were predictive of MAP response.

Conclusion.—Fifty-eight percent of patients with MS were unable to increase arterial pressure in response to isometric handgrip exercise. Eighteen of 104 patients with MS were unable to increase MAP by more than 15 mm Hg, which is evidence of a profoundly abnormal pressor response to exercise. This may be because MS lesions located in the hypothalamic nuclei or areas of the spinal cord are on or near neurons associated with autonomic control of cardiovascular reflexes. The significant between-group difference in age was not a likely factor in MAP scores.

▶ We tend to think of the limitation of performance in MS as attributable simply to a loss of muscle function, and this paper provides a useful reminder that sclerotic plaques can also affect the autonomic system, giving an impaired cardiovascular response to exercise. Nevertheless, the proportion of patients with autonomic lesions may be less than the present figures would suggest, because a part of the stimulus to the rise of blood pressure during isometric contraction is a stimulation of metaboreceptors within the active muscles, and in MS muscle weakness may limit the force of contraction and thus the accumulation of peripheral stimulants of the cardiovascular system.

R.J. Shephard, M.D., Ph.D., D.P.E.

Does Physical Activity Reduce Risk of Estrogen-dependent Cancer in Women?
Kramer MM, Wells CL (Arizona State Univ, Tempe)
Med Sci Sports Exerc 28:322–334, 1996   8–44

Background.—Cancers of the breast, ovaries, and endometrium are sometimes classified as estrogen-dependent cancer. Mortality, from cancer as well as from all causes, is significantly reduced with a moderate level of cardiovascular fitness. Research on the link between physical activity and prevention of estrogen-dependent cancers in women was reviewed.

Physical Activity and Estrogen-dependent Cancer.—Ten published studies support the hypothesis that physically inactive women are at higher risk of breast, endometrial, and ovarian cancers. Another 3 studies do not support this hypothesis. Vigorous occupational activity may have a greater protective effect than vigorous nonoccupational activity, perhaps because occupational activity is more regular. Body mass or body fat is an important confounding variable in this relationship. There is considerable evidence to suggest a link between excess body mass, adult weight gain, and estrogen-dependent cancers.

Possible Mechanisms.—The main mechanism for the ability of physical activity to influence the incidence of estrogen-dependent cancer may be maintenance of low to moderate adipose tissue and, thus, of extraglandular estrogen. The intensity of physical activity appears to have a major role in maintaining favorable levels and distribution of body fat. Breast cancer risk may be related to the cumulative number of ovulatory menstrual cycles. Higher gynecologic age has also been linked to endometrial and ovarian cancer. Physical activity may protect against estrogen-dependent cancer by reducing the total number of ovulatory cycles, thus inducing hypoestrogenism. Another possibility is that exercise enhances immune resistance to carcinogenesis, although the evidence for this theory comes from animal studies. Finally, it may be that people who are physically active have other healthy life style habits as well. However, causal relationships have yet to be determined.

Discussion.—The available evidence suggests that low to moderate physical activity may help to prevent estrogen-dependent cancers in women. An active lifestyle to maintain low body fat levels can be recommended for reducing breast cancer risk, particularly postmenopausal breast cancer.

▶ The suggestion by 2 investigators quoted in this review that reproductive cancer risk can be decreased by increasing physical activity until a girl or woman becomes hypoestrogenic[1, 2] completely ignores the fact that decreased levels of endogenous estrogen in active women are associated with a decrease in bone density and a potential risk for osteoporotic-type fractures. To suggest that "...high levels of habitual physical activity may protect women from estrogen-dependent cancer by reducing the total number of ovulatory cycles and inducing hypoestrogenism" is treading on thin ice.

B.L. Drinkwater, Ph.D.

References

1. Bernstein L, Ross RK, Lobo RA, et al: The effects of moderate physical activity on menstrual cycle patterns in adolescence: implications for breast cancer prevention. *Br J Cancer* 55:681–685, 1987.
2. Frisch RE, Wyshak G, Albright NL, et al: Lower prevalence of breast cancer and cancers of the reproductive system among former college athletes compared to nonathletes. *Br J Cancer* 52:885–891, 1985.

The Influence of Physical Activity on Lung-cancer Risk: A Prospective Study of 81,516 Men and Women
Thune I, Lund E (Univ of Tromsø, Norway)
Int J Cancer 70:57–62, 1997   8–45

Background.—Physical activity has been found to be related inversely to death resulting from respiratory disease, including lung cancer. Although physical activity improves pulmonary function, its effect on the risk for lung cancer has not been studied thoroughly.

Methods.—Data were obtained from a population-based health survey conducted between 1972 and 1978. A total of 53,242 men and 28,274 women, aged 20–49 years, participated in that study. Follow-up extended through 1991.

Findings.—Lung cancer developed in 413 men and 51 women. Leisure activity but not work activity was inversely associated with the risk for lung cancer in men after adjustment for age, smoking habits, body mass index, and geographic residence. Risk for lung cancer was lower in men who exercised at least 4 hours a week than in those who did not exercise. The reduction in risk was particularly pronounced for small-cell carcinoma and adenocarcinoma. There was no apparent effect on squamous-cell carcinoma. Among women, no consistent association was seen between physical activity and risk for lung cancer (Table 2).

Conclusions.—Leisure-time physical activity appears to have an effect on the risk for lung cancer in men. The small number of incident cases and

TABLE 2.—Adjusted Relative Risk for Lung Cancer With 95% Confidence Intervals Related to Categories of Occupational and Recreational Physical Activity at the First Screening (1972–1978) Among Men and Women

Physical activity (PhA)	Men			Women		
	Number of cases	RR*	95% CI	Number of cases	RR*	95% CI
Occupational PhA						
Sedentary (O1)	139	1.00	(Ref)	8	1.00	(Ref)
Walking (O2)	119	1.15	(0.90–1.47)	34	0.81	(0.37–1.76)
Lifting (O3)	97	1.13	(0.87–1.47)	8	0.79	(0.30–2.12)
Heavy manual (O4)	47	0.99	(0.70–1.41)	0	—	
Trend test		$p = 0.71$			$p = 0.30$	
Recreational PhA						
Sedentary (R1)	123	1.00	(Ref)	14	1.00	(Ref)
Moderate (R2)	217	0.75	(0.60–0.94)	32	0.91	(0.48–1.71)
Regular training (R3 + R4)	62	0.71	(0.52–0.97)	5	0.99	(0.35–2.78)
Trend test		$p = 0.01$			$p = 0.88$	
Total PhA (occupational + recreational)						
Sedentary (O1 + R1)	52	1.0	(Ref)	2	1.0	(Ref)
Active	349	0.73	(0.54–0.98)	48	0.87	(0.21–3.62)

*Adjusted for age at entry, geographical region, smoking habits (ex-smoking, pipe/cigar smoking [men only], number of cigarettes smoked, years smoked) and body mass index.
Abbreviations: CI, confidence interval; O, occupational; R, recreational; RR, relative risk.
(Courtesy of Thune I, Lund E: The influence of physical activity on lung-cancer risk: A prospective study of 81,516 men and women. *Int J Cancer* 70:57–62, 1997. Reprinted by permission of Wiley-Liss, Inc., a subsidiary of John Wiley & Sons, Inc.)

the narrow range of physical activity reported may have limited the ability of the current research to detect such relationships among women.

▶ Good evidence now shows an association between physical activity and protection against colon cancer, and there have been suggestions that this protection may extend to other body regions, including the lungs. Lung cancer is particularly interesting, because any benefit would presumably reflect a direct influence on immune defenses, rather than some incidental factor such as a speeding of gastrointestinal transit or a reduction in body fat content. The big problem with analyzing epidemiologic data on bronchial tumors is the overwhelming influence of cigarette smoking. Thune and Lund have been careful to covary their data for such findings as years of smoking, number of cigarettes consumed, and ex-smoking, but the nagging problem remains as to whether sedentary smokers take more or deeper puffs per cigarette, smoke cigarettes with a higher tar content, or are exposed to other carcinogens that act synergistically with cigarette smoke.

R.J. Shephard, M.D., Ph.D., D.P.E.

Leisure and Occupational Physical Activity and Risk of Colorectal Adenomatous Polyps

Neugut AI, Terry MB, Hocking G, et al (Columbia Univ, New York; Univ of Michigan, Ann Arbor; Mt Sinai School of Medicine, New York)
Int J Cancer 68:744–748, 1996   8–46

Background.—Research has demonstrated that physical activity protects against colorectal cancer. However, few studies have investigated the

TABLE 3.—Relationship Between Incident and Metachronous Adenomas and Occupational Physical Activity*

	Incident adenomas		Metachronous adenomas	
	Cases/controls	OR (95% CI)	Cases/controls	OR (95% CI)
Males				
Low activity	85/78	1.0	38/55	1.0
Average activity	86/136	0.6 (0.4–0.9)	96/137	0.9 (0.5–1.6)
High activity	2/11	0.2 (0.0–0.9)	4/4	1.2 (0.2–5.9)
p for trend†		p = 0.003		NS
Females				
Low activity	45/89	1.0	17/51	1.0
Average activity	79/194	0.9 (0.6–1.6)	41/96	1.2 (0.7–3.3)
High activity	3/0	Combined w/average	1/2	3.6 (0.3–53.9)
p for trend†				NS

*All estimates are adjusted for age, years of education, body mass index, total caloric intake, dietary fiber intake, dietary fat intake, and cigarette smoking (men only).
†*P* test for linear trend.
Abbreviations: NS, not significant at *P* = 0.05; *OR,* odds ratio.
(Courtesy of Neuget AI, Terry MB, Hocking G, et al: Leisure and occupational physical activity and risk of colorectal adenomatous polyps. *Int J Cancer* 68:744–748, 1996. Reprinted by permission of Wiley-Liss, Inc., a subsidiary of John Wiley & Sons, Inc.)

association between physical activity and incident adenomas, and none has determined the association of activity with metachronous adenomas.

Methods.—A total of 2,001 patients undergoing colonoscopy in 3 New York City practices between 1986 and 1988 were interviewed. Two hundred ninety-eight patients had a first diagnosis of adenomas; 197, metachronous adenomas; 345, normal colonoscopic findings with a history of adenomas; and 506, normal findings on colonoscopy.

Findings.—After adjustment for age, years of education, body mass index, total energy intake, dietary fiber intake, dietary fat intake, and years of cigarette smoking, leisure-time physical activity had borderline-significant protective effects against metachronous and incident cases among men. Among men, occupational physical activity also had a significant protective effect. No protective effects were found among women (Table 3).

Conclusions.—Incident and metachronous cancers were reduced among men with increased levels of either occupational or leisure-time activity. Such activity did not have a protective effect among women.

▶ The association between exercise and protection against colon cancer is now fairly well established. A similar association should thus be seen for the precursor of such cancers—adenomatous polyps. This study by Neugut and colleagues examines this question. As in many of the studies of colon cancer, benefit seems stronger for occupational than for leisure activity and stronger for men than for women. It is not clear whether this is because few people participate in leisure activity, whether leisure activity is difficult to measure, or whether benefit is associated mainly with the sustained moderate-intensity effort that occurs in many of the physically active jobs that are performed mainly by men.

Most features of the experiment, including the blinding of job categorization and control for interfering variables, seem well conceived and conducted. The one question mark is the estimated food intake, which is suspiciously low for both active and inactive participants.

R.J. Shephard, M.D., Ph.D., D.P.E.

Effect of Exercise on Mouth-to-Cecum Transit in Trained Athletes: A Case Against the Role of Runners' Abdominal Bouncing
Kayaleh RA, Meshkinpour H, Avinashi A, et al (Univ of California, Irvine)
J Sports Med Phys Fitness 36:271–274, 1996   8–47

Introduction.—Reports are not in agreement concerning the role of physical exercise in gastrointestinal motor function, particularly its impact on transit time. It has been suggested that running may have a different effect on mouth-to-cecum transit than exercises performed in a stationary setting because of the jostling of the abdomen. A group of well-conditioned athletes were evaluated after resting and after running to determine the effect of exercise on mouth-to-cecum transit.

Methods.—The mean age of the 8 healthy male athletes was 25 years. After ingesting 10 of lactulose in 100 mL of water, the subjects were randomly assigned on separate days to either relax on a couch for 180 minutes or run on a treadmill at a maximum speed of 9.6 km/hr for 1 hour; the running was followed by 30 minutes of rest. During both sessions, exhaled gas was measured every 10 minutes for volume, minute ventilation, and hydrogen concentration.

Results.—During exercise and rest, the mean oxygen consumption was 36.8 mL/min/kg and 4.7 mL/min/kg, respectively. The postlactulose rise in hydrogen concentration occurred at a mean of 85 minutes for the resting session and 84 minutes for the exercise session.

Conclusion.—Mouth-to-cecum transit time was not significantly affected by short, intense exercise in well-conditioned athletes. It is likely that bouncing of the abdominal content in running does not affect transit time. Mouth-to-cecum transit is not influenced by fitness stage.

▶ The influence of exercise upon gastrointestinal transit has a number of important practical applications. Perhaps the most important is the suggested link between accelerated transit and a decreased risk of bowel cancer. This study provides good data showing that there is no effect of quite vigorous exercise on mouth-to-cecum transit time, but there could still be an effect on colonic transit; the main beneficial effect of exercise is on the incidence of cancer in the descending colon.

R.J. Shephard, M.D., Ph.D., D.P.E.

Subject Index*

A

Abdomen
  bouncing in runners, effect on
      mouth-to-cecum transit, 97: 439
  pain, acute, assessment of, 97: 108
  trauma, blunt, spleen injury from, in
      children, CT of, 96: 303
Abduction
  -adduction moments at knee during
      stair ascent and descent, 97: 139
  shoulder, in scapular plane, kinematics
      of, 96: 82
Abductor
  strength characteristics of professional
      baseball pitchers, 96: 29
Absorptiometry
  x-ray, dual energy, for body
      composition evaluation, 96: 305
Abuse
  of corticosteroid injections, 95: 33
  drug, 97: 279
  stanozolol, severe cholestasis and acute
      renal failure after, in athletes,
      95: 390
  steroid (see Steroids, anabolic)
Accidents
  squash ball, causing retinal
      detachments, 97: 28
Accu-Chek Easy
  performance, effect of simulated altitude
      on, 97: 287
Acetabular
  labral lesions causing hip pain, 97: 116
Achilles tendon
  injuries
    in athletes, 95: 193
    overuse, surgery of, long-term
        follow-up, 95: 194
  rupture
    acute, immediate free ankle motion
        after surgical repair of, 95: 195
    repair, late vs. early, clinical and
        biomechanical evaluation, 96: 192
    repair, new method, and early range
        of motion and functional
        rehabilitation, 96: 193
    repair, polypropylene braid
        augmentation in, 95: 197
    risk of, clinical and sonographic
        evaluation of, 97: 202

Acidosis
  gastric mucosal, exercise-induced,
      96: 296
Acromegaly
  octreotide in, cardiopulmonary
      performance during exercise after,
      96: 402
Acromioclavicular
  joint
    dislocation, conservative treatment,
        long-term results of, 97: 54
    injection technique, 97: 22
    separations during alpine skiing,
        97: 11
  osteoarthrosis, primary, results of
      operative resection of lateral end of
      clavicle for, 97: 60
ACSM
  cycle ergometry equation for young
      women, accuracy of, 95: 291
ACTH
  levels in indoor Olympic cyclists, effects
      of training intensity on, 97: 415
Adduction
  -abduction moments at knee during
      stair ascent and descent, 97: 139
Adductor
  strain, groin pain signaling, 96: 129
  strength characteristics of professional
      baseball pitchers, 96: 29
Adenoma
  colon, risk, physical activity and obesity
      in, 96: 291
Adenomatous
  polyps, colorectal, risk of, and leisure
      and occupational physical activity,
      97: 438
Adhesion
  abdominal pain due to, acute, 97: 109
  molecules, cell, in middle-distance
      runners under different training
      conditions, 95: 392
Adipose
  tissue lipoprotein lipase responses in
      silent myocardial ischemia in older
      athletes, 95: 418
Adolescent
  burner syndrome in, recognition and
      rehabilitation, 97: 69
  chest pain in, training room evaluation,
      96: 237

---

* All entries refer to the year and page number(s) for data appearing in this and the
previous edition of the YEAR BOOK.

Ejection fraction
   left ventricular, in coronary artery
      disease, efficacy of high-intensity
      exercise training on, 96: 247
Elbow
   injury, throwing, pathomechanics of,
      97: 37
   ligaments
      medial, collateral complex,
         arthroscopic assessment, 96: 112
      medial, stress radiography of, 95: 68
      ulnar collateral, histology and
         arthroscopic anatomy of, 95: 70
   Little League, treating and preventing,
      95: 72
   osteochondritis dissecans of, 97: 147
   pain and stiffness after trauma,
      arthroscopic treatment, 95: 71
   in sports, clinical anatomy and
      pathomechanics of, 96: 111
   tennis, 96: 115
   ulnar neuropathy at, and operative
      treatment of epicondylitis, 96: 119
Elderly
   altitudes and, moderate, 96: 408
   bone mineral density in, in women
      additive effects of weight-bearing
         exercise and estrogen on, 96: 339
      dynamic muscle strength as predictor
         of, 96: 342
   circulatory responses to weight lifting,
      walking, and stair climbing in, in
      males, 97: 370
   colonic transit time in, brief physical
      inactivity prolonging, in men,
      95: 426
   exercise in
      antecedents and consequences of,
         96: 346
      resistance, muscle strength response
         to, effect of recombinant growth
         hormone on, 95: 365
      water, nonswimming, 95: 361
   functionally impaired, role of strength
      in rising from chair in, 97: 249
   insulin-like growth factor-1 in, effect of
      endurance training on, 95: 412
   knee of, in level walking, alignment,
      kinematic and kinetic measures of,
      95: 83
   lipids in, serum, effects of endurance
      exercise and hormone replacement
      therapy on, in women, 97: 329
   muscle mass and composition in, thigh
      and leg, effects of strength and
      endurance training on, in women,
      96: 354

   neuromuscular function and muscle
      cross-sectional area in, and gender,
      97: 247
   physical activity in
      antecedents and consequences of,
         96: 346
      physical functioning and,
         performance-based and
         self-reported, in men, 96: 351
      risk of severe gastrointestinal
         hemorrhage and, 95: 428
      resistance training program in,
         year-long, muscle strength and fiber
         adaptations to, 95: 352
      skeletal muscle weakness in, underlying
         mechanisms, 95: 353
      sports injuries in, common, 96: 345
      strength conditioning in, effects on
         women's ability to perform daily
         tasks, 96: 357
      torque production in, voluntary and
         neuromuscular electrical
         stimulation inducing, 95: 268
      walking endurance in, effect of weight
         training on, 97: 243
Electrical
   capacitive coupling in long bone
      nonunion, 95: 203
   evoked myoelectric signals in back
      muscles, effect of side dominance
      on, 95: 220
   fields, capacitive coupled, in stress
      fracture, 96: 392
   stimulation
      in cruciate ligament reconstruction,
         anterior, 96: 141
      effect on triceps surae mechanical and
         morphological characteristics,
         95: 269
      -induced torque production,
         voluntary and neuromuscular, in
         elderly, 95: 268
      motor unit activation during, twitch
         analysis of, 95: 266
Electrocardiography
   exercise
      in coronary artery disease, 96: 233
      exercise and recovery phases of,
         accurate detection of coronary
         artery disease by integrated analysis
         of ST-segment depression/heart rate
         patterns during, 97: 386
   for monitoring during cardiac
      rehabilitation, 96: 235
Electrolyte
   alterations after 100-km run, 95: 282
Electromyography
   activity(ies)

Author Index